QUEEN MARGARET UNIVERSITY

100   222   741

KU-529-629

Withdrawn from
Queen Margaret University Library

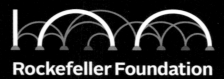

Rockefeller Foundation

Innovation for the Next 100 Years

HEALTH & WELL-BEING

SCIENCE, MEDICAL EDUCATION, AND PUBLIC HEALTH

By Angela Matysiak, Ph.D., M.P.H.

Innovation for the Next 100 Years
Rockefeller Foundation Centennial Series

QUEEN MARGARET UNIVERSITY LRC

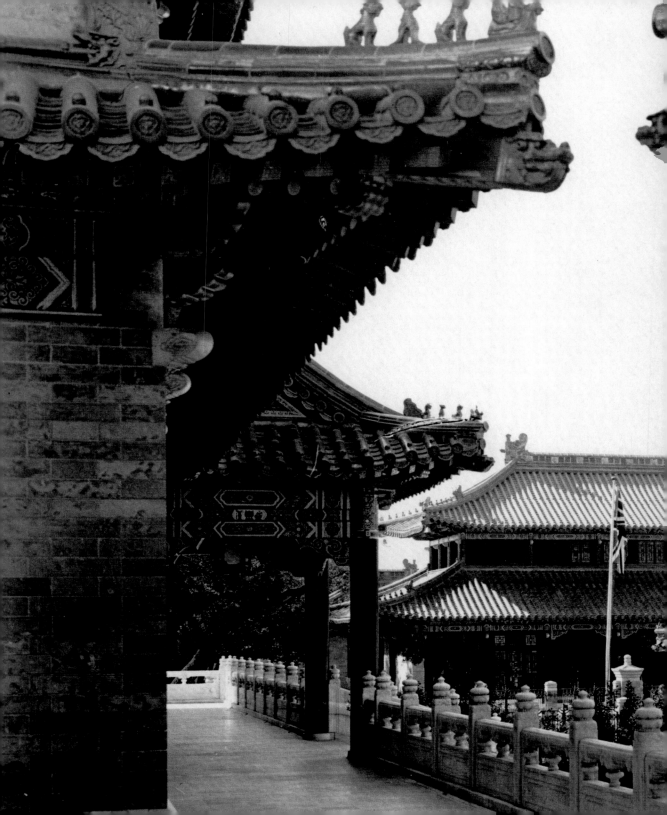

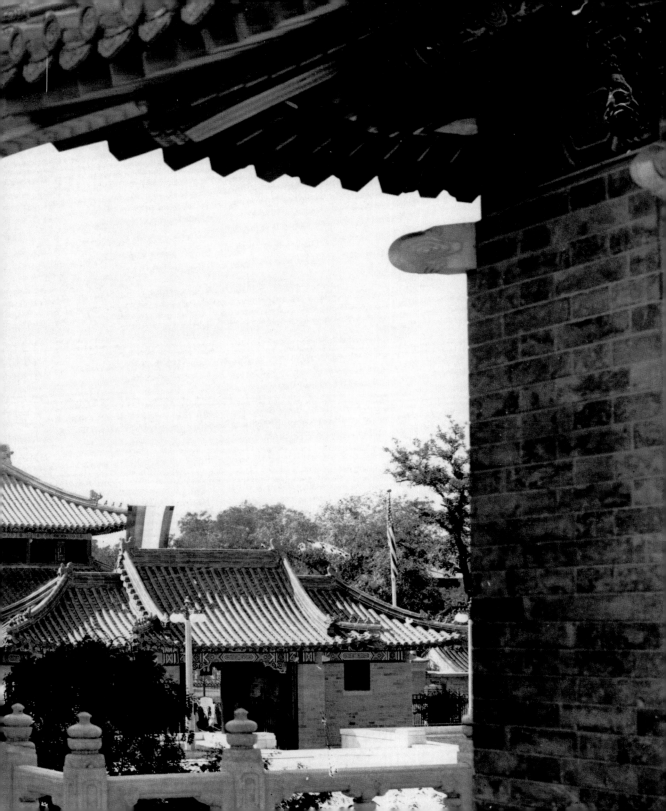

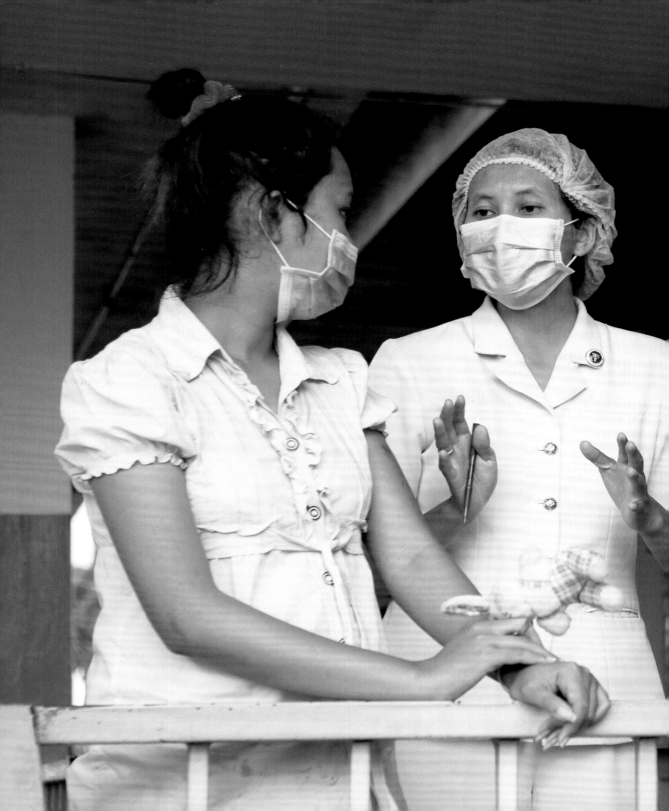

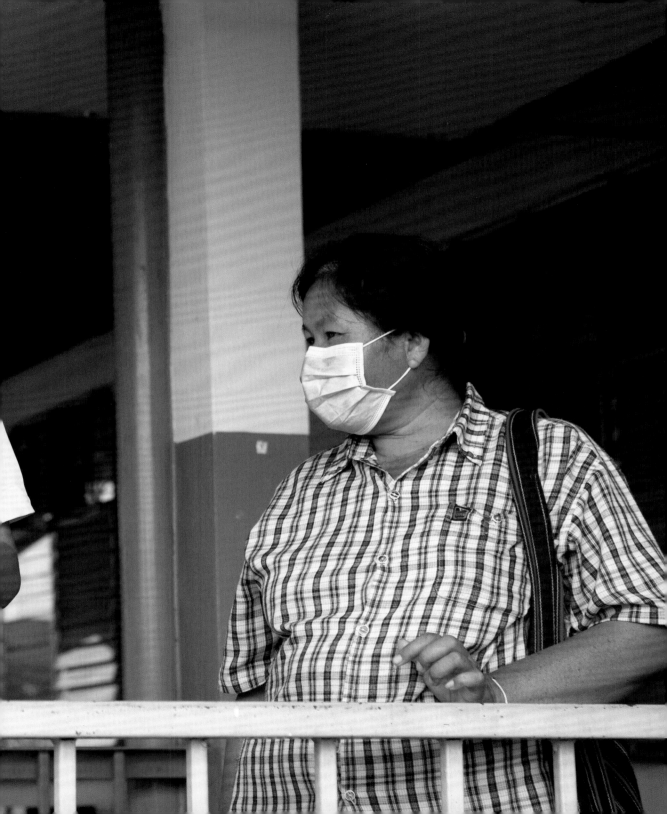

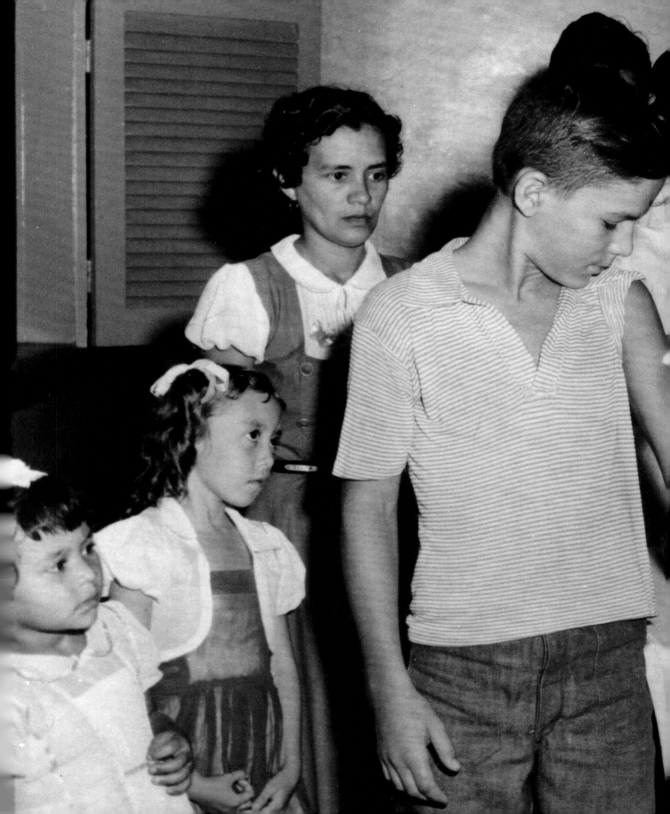

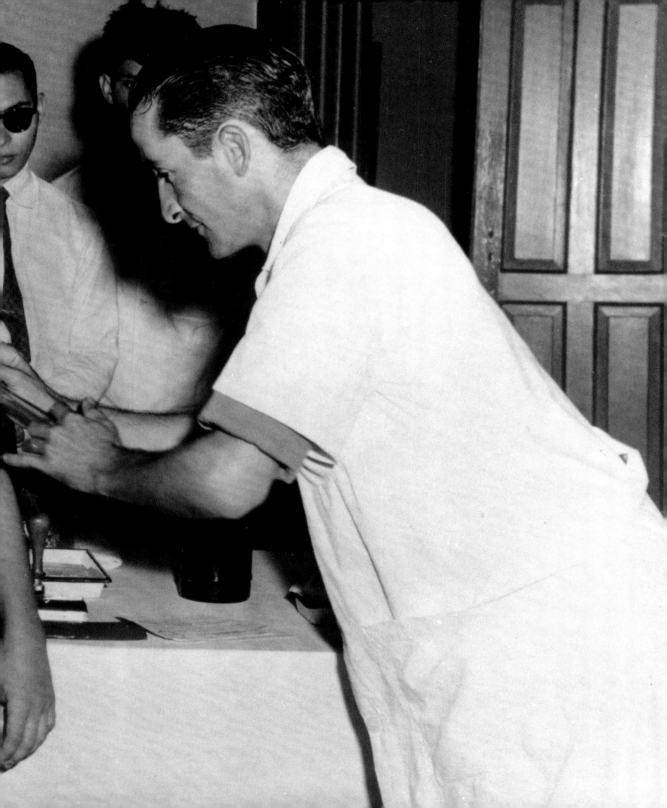

© 2014 by
The Rockefeller Foundation
Foreword copyright Paul Farmer, 2014
All rights reserved.

Cover:
Top: Inoculation to prevent
yellow fever, Brazil, 1938.
(Rockefeller Archive Center.)
Bottom: Photo by Shaen Adey.
Getty Images.

Book design by Pentagram.

*Health & Well-Being
Science, Medical Education,
and Public Health*

Printed in Canada.

Published by
The Rockefeller Foundation
New York
United States of America

In association with Vantage Point
Historical Services, Inc.
South Dakota
United States of America

ISBN-13: 978-0-9796389-5-4
ISBN-10: 0-9796389-5-X

Rockefeller Foundation Centennial Series

Books published in the Rockefeller Foundation Centennial Series provide case studies for people around the world who are working "to promote the well-being of humankind." Three books highlight lessons learned in the fields of agriculture, health, and philanthropy. Three others explore the Foundation's work in Africa, Thailand, and the United States. For more information about the Rockefeller Foundation Centennial initiatives, visit centennial.rockefellerfoundation.org.

Notes & Permissions

The Foundation has taken all reasonable steps to ensure the accuracy of the information provided in the book; any errors or omissions are inadvertent. This book is published without footnotes or endnotes. A manuscript version with citations and references for all sources used is available at centennial.rockefellerfoundation.org.

Captions in this book provide information on the creator and the repository from which the images in this book were obtained. The Foundation has made its best efforts to determine the creator and copyright holder of all images used in this publication. Images held by the Rockefeller Archive Center have been deemed to be owned by the Rockefeller Foundation unless we were able to determine otherwise. Specific permission has been granted by the copyright holder to use the following works:

Patrick de Noirmont: 4-5, 17, 292
Jonas Bendiksen: 76-77, 194-195, 242-243, 278, 282-283, 288-289, 295, 298
The John Hopkins Bloomberg School of Public Health: 31
Tom Perry: 106-107
Tennessee State Library and Archives: 117
Pach Brothers: 123
Merck & Co., Inc.: 130
United Nations: 132-133, 163, 209, 216-217, 221, 236, 241, 245, 249, 258
Montclair Historical Society: 136 (top)
New York Times: 136 (bottom)
Alan Mason Chesney Medical Archives of the Johns Hopkins Medical Institutions: 142, 158
Arne Hoel: 160-161
World Bank: 174-175, 293
Succession Raghubir Singh: 182
Tibor Farkas/WHO: 201
Matt Herron/Take Stock/The Image Works: 205
D. Henrioud/WHO: 207, 227
Wendy Stone: 212
Romina Rodríguez Pose: 228
McMaster University/FCIHR: 232
Antony Njuguna: 263
Courtesy of International AIDS Vaccine Initiative: 272
Ralph Alswang: 274
Vanessa Vick: 277
Chong Fat: 285
Sokomoto Photography: 301
John D. and Catherine T. MacArthur Foundation: 304
Athit Perawongmetha: 308-309

DR. JUDITH RODIN

PRESIDENT, THE ROCKEFELLER FOUNDATION

Long before he came to work for John D. Rockefeller as a philanthropic advisor, Frederick Gates was a genial, but sometimes irascible, Baptist preacher in Minneapolis, Minnesota. At the end of the nineteenth century, as he tells it, he had "the usual quota" of physicians and faith healers in his congregation. One of these men was a prominent doctor who quietly confessed that with nine out of ten of his patients he could do nothing but let illness run its course. With most of the others, he might be able to assist in the healing or recovery or make the patient more comfortable. But in only one case in a hundred was he able to use science to effect a cure. This conversation helped convince Gates "that, if there was a science of medicine, that science was not being taught or practiced in the United States."

After he joined Rockefeller's staff, Gates encountered others who believed that a scientific revolution was underway, led by Louis Pasteur and Robert Koch, who showed that micro-organisms were often responsible for disease. These new scientific insights suggested the need to transform medical education. Coupled with John Snow's work in Paris and London, which demonstrated the relationship between poor sanitation, water supplies, and outbreaks of cholera, the new science also presented an opportunity to develop the field of public health.

On the eve of the establishment of the Rockefeller Foundation, the excitement over these opportunities was palpable. At Gates's urging, Rockefeller had created and endowed the Rockefeller Institute for Medical Research in New York in 1901, the first institution in the United States dedicated exclusively to understanding the bioscience of disease. He had also established the Rockefeller Sanitary Commission for the Eradication of Hookworm Disease to launch a massive public health campaign in the American South. With the founding of the Rockefeller Foundation in 1913, the newly formed board of trustees hoped to support medical science and research and reform and invigorate medical education and public health around the world.

Over the last hundred years, as *Health and Well-Being* describes, we have remained remarkably true to this vision. We helped to build and develop schools of medicine and public health on nearly every continent. Grants provided for basic research and work done in our own laboratories led to new medicines and treatments that helped or cured patients and earned Nobel Prizes. Along the way, we helped train new generations of scientists, physicians, nurses, and technicians whose dedication to their patients and their communities inspired the world around them.

At any given point in our history, we can see the officers of the Foundation and the members of the board working with grantees to strike the right balance in the allocation of the Foundation's funds between scientific research, medical education, and public health training. We can also see them struggling with concepts that in later years would crystalize around the idea of health equity—how to allocate precious resources in ways that will provide the greatest benefits for the largest share of humankind, and particularly address the needs of the poor and vulnerable.

Prior to World War Two, the Foundation's International Health Division was virtually the only global agency focused on the physical well-being of the world's population. We collaborated closely with governments and local agencies to develop schools and public health programs. As historians of the Foundation and of global health have noted, it was a two-way learning process that benefited local communities in countries ranging from Brazil to China, and also reshaped the Foundation's perspective and methods of operation. At every step of the way, we learned by doing.

Since World War Two, thankfully, a host of multinational agencies, including the United Nations and the World Health Organization, have joined us and other philanthropies in the effort to promote global health. And, equally important, governments, especially the United States, began to invest heavily in biomedical research. Beginning with the creation of the International AIDS Vaccine Initiative, we have also worked to bring businesses and private capital into the work of global public health. These new models for public/private collaboration are needed if we hope to stop the spread of HIV/AIDS, tuberculosis, malaria, dengue fever, and other tropical diseases that overwhelmingly affect developing countries.

The Foundation's efforts to advance human understanding of health and well-being have always been linked to programs designed to transform the systems that provide health care to the people who need it. In the early years, these efforts were largely focused on disease eradication campaigns, the development of vaccines, and the training of health care professionals. Our work on the development of population-based medicine and selective primary care in the 1970s and 1980s highlighted the need to focus resources where they could save the greatest number of lives. These initiatives helped us recognize an urgent need to help ministries of health and health care providers take advantage of new information technologies to monitor disease patterns and improve delivery systems and health financing to achieve the goal of providing universal health coverage.

Our long history has given the Rockefeller Foundation a unique place in the field of global health. We have the ability and the privilege to convene and to catalyze new initiatives, to work with others to identify new opportunities to innovate in high-tech laboratories, as well as in rural health clinics. Today, we are especially attuned to the risks to human health posed by climate change and rapid human migration in an increasingly global society.

Just as our history calls us to carry on the process of innovation, it also gives us great confidence in the powers of imagination and ingenuity. For over one hundred years, the works of our grantees and staff have helped to save millions of lives. As we move forward into our second century, we seem to be living in an era when new technologies and scientific discoveries hold even greater promise for health and well-being. Our goal remains clear—to identify and develop innovations to improve the health and quality of life for people throughout the world.

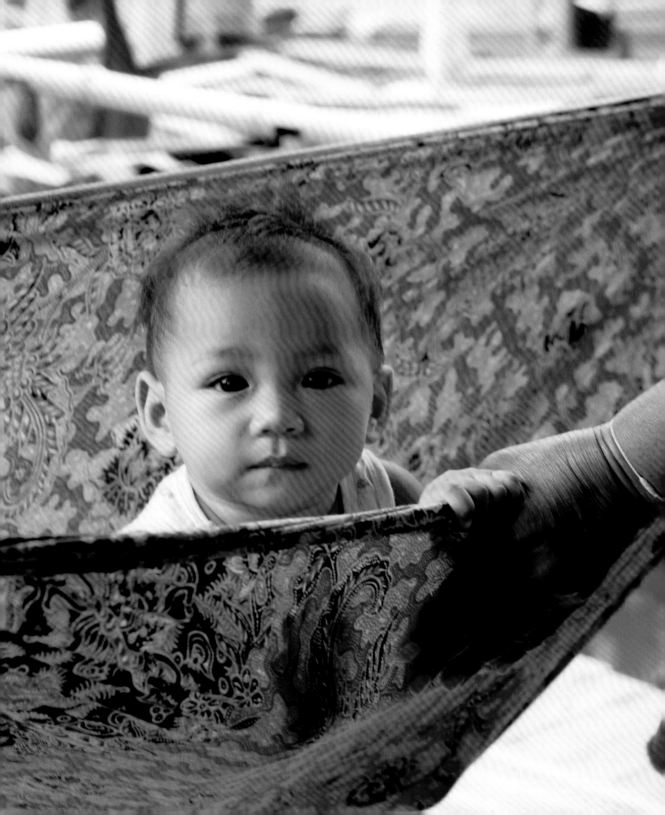

FOREWORD

By Dr. Paul Farmer

Harvard Medical School,

Brigham and Women's Hospital, Partners in Health

The centennial of the Rockefeller Foundation offers a chance to reflect on a century of progress in the quest to promote health and well-being. These vague terms are not always complementary; they are also contingent and contested. Even as medical progress occurs, we need to understand when and why it fails to reach those in greatest need.

Born at the dawn of what many would call modern medicine, the Foundation sought to promote scientific progress of uncontested significance. This history chronicles milestones in medical science, education, public health, and clinical care. Through the prism of institutional history it also informs debates now facing an even more ambitious enterprise: achieving global health equity.

The Foundation's work began early in the twentieth century, when the grand projects of medical science and "social reform" collided in efforts to tackle the greatest public health dilemmas of the day. In its scope and ambition, the Foundation was, in the terms of this account, a "philanthropic colossus."

Health and Well-Being offers an illuminating and useful review of the Foundation's signature efforts, as well as some of the key disputations within the institution. From the early days, staff and directors debated abiding issues in medicine and public health. Should the Foundation's programs invest primarily in education, research, or care delivery? With what institutions should it build enduring partnerships? What were the ranking health problems of the poor and how might these become priorities?

The campaign to eradicate hookworm, launched in 1909 by the Rockefeller Sanitary Commission (a precursor of the Foundation) shaped the trajectory of the Foundation's work in health. Hookworm was a significant cause of debility (and, sometimes, death) in the American South. At the time, hookworm could be diagnosed and treated, if imperfectly. It could be prevented through improvements in basic sanitation, such as the construction of latrines. But it was not southern latitudes alone that determined risk for this or any other "tropical" disease. Race and class usually governed who had access to modern sanitation, just as they determined who was diagnosed and treated.

In this vivid account, we meet the campaigners and evangelists, like Wickliffe Rose, who sought to prevent infection and to treat rural people affected by hookworm. Many of the early Rockefeller leaders, including Rose, were looking for a vertical "wedge," a campaign against a specific disease, that would lead to more integrated or "horizontal" initiatives. They hoped the hookworm campaign would improve access to health care and establish public-health bureaus in states and counties that did not have them.

In its first year of operations in the American South, the hookworm program brought some 3,400 physicians—an estimated 17 percent of all doctors in the region—into the campaign. These efforts led to unprecedented commitments of federal and state dollars to create local and regional public-health institutions. This success prompted an expansion of the campaign to subtropical regions around the world.

The history of the Rockefeller Foundation, an American institution, shows the global reach of science and evidence-based medicine. From the outset, however, there was brisk debate about *how* to proceed in the battle to control or eradicate hookworm and other diseases. While one set of campaigners sought to concentrate on disease-specific campaigns focused on diagnosing and treating hookworm, another group pointed to the social determinants of hookworms' persistence, or recurrence, including a lack of shoes, sanitation, schools, and jobs, as well as, execrable housing. The affliction was caused by an intestinal parasite, the campaigners agreed; but wasn't poverty itself the cause of such conditions? These quandaries, basic to social medicine as laid out by Rudolf Virchow in a previous century, signaled growing convergences, as American progressives turned towards the problems spawned or worsened by rising inequalities.

And there were always unintended consequences. The treatment then used, thymol, was more toxic than hoped or advertised. When more than 200 died as a result of therapy, almost half of them children, staffers and trustees proposed a sharper focus on basic scientific research that would lead to better and safer therapies, or maybe even a vaccine. The internal organizational struggles over these issues raised almost all of the challenges and struggles encountered in public health and medicine to this day.

SCIENCE, EDUCATION, AND CARE

ealth and Well-Being portrays an institution struggling to define and redefine itself in the face of rapid change in three important realms of global health: basic science, education, and care.

Before the rise of significant federal or private pharmaceutical commitments to biomedical research, many of the Foundation's investments, though relatively small in size, turned out to be prescient. The Foundation participated in the discovery of tools ranging from penicillin to polio vaccines, focusing on what today might be called "translational research," with enough discernment to support researchers who later became Nobel Laureates.

The story of the struggle to create a yellow fever vaccine, retold with affecting detail in *Health and Well-Being*, began in the first years of the Foundation and endured for four decades, in spite of the fact that at least five of those working on a vaccine died of accidental exposure to the causative virus. These sacrifices, coupled with improved laboratory safety and scientific breakthroughs, led eventually to the creation of a vaccine—an accomplishment recognized with a Nobel Prize.

From the outset, the Foundation's efforts in medical education were, like its early eradication campaigns, global in aspiration. The Foundation helped to found the first schools of public health in the United States and in Asia and Latin America. It also worked to bridge the "know-do" gap in many arenas, to broaden the impact of much of the basic science it funded. This universalism reflected the idea that the fruits of science should be for everyone. Once it was clear how malaria transmission might be stopped, for example, Foundation teams joined many others in southern Europe, Asia, and Latin America in seeking to do so. Again, the sheer scale of such projects was remarkable, if in some places (southern Europe) more than others (most of Africa). At one point, this effort employed—in Sardinia alone—38,000 people. This was in 1949.

Health and Well-Being brings into view the tensions between progressive universalism and the goal of most public health authorities, which is to promote the health and well-being of the citizens of distinct polities (county, district, state, nation, region, empire, et cetera). Throughout much of the twentieth century, however, global health equity—with the best tools focused on the needs of the most vulnerable—was not a priority for most foundations, universities, and standard-setting bodies. Otherwise, how to explain the relative neglect, say, of malaria control efforts in Africa and other places where health systems were weak or absent and opportunities for professional training or research few and far between?

For many years, Foundation debates focused on how best to deliver research, training, or care in settings of poverty and inequality. Programs tended to work best in settings of rising affluence (Thailand, Colombia, and even China) and to falter in settings of greater poverty (Uganda, say, or elsewhere in sub-Saharan Africa). When rural regions of poor countries were considered, the impact of some of the Rockefeller Foundation's global health programs was often negligible.

Negligible, that is, unless one takes the long view. For years the Foundation emphasized the links between research, training, and service delivery. In 1961, for example, it provided support to a university in Colombia for social medicine programs with goals as sophisticated as any floated today. But as a recessionary U.S. economy sapped the Foundation's endowment, the Foundation's ability to fund such ambitious endeavors waned in the 1970s, and so did its influence. Once the only show in town, the Rockefeller Foundation became, within 60 years of its founding, one among dozens of entities supporting medical research. Even its largest grants were dwarfed by some of the international health programs of what would be termed "aid organizations," most of them sponsored by governments. Funding a smorgasbord of programs might be possible for a colossus of philanthropy, but internal Foundation assessments reveal fears that the influence of this once-great colossus was reduced, by 1962, "to a barely detectable ripple."

As the Foundation wrestled with ways to "leverage" its resources, it joined a growing debate about setting priorities in global health. Building health systems in settings of poverty, whether relative or absolute, is hard work. This was especially true when such delivery systems sought to incorporate training and research, a goal much discussed but rarely seen outside of academic medical centers. Trustees and leaders were of course called to set priorities and be selective. In 1972, when the Foundation chose as its new leader a Harvard medical professor John Knowles, they picked a strong advocate for reform who helped turn the Foundation towards community health and primary care.

Various stakeholders define "primary care" in different ways. In the United States, the term refers to care provided by first-line clinicians, including specialists in internal medicine and nurse practitioners. In settings of poverty and privation, where the leading cause of destitution was, and remains, catastrophic illness, many people lived and died without ever seeing a well-trained doctor or nurse. Meanwhile, their meager resources were frittered away in ineffective care for preventable and treatable diseases.

In the 1970s and later, there was great pressure to identify or "select" interventions that were "cost-effective." Some of the ascendant voices in international health were proposing a set of interventions called "selective primary care." This was in contrast to the "unrealistic" and "wasteful" non-selective interventions that were very much the rule in the United States.

Public and private funders often preferred interventions that were cheap and effective by any criteria. In the developing world, they focused on measles, polio, and other vaccine-preventable illnesses and elevated family planning and oral rehydration for infants sick with diarrheal disease. But "selective" primary care was also in contrast to the comprehensive primary health care ideal advanced in Alma Ata in 1978, and it raised questions about caring for people with other health needs. What about tuberculosis treatment, for example, which required (after effective diagnosis) a multidrug regimen for the better part of a year? What about surgical care for illnesses ranging from obstructed labor to abscesses or cancer, or therapy for diseases like epilepsy or schizophrenia, or even treatment for trauma caused by road traffic accidents? Why would these pathologies not be characterized as "primary care" if they are among the primary problems requiring medical attention in many of the poor and disrupted settings in which the Foundation funded important efforts in research, training, and service?

All of the above questions were posed in the early 1970s, as they have been in every year since. A decade before the term "AIDS" was coined, and a quarter of a century before the advent of SARS—both of which figure prominently in

Health and Well-Being—these key questions of global health equity were posed lucidly and debated fiercely within the Foundation.

One of the saving graces, during these decades of selective attention to some ranking problems of the poor and not others, was that the Rockefeller Foundation continued to invest in training. The legacy of this investment, according to *Health and Well-Being*, "was a cadre of well-trained scientists capable of training future generations to conduct research in population stabilization, agriculture, neglected diseases, and epidemiology at the international level."

INSIGHTS FROM THE PAST

Reading *Health and Well-Being* makes clear that not all of these debates in the past were smart ones. Tension between minimalist and optimalist approaches did not recede since, with rare exceptions such as smallpox, the pathogens would not go away. When, in 1980, the Foundation launched, with some fanfare, a new initiative on "Great Neglected Diseases," for example, one of these diseases was none other than hookworm. Even today, when these issues are, or should be, informed by an almost immeasurably larger body of evidence, they are often marred by a series of false debates framed around choosing one course over another. Even within institutions concerning themselves with transnational populations, the walling-off or "stovepiping" of certain aspects of general or systemic problems continues.

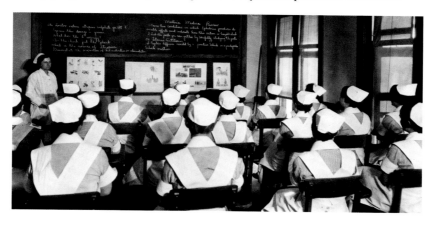

Reading an honest historical account, such as *Health and Well-Being*, makes clear the limitations of such siloed approaches. They arise for reasons ranging from increased disciplinary specialization, which has brought mostly handsome returns on investment in the biomedical sciences, to the decreased latitude seen with most forms of bureaucratization. A division of labor is needed to create new fields of knowledge, but it is also true that specialization sometimes comes with a cost, as revealed in histories like this one.

Five of these false debates are limned in the pages of this book. First, basic discovery science, increasingly conducted in laboratories, is too often pitted against clinical practice and the delivery of services. Attempts to eradicate hookworm, for example, depended on advances in parasitology and pharmacology, which led to new and better diagnostics and treatments. It's not that one institution, even a colossus, can do any of this alone. Proponents of global health equity must *collectively* support basic discovery science to develop new tools and advance ways to deliver care to those in greatest need.

A second false debate is in the medicine-versus-public-health discussions that have smoldered for more than a century. The tensions are evident in the debate over clinical care versus population-based efforts; they're also evident in a more draconian, but still commonly encountered view that pits prevention against care. In reality, the integration of prevention and care almost invariably advances the cause of global health equity.

Third, the pitting of the education of one cadre or profession against another has stalled development of human resources for health. In the early years of public health, this debate often focused on doctors versus nurses; community health workers were rarely central to the discussion.

Fourth, the "new international health" agenda of the last decades of the twentieth century, when based on overly confident claims about both cost and effectiveness, swerved away from global health equity. It also tarnished the value of delivery of *care* for complex illness ranging from major mental illness to AIDS to road trauma. This debate can never be settled when cost is so often conflated with price, and price can vary by a factor of hundreds (sometimes thousands) on the same day for the same commodity. Think of antiretroviral therapy, which cost $20,000 per patient per year in one corner of the global political economy and less than $100 in another. The entire history of the

Foundation offers a cautionary tale about undue confidence in claims of cost effectiveness, as well as the potential of a new technology, whether a vaccine or a therapy, to change our notion of what's effective and what's not.

Fifth, making sure innovation reaches the poorest and most vulnerable—those most likely to benefit—remains a challenge. Some would argue that all diseases afflicting primarily the poor are by definition neglected. If this is true of hookworm and other communicable diseases, what might be said of complex pathologies such as leukemia or roadside trauma? Or about new pandemics, not simply those "caused" by microbes, but also those associated with changing and noxious social conditions, including obesity and diabetes?

If an understanding of the burden of disease among the poor might be linked to knowledge of gaps in attention and delivery, what would be wedge strategies like those advanced by Wickliffe Rose over a century ago? In the end, only *global health equity* is left as the surest goal, and history, it seems, will absolve those who invest in reaching it. I first heard the term from Bill Foege, one of the protagonists in this book. Foege worked on what many think of as global health's greatest achievement—smallpox eradication—and later founded the Task Force on Child Survival. The Task Force, supported by the Rockefeller Foundation and others, sought to ensure that the *least* we might do is roll out vaccines known to be effective. This effort required substantial funding from public and private partners. It reflected an attempt to link knowledge of the burden of disease with an understanding of how to close the know-do gap. This focus on delivery helped lead to the revolution in child survival, but it did not close the door on other ranking problems, including those sure to emerge when efforts to cull low-hanging fruit are met with success.

Public health is not a discipline so much as a collection of problems. Threats to health change, as does their relative rank in any given place. And the tools on hand change. As the pace of technological and social innovations quickens, those who cherish the goal of healthier societies need to take stock, to look back at what has worked and what has not worked in the past. For this reason alone, we have cause to be grateful to those who compiled and shaped this important volume. The goal of "global health equity" may sound vague, but setting goals to achieve it, and linking it to policies to foster it, are among the most urgent tasks before us.

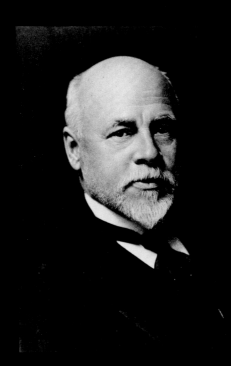 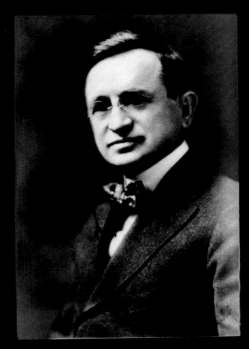

William Welch and Wickliffe Rose were instrumental in creating the field of modern public health. While they differed in their views on public health training, and on whom that training should include, both men can ultimately be credited with helping to create the world's first university-based public health programs. (Rockefeller Archive Center.)

William Welch was late, and Wickliffe Rose was growing increasingly anxious. The two men had promised to co-author a plan to create the first school of public health in the United States, and their deadline was fast approaching. Welch had agreed to write the first draft, but so far, Rose had not received anything. They were both busy men. Welch, with his silver goatee and bushy moustache, was the dean of the Johns Hopkins University School of Medicine. Sixty-four years old, he was a popular teacher, nicknamed "Popsy" by his students. In 1915 he was also widely regarded as one of the foremost physicians in the United States.

Rose was 12 years younger. A dapper man who favored bow ties and wireless spectacles, he had been a professor of philosophy and a leading advocate of education reform in the American South. He was now the director of the Rockefeller Foundation's International Health Commission, which had been established to fight hookworm in tropical regions around the world.

These were momentous times in the history of medical education, medical science, and public health as John D. Rockefeller, the founder of Standard Oil, created and endowed a series of philanthropic organizations to promote science, education, and the well-being of humanity. In 1901 he had launched the Rockefeller Institute for Medical Research, the first major scientific research facility in the United States devoted to medical science. In 1903 he created the General Education Board (GEB) to reform teaching in the American South and bolster higher education in the United States. Six years later, in 1909, he founded the Rockefeller Sanitary Commission for the Eradication of Hookworm Disease, the first broad-based, multi-state public health campaign in the history of the United States. Then, in 1913, he established the Rockefeller Foundation to act as the major vehicle for his philanthropy. The Foundation, in turn, worked with the GEB to transform medical education in the United States based on the recommendations of a newly released report commissioned by the Carnegie Corporation of New York and written by Abraham Flexner.

Welch and Rose had been key players in all of this work. At Johns Hopkins, Welch had trained a generation of physicians interested in research pathology, which was at the cutting edge of innovation in medicine at the beginning of the twentieth century. Known as "Welch rabbits," these doctors had gone on to teach at medical schools across the United States and become advocates of reform. Meanwhile Rose had directed the work of the Rockefeller Sanitary Commission. In this position he had come to see the need for public health workers in every county in the United States. After the Rockefeller Foundation was established in 1913, he had been asked to launch a global campaign to battle hookworm and other diseases as the head of the Foundation's International Health Commission. In 1915 Welch and Rose were also at the center of an effort, led by the Rockefeller Foundation and the GEB, to essentially create and define the modern field of public health in the United States—and eventually throughout the world.

This effort had begun with Rose 18 months earlier. After traveling abroad to evaluate the prevalence of hookworm, he had returned to the United States in the fall of 1913 to meet with the board of the International Health Commission. During that meeting, the board passed a resolution suggesting that the Rockefeller Foundation work with the GEB to train public health service workers. Abraham Flexner, who was a member of the GEB's board and whose brother Simon directed the Rockefeller Institute for Medical Research, was assigned the task of developing this initiative.

Flexner organized a meeting on October 16, 1914, in the offices of the GEB at 17 Battery Place in New York City. It was a difficult time for decision making. As they arrived that rainy morning, trustees selected from the GEB and the Rockefeller Foundation were well aware that war and panic raged in Europe. The headlines on the front page of the *New York Times* declared that the Allies had repelled the German Army the day before, but Americans in London were worried that an invasion was imminent. A day earlier, former President William Howard Taft and philanthropist Andrew Carnegie had praised President Woodrow Wilson for pledging that the United States would remain neutral. In Belgium refugees were desperate for food and shelter.

The twenty-odd men assembled for the meeting represented some of the leading lights in medicine, medical education, and public health in the United States. They included the health commissioner for the state of New York and professors of bacteriology from the University of Pennsylvania, the University of Chicago, and Columbia University. Harvard University had three delegates, including Dr. Milton J. Rosenau, professor of preventive medicine, because it hoped to edge out Columbia and receive funding from the Rockefeller Foundation to establish the first school of public health in the United States. William Welch, of course, hoped that Johns Hopkins would get the nod. Among these giants and rivals, Wickliffe Rose waited to see what kind of vision would emerge for the future of public health.

Frederick Gates, John D. Rockefeller's leading philanthropic advisor and a member of the boards of both the GEB and the Rockefeller Foundation, chaired the meeting. Trained as a Baptist minister, he believed in the tremendous power of science and the scientific method. As the oil king's advisor, Gates had systematized Rockefeller's philanthropy. He believed that disease represented the greatest threat to human well-being, and he had persuaded Rockefeller to devote unprecedented resources to medical research and public health.

Gates presided as the meeting began, but it was Abraham Flexner who orchestrated the conversation. He began by asking what sorts of skilled individuals were needed to create an effective system of public health in the United States. The New York State health commissioner said there were three: executives, technical experts, and field workers. Flexner then asked how each of the three should be trained. As the discussion progressed, the debate focused increasingly on how to create a system for training public health workers. Some at the table favored focusing on individuals who had already graduated from medical school. Others empha- sized the need to train a cadre of professionals separate from those receiving medical training.

Welch argued that students in a new public health program should be medical doctors. He suggested a program that would em- ulate the British Diploma in Public Health. In Britain participants had completed their medical training and a year of clinical practice before they were admitted to the program in public health. Welch was certain that this work would be attractive to doctors.

Gates was not convinced. At the time, many doctors in the United States and elsewhere were poorly trained. They had little lab experience and a weak knowledge of science. He resisted the idea that only doctors should be enrolled and feared that the only doctors who would be interested would be those who had failed in private practice. The health commissioner for the state of New York echoed Gates's concerns. Providing training only to doctors would slow the process of building a strong corps of public health officials. Theobald Smith, who would soon join the Rockefeller Institute and become one of its most famous scientists, supported Welch. He asserted that public health officials would need to hold a medical degree so that physicians would respect them as peers.

Rose listened to the debate for a long time before he spoke. Then he outlined a very different concept. As Rose's biographer, Roy Acheson, has written, "Rose saw the medical profession as essential contributors to the practice of public health, but did not consider public health to be a specialty of medicine." In great detail he described the country's need for a labor force in public health with varying degrees of expertise. He imagined a series of institutions across the country, akin to state teachers' colleges, devoted to the cause. These programs would be related to medical schools, if possible, but they should accommodate the training needs of people headed for careers as sanitary engineers, public health nurses, engineering technicians, and other rank-and-file members of the nascent profession. They should also offer in-service short courses for people working in related fields. These state institutions would look to a new national institute of hygiene for leadership. This institution would be at the center of a vast new system of public health.

Rose's vision was revolutionary and eagerly embraced by the other men in the room. The New York health commissioner called it "admirable." Theobald Smith declared it "magnificent." Even Welch conceded that it was "stirring and inspiring." But there was also a general recognition that Rose's vision was very large. Moreover, it seemed to slight the importance of scientific research, work that many in the room felt was vital to the business of developing cures for disease. To implement Rose's plan, the Rockefeller Foundation would have to start smaller, probably with one school. In making this start, Welch's emphasis on the importance of training an elite corps of public health doctors would have to be reconciled with Rose's idea of building a system for training many kinds of public health workers.

Wallace Buttrick, president of the General Education Board, who had been silent for most of the meeting, suggested that Welch and Rose, the two leading visionaries in the group, should be given the job of reconciling their ideas. The goal would be to strike a balance among basic medical research, medical education, and the development of the field of public health.

It's unclear how Rose and Welch felt about the assignment, but they were gentlemen and both were passionately committed to improving public health, so they accepted the task. The following week, according to Acheson, Rose rode the train from New York to Baltimore to meet with Welch at Johns Hopkins. They had dinner in the Maryland Club. While other members and guests played billiards or cards, Welch and Rose discussed plans for the first school of public health in the United States. When they were done, Welch agreed to write the first draft of their proposal.

Rose was soon sidetracked by other events. As the plight of war refugees in Belgium deteriorated, he was asked to lead a Rockefeller Foundation-sponsored commission to Europe to assess the critical civilian need for food. When he returned to the United States weeks later, however, he discovered that the esteemed dean from Johns Hopkins had not made any progress on the document. Rose expressed his concern. In the meantime, the date for the next meeting of the GEB's trustees—May 27, 1915—grew closer.

Welch told Rose in March that he would have a draft soon, but Rose still had received nothing by April. Several more weeks passed. Finally, Rose drafted a memorandum on his own. It reflected much of what he had said during the dinner at the Maryland Club in October. It's unclear how faithfully it represented the discussion he had had with Welch. It was a broad vision that aimed to build a robust public health system across the nation. In Rose's words, it recognized that "the science of protection is quite different from the science of cure."

Unfortunately for Rose, it was not a vision that Welch shared. When the trustees of the GEB and the Rockefeller Foundation met weeks later, the conversation would turn in a different direction. The outcome would shape the future of public health in the United States and reflect fundamental issues at stake as the Rockefeller Foundation tackled problems in medical science, medical education, and public health in the century ahead.

The history of the Foundation's work in health over the next century would often be shaped by profound questions of strategy and values that would have seemed all too familiar to Wickliffe Rose and William Welch. Always they revolved around an age-old tension between technology's promise to find a cure for disease and society's hope that sickness and ill health might be prevented in the first place. Battling epidemics from yellow fever to HIV/AIDS, and endemic health problems from hookworm to malaria, trustees and staff at the Foundation would wrestle with decisions about how to prioritize the use of the Foundation's finite resources in order to promote the health and well-being of humanity.

Overview

This book explores the history of the Rockefeller Foundation and its predecessor and sister organizations in the field of global health. It looks at disappointments as well as triumphs. It highlights the ways in which lessons learned from one initiative helped propel innovation for the next.

The book begins in the first decades of the twentieth century with the development and expansion of the campaign against hookworm from the American South to the equatorial regions of Africa, Latin America, and Asia. Over the course of this fight, for the first time the Foundation had to reconcile its ambition to eradicate disease with the realization that in many cases amelioration was the more achievable outcome. Rockefeller philanthropists also learned to work with local and state governments, local physicians, native healers, tribal elders, and colonial authorities.

The campaign against hookworm underscored the need to develop the field of public health. New institutions had to be created to channel an enormous investment in human capital to make prevention as important as treatment in the battle against disease. For decades the Rockefeller Foundation was the preeminent international leader in public health. Its grants enabled the establishment of the first schools of public health in the United States, and financed the development of similar institutions around the world. The Foundation played a pivotal role in the development of education for doctors, nurses,

Founded in 1916 with a $6 million endowment from the Rockefeller Foundation, the Johns Hopkins School of Hygiene and Public Health was the first institution to offer public health education in the United States. The university was chosen in part for the quality of its medical school and its promising faculty. (Johns Hopkins Bloomberg School of Public Health. Rockefeller Archive Center.)

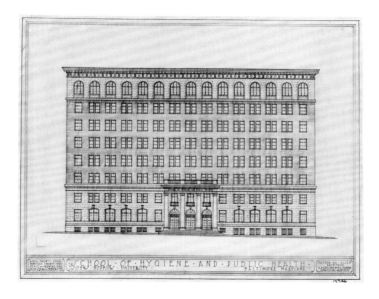

and other health professionals in North America, Asia, Europe, Latin America, and Africa. The Foundation helped shape these institutions within a framework anchored in the natural sciences and, to some extent, the social sciences.

Even as it worked to reshape the institutional landscape for medical training and public health, the Rockefeller Foundation continued to invest in basic research with the hope that break-through discoveries might lead to cures for disease. The Foundation's efforts to develop a vaccine for yellow fever saved millions of lives and earned a Nobel Prize for Foundation researcher Max Theiler. Meanwhile the Foundation's leadership in developing what would become the field of molecular biology paved the way for a host of treatments and cures based on biotechnology.

All of these initiatives were shaped by the era and by the experiences of the individuals who led the Foundation. Nowhere is this more clear than in the Foundation's pathbreaking approach to mental illness. By the 1930s, psychoanalysis dominated the effort to address problems of human behavior and mental illness, but the Foundation took a dramatically different path, searching for under-standing in the science of human physiology and brain chemistry. The Foundation's fundamental policy decisions during this period were influenced by painful tragedies in the lives of two Rockefeller Foundation presidents, who lost spouses and family members to mental illness but emerged from their grief determined to expand humanity's understanding of the brain and human behavior. At times, this research was unsuccessful. At other times, the research was highly controversial. But as with other Foundation initia-tives that had far-reaching consequences, the efforts to build a field focused on the physiology of human behavior would lead to breakthrough discoveries by others and a revolution in treatment for mental illness that materialized in the 1970s.

Throughout the pre-World War Two era, the Rockefeller Foundation played a leading role in funding innovation in medical science, medical education, and public health around the world. There were no other institutions at that time with a global vision for health. After the war, the institutional landscape was transformed with the establishment of the United Nations, the World Health Organization, the World Bank, and other transnational agencies. In the United States, the creation of the National Institutes of Health and the National Science Foundation brought government funding of medical research on a scale that dwarfed the resources of private philanthropy. In this new environment, the Foundation had to learn to work with these new institutions and develop new strategies to address unmet needs in the field of health.

The development of a new strategy was not easy. Through the 1960s, the Foundation's work in health reflected the trajectory of the past, including continued support for virus research and population control. In the context of its major effort to launch a green revolution to increase food production in developing countries, the Foundation focused increasingly on the relationship between nutrition, health, and development.

The selection of a physician as president in 1972 rejuvenated the Foundation's attention to health and directed it in a powerful and innovative new direction—community health. Under John Knowles, the Foundation became a catalyst for international cooperation guided by the idea that basic interventions could produce the biggest improvements in public health and well-being.

Building on the fundamental turn toward community medicine, the Rockefeller Foundation became increasingly interested in the ability of epidemiology to affect health outcomes. In some sense, this represented a return to the Foundation's roots. Disease surveys had been a cornerstone of methods developed by the Rockefeller Sanitary Commission and the International Health Commission. This time, however, the efforts were anchored in broad alliances. The Foundation helped build an international coalition to address Great Neglected Diseases of Mankind that affected primarily the poor and disenfranchised around the world. The Foundation also played a key role in launching the International Clinical Epidemiology Network (INCLEN).

This work on neglected diseases and epidemiology highlighted the need for international collaboration in vaccine research and the prevention of childhood illnesses. It led to major new initiatives, including the Task Force for Child Survival, the Universal Childhood Immunization program, and the Children's Vaccine Initiative. These efforts furthered the Foundation's broad strategy of building scientific capacity in the developing world.

With the appearance of HIV/AIDS, the world faced a growing crisis. Like many organizations, the Foundation struggled to understand this horrible new disease and then define the arenas in which it could make a meaningful contribution to treat those who were afflicted and prevent others from being infected. In some sense, the Foundation took the riskiest path—one that others were afraid to follow because the odds were long—to develop a vaccine. The vaccine itself has continued to elude medical researchers, but the broad-based coalition the Foundation helped create represented a significant institutional innovation in the field of medical research.

HIV/AIDS made it clear that, with increasing globalization and travel, new diseases could appear and spread very quickly. In 2003 the appearance of SARS in China sparked new fears of a global pandemic. With SARS, however, alert, comprehensive health information systems shared among nations and agencies proved critical to the ability to stop the spread of this new pathogen quickly. These new health information systems—a primary focus of Rockefeller Foundation health funding in the 1990s and the early years of the twenty-first century—also played a critical role in reducing the overall cost of health care delivery, especially for the poor and vulnerable.

For more than a century, the Rockefeller Foundation's role in developing medical science, medical education, and public health has been enormous. It has also reflected an ongoing tension between the desire to find cures and the impulse to promote social development that creates the conditions for good health. At times, the Foundation has leaned in one direction more than the other. Most often, it sought to find the right balance based on the institutional landscape, the partners available, the social conditions, and the resources at hand. Throughout its history, the Foundation has aimed to fulfill Frederick Gates's notion that the most important contribution philanthropy can make to humanity's well-being is to promote health. But as Wickliffe Rose discovered in 1910, attacking even the smallest parasite could be enormously complicated.

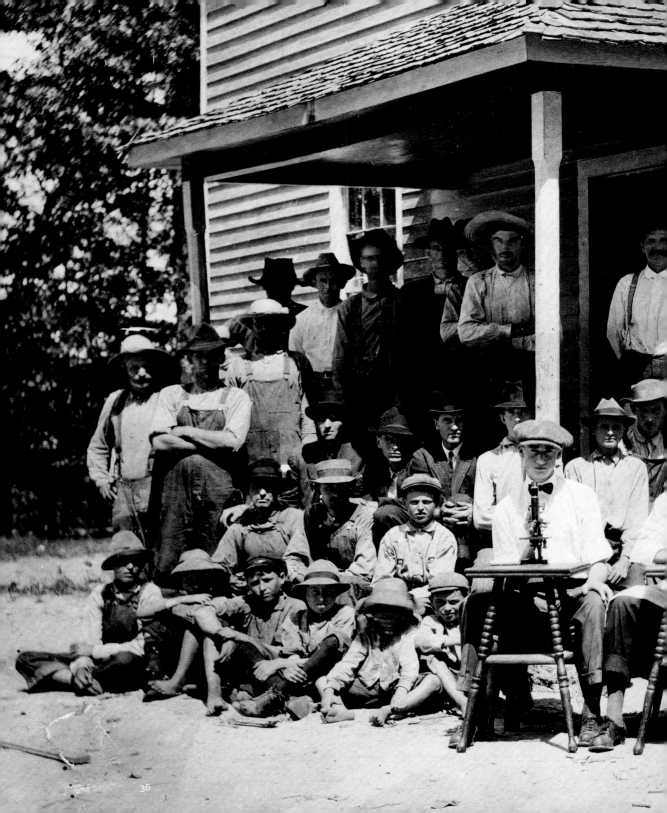

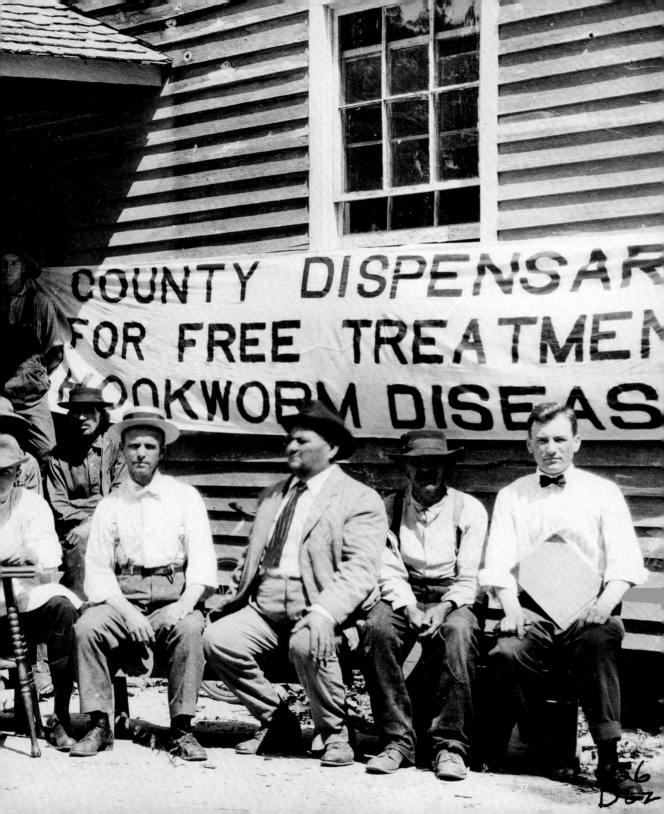

A WEDGE THAT LEADS TO PUBLIC ACTION

One morning in the winter of 1908, Charles Stiles, a zoologist with the U.S. Public Health Service, traveled by train to New York City. Weighing heavily on his mind was the "American murderer" known as *uncinariasis*, or hookworm, a tiny intestinal parasite that left its victims anemic and confused, making it difficult for them to work or learn. Hookworm afflicted mostly poor people, in the American South and in equatorial regions around the world, who worked barefoot on soil polluted with larvae that had been shed in human feces. Millions of people in the United States, many of them school-age children, were infected. How many more worldwide was unknown. But for Stiles, this much was certain: efforts by the U.S. Public Health and Marine Hospital Service to target cotton mills where hookworm was widespread were insufficient. Hookworm disease, he believed, could be eradicated—or at the very least controlled—only with a population-level campaign combining treatment of everyone infected and wholesale improvements in sanitation to prevent reinfection. Nothing of this magnitude had ever been attempted by government public officials or nonprofit institutions in the United States.

In fact, the field of public health was still largely undeveloped in the United States and abroad at the beginning of the twentieth century. In the U.S., public health, if it was addressed at all by government, was largely a local issue. The federal government had established marine hospitals under President John Adams in 1798 to address the needs of officers and sailors in

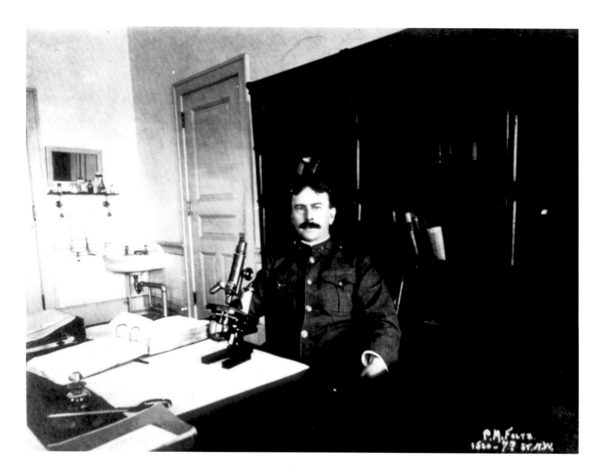

the U.S. Navy. After the Civil War, administration of these hospitals was centralized in Washington, D.C. under the management of the supervising surgeon (later called the Surgeon General). As immigration increased at the end of the nineteenth century, Congress passed the National Quarantine Act in 1878 and gave the Marine Hospital Service responsibility for preventing the introduction of contagious and infectious diseases and, later, for preventing epidemics from spreading among the states. In 1902 this service was renamed the Public Health and Marine Hospital Service. Although the service launched efforts to fight hookworm in the South and Puerto Rico, its staff remained limited and was assigned primarily to immigrant stations like Ellis Island in New York Harbor. In 1908 Stiles envisioned a public health system much more deeply embedded in local communities throughout the American South.

Charles Stiles was instrumental in eradicating hookworm disease in the American South. An expert in parasites, Stiles conducted research that led to the discovery of the unique American species of hookworm. In cooperation with the Rockefeller Sanitary Commission, Stiles helped to cure patients as well as educate the public on the disease and its relation to sanitation. (P.M. Foltz. National Library of Medicine.)

Over the weeks and months following his arrival in New York City, in an effort to drum up support for the eradication of hookworm, Stiles sought out the most important people in philanthropy and science at the time. Although he did not gain a direct audience with John D. Rockefeller, the richest man in the world, Stiles met with Frederick Taylor Gates, Rockefeller's most important philanthropic advisor. Gates had entered Rockefeller's orbit during the oil tycoon's creation of the University of Chicago, and he was now advocating that Rockefeller provide financial support for medicine. Stiles also met with Rockefeller's administrator, Wickliffe Rose, and the renowned pathologist Simon Flexner.

This was a time of extraordinary scientific optimism in America. Medicine had been revolutionized as a result of biological discoveries and advances in bacteriology. This new science built upon the discoveries of Louis Pasteur (1822-1895) and Robert Koch (1843-1910) in Europe. With the breakthroughs in bacteriology, the causes of numerous diseases were being discovered for the first time in human history. Sources were uncovered for tuberculosis, typhoid fever, and dysentery, which in 1900 accounted for 100,000 deaths in the United States. By then knowledge of disease vectors was accumulating. Healthy human carriers spread infectious diseases such as cholera, meningitis, and poliomyelitis. Animals transmitted diseases such as dengue, malaria, and yellow fever. Mosquitoes carried malaria plasmodia in their guts. The disease-causing parasite, which was endemic in the American South, had an annual mortality rate of 7.9 per 100,000.

With the emergence of this new scientific understanding, rational treatment and prevention of infectious diseases became possible. Clinicians could bridge the gap between the discoveries of pure science and their successful clinical application throughout the world. The developments in bacteriology made laboratory training for medical students of paramount importance. The new tools and knowledge could be used to institute public health and sanitary reforms. Physicians demonstrated how medical research could directly benefit their patients and the public.

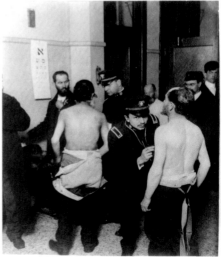

Doctors from the U.S. Public Health and Marine Hospital Service (later Public Health Service) examine a group of immigrants at Ellis Island. In the early twentieth century the U.S. government played a limited role in public health, and resources were directed at stations like Ellis Island in an effort to prevent the spread of contagions. The Rockefeller Sanitary Commission's hookworm campaign helped to change public opinion on the government's role in promoting health. (Library of Congress.)

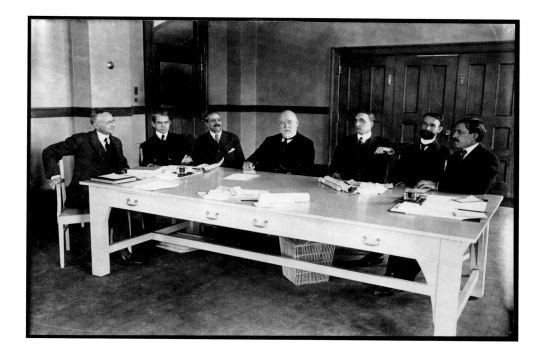

The original Board of Scientific Directors at the Rockefeller Institute for Medical Research. Seated from left are Drs. Simon Flexner, L. Emmett Holt, T. Mitchell Prudden, William Welch, Christian Herter, Theobald Smith, and Hermann Biggs. (Rockefeller Archive Center.)

Knowing all this, Stiles carried with him a specimen case, a microscope, drawings, photographs, lantern slides, and pages of statistics. He had demonstrated the need for hookworm eradication to professional and lay audiences throughout the Southern states. His photographs depicted dwarfed and hunched victims with yellowish, parchment-like skin. Lantern slides showed graphic pictures of the parasite's eggs found in human feces. The microscope revealed tiny wriggling pathogens that had been shed from the human body. Statistics revealed the percentages of infection by sex and age. "It seems to me," Frederick Gates remarked, when first presented with the idea for an eradication program, "that the all-important question to be solved is 'How many lives will be saved?'"

Like much of the lay public, Gates was concerned about the state of contemporary medicine, but optimistic about its potential. Driven by discoveries and progress in medicine and science, Gates had already been urging John D. Rockefeller to shift the bulk of his philanthropy from religious charities to more secular medical research and education programs. In 1901 Gates had encouraged him to establish the Rockefeller Institute for Medical Research, followed in 1903 by the General Education Board (GEB), to support higher education and medical schools in the United States and to help rural white and African-American schools in the South modernize farming practices. But in the fall of 1908, Gates saw hookworm eradication as a test case for the ability of Rockefeller philanthropy to address not only disease but also social and economic development.

Gates initially offered Stiles $50,000 for his hookworm campaign. But given the significance of the problem—the physical and educational abilities of more than two million Southerners had been hampered by hookworm—this was a mere drop in the bucket. Stiles said he would need much more. "He asked me to name a sum," Stiles reported, "and I suggested one million dollars." ($24 million in 2013 dollars.)

Rockefeller agreed to finance this massive effort. On October 28, 1909, he announced that he would give one million dollars over a period of five years to treat two million people affected by hookworm disease in the United States and Puerto Rico. The money would be given to a newly created entity—the Rockefeller Sanitary Commission for the Eradication of Hookworm Disease—to carry the battle forward. Everyone involved believed it surely would be enough.

The Southern Campaign

Wickliffe Rose wondered if hookworm was really as bad as Charles Stiles estimated. A professor of history and philosophy, Rose was teaching at the University of Nashville in 1910 when another Rockefeller advisor, Wallace Buttrick, contacted him with an extraordinary request.

Buttrick was the head of the GEB. After listening to Stiles talk about hookworm, he had become convinced that educational reform depended on eliminating the public health problems that limited the ability of children to concentrate in school, and, in turn, eradicating hookworm depended on health education. As Buttrick explained, people had to understand how this parasite worked. They needed to learn how to get rid of hookworms that had inhabited the body. Most of all, they needed to know what to do to prevent infection and reinfection. Buttrick believed that this public campaign needed a leader who was an educator, and Buttrick wanted Rose to do the job.

Rose was a Southerner. Born in Tennessee, he was an educator and academic by training, and he had considerable experience in planning and administration. With degrees from the University of Nashville and Harvard, he had been a professor of philosophy at Peabody Normal College. In 1902 he joined the Southern Education Board's Bureau of Investigation and Information at the University of Tennessee. Five years later, he became general

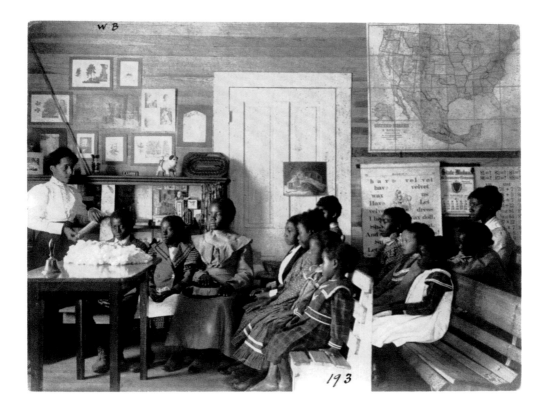

agent of the Peabody Education Fund, which promoted education in the Southern states. As part of his work with the fund, Rose collaborated with Buttrick on some of the GEB's initiatives. He had emerged as a powerful advocate for education reform. He understood what Buttrick wanted, and he agreed to take the job.

The Rockefeller Foundation's campaign against hookworm in the American South was one of modern philanthropy's first forays into public health. It entailed the application of science to a population-wide issue, and it required the education of medical personnel as well as the lay public and government officials to ensure their cooperation. At stake was the health and welfare of millions of people, many of them poor and African-American, many of them children—all innocent victims, directly or indirectly, of poverty.

As he traveled through the American South in the spring of 1911, Rose was overwhelmed by the evidence. In one county, infection rates were as high as 90 percent. Entire families were sick. In three of the schools he visited, only

At the turn of the last century, public education in the Southern United States was wholly inadequate and contributed to high rates of illiteracy, poverty, and poor health in the region. In 1903 the General Education Board (GEB) was created with the goal of reforming education and bettering the lives of African Americans and poor whites. The GEB helped launch the hookworm campaign and provided major grants to reform medical education. (Francis Benjamin Johnston. Library of Congress.)

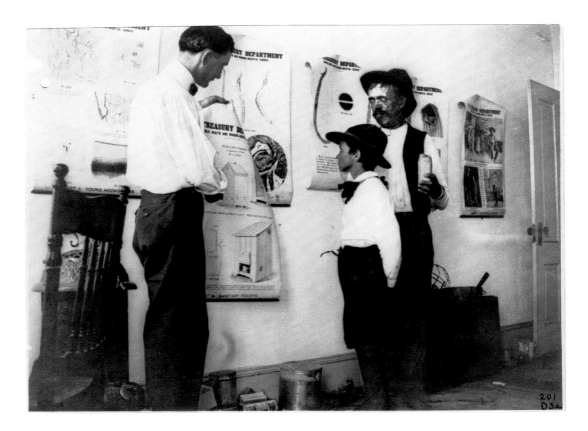

one child was healthy. He saw a 62-year-old woman who, after a lifetime of suffering from the infection, looked as though she was 90. "Her anemia was so extreme she was merely existing," Rose wrote. And yet there was hope; people were beginning to understand the connections among poverty, unsanitary conditions, infection, their lack of vitality, and the dire possibility of passing this all on to the next generation.

Hookworm disease was easy to explain, treatable, and preventable, providing an ideal way to educate Americans on the tenets of public health. Scenes like this, in which a doctor educates a father and son on the use of privies to halt the spread of hookworms, became a familiar part of the campaign to eradicate the disease. (Rockefeller Archive Center.)

Indeed, eradication of hookworm in the South was a tall order. At the beginning of the twentieth century, the Southeastern United States was still recovering from the Civil War. Public education was racially segregated and largely inadequate for both white and black children. Illiteracy was as high as 12 percent in the South, compared to a national average of 4.5 percent. Among African Americans it rose to more than 50 percent. Eighty percent of the population in the South relied on subsistence farming and lived in shanties—rural homes with primitive or no sanitation. The public health infrastructure was weak or nonexistent.

Chapter One: A Wedge That Leads to Public Action

Hookworm imposed a significant economic and social burden on the Southeastern United States. In 1909 Stiles had calculated that hookworm disease affected as many as two million persons. By 1910 he realized that the situation was worse than he had thought. He estimated that 43 percent of North Carolinians and more than six million residents of eight other Southern states were infected. The disease was especially widespread among African Americans in Alabama, Georgia, Florida, and North and South Carolina. Parasite-induced anemia made work difficult for its victims, who were unfairly charged with "laziness." Hookworm was the main cause of "sluggish" productivity among Southeastern agricultural workers and was associated with reduced intelligence in adults and children—by up to one-third and one-fourth, respectively, relative to their uninfected peers.

Fortunately, hookworm could be readily diagnosed and treated, and prevention methods were well known. Hookworm larvae enter the human body through the skin of the feet and migrate to the intestinal lining, where they feed on blood in the capillaries and lay eggs. The eggs are passed in feces and, where sanitation is inadequate, they enter the soil, where they develop into larvae to repeat the cycle. Because the parasite in both its egg and worm form can be seen through a microscope, infected people can be readily identified. Thymol, administered orally, can dislodge the worms after they attach to the small intestine. And actions as simple as using a toilet and wearing shoes (to keep larvae from entering the body) are enough to break the cycle.

Because hookworms could be detected in humans, eliminated with drugs, and prevented by improvements in sanitation, and because treatment quickly led to relief and thus increased productivity, it was the perfect candidate for the first major, widespread public health campaign in American history. Indeed, it would be the test case for the development of the field of public health.

Rose's Wedge

Frederick Gates and Wickliffe Rose disagreed about how best to deal with hookworm in the South. Gates argued for total eradication of the parasite and contended that the Rockefeller Sanitary Commission (RSC) should stay in the South until hookworm was eliminated. Rose, fearful that Southern health agencies would become dependent on Rockefeller resources, cautioned that the program should be funded only up to the point where other public agencies could take over. "If the infection is to be stamped out," Rose wrote in his diary, "the State in which it exists must assume the responsibility. An outside agency can be helpful only in so far as it aids the States in organizing and bringing into activity their own forces."

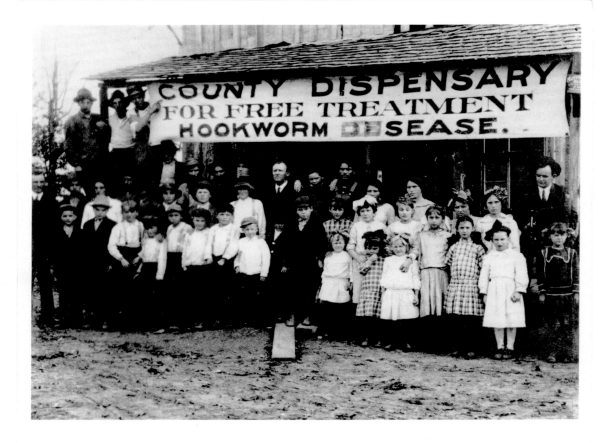

Indeed, Rose envisioned that the hookworm campaign would lead to the development of a whole new system of public health in the United States. From Rose's perspective, each step in the campaign—including diagnosis, drug treatment, sanitation improvements, and training—was a potential "entering wedge" that would eventually lead government agencies to accept responsibility for "the whole question of medical education, the organizing of systems of public health, and the training of men for the public health service."

County dispensaries, like the one pictured here in Alabama, offered free testing and treatment for hookworm disease. While treatment for adults was on a voluntary basis, infected children were required to receive treatment as a condition of school attendance. (Rockefeller Archive Center.)

Thus Rose organized the RSC's work with three main tasks in mind: to assess the spread of the disease in the Southern states, to treat the afflicted, and to establish a sanitation system to prevent reinfection. The first campaign began in January 1910. It was organized vertically; direction flowed from the board at the top, down through subordinate bureaus or their expert advisers,

Chapter One: A Wedge That Leads to Public Action

and on to the local directors and fieldwork personnel. But in the spirit of Rose's vision, it also proceeded collaboratively, with Rockefeller funding priming the pump of state public health systems.

From the start, the commission cooperated closely with state boards of health, allotting funds for increased personnel, promoting physician-training programs to help doctors diagnose and treat the disease, and sponsoring the purchase of equipment that would allow state laboratories to identify the hookworm parasite. A system of collaboration developed between the RSC and the state boards of health along with the state laboratories through a contingent of newly appointed directors of sanitation. Each director worked with a team of health inspectors, microscopists, and laboratory technicians who were paid by the state boards. In the first year alone, the commission enlisted 3,400 doctors in the eradication effort—17 percent of the region's medical force.

Local outpatient dispensaries for hookworm, pioneered by the U.S. Public Health and Marine Hospital Service in Puerto Rico in 1904, played a key role in much of this work. Frequently organized as tent clinics, and staffed by doctors, nurses, and diagnosticians with microscopes, the dispensaries often resembled a religious tent revival. Local residents came for the speeches delivered by physicians and scientists. They stared into microscopes to observe hookworms. People were called to provide stool samples the way a religious leader might exhort them to declare their faith. And once they had been diagnosed, they received doses of thymol to treat the infection.

Dr. C.J. Cully opened the first dispensary for the hookworm campaign in Columbia, Mississippi, on December 15, 1910. Typically, three to five dispensaries were set up per county. They were usually open one day a week for three to eight weeks, depending on the local need. Treatment—paid for by

The *Story of a Boy* was a picture book created to educate children and illiterate adults regarding the cause and cure of hookworm disease. The cartoon depicts bright red hookworms infecting the soil surrounding the boy and the dog. Public education—using posters, lectures, and demonstrations with microscopes—played an important part in the effort to eradicate hookworm. (B. Stephany. Rockefeller Archive Center.)

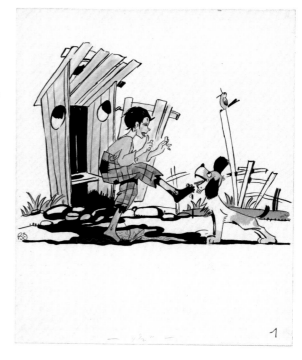

the commission and sometimes by the county, thus free of charge to the recipients—was voluntary for adults but compulsory for all schoolchildren. In the first year, more than 100,000 Southerners were examined for hookworm parasites. Nearly 45,000 were found to carry the disease, and of those, more than 38,000—84 percent—received treatment. By the middle of 1911, in Mississippi alone, 11,456 persons had been treated in 38 free dispensaries in seven counties. The progress was mirrored in other Southern states, including Virginia, North Carolina, and Kentucky.

Statistics developed to track the incidence of hookworm, the number of patients treated and cured, and the rate of re-infection proved critical to the work of the Rockefeller Sanitary Commission. In 1911 the RSC introduced a more uniform record-keeping system to increase the campaign's effectiveness. The system focused on local schools because they represented an important cross-section of the community and helped to standardize the sampling process. The diagnostic process was standardized to include microscopic examination of stool samples, eliminating variations based on less scientific evidence. Record keeping was also made uniform so that statistics in one county could be easily compared with others. This early disease surveillance system would provide the model for other public health campaigns in the future.

Education's Role

"This whole work is essentially educational," Rose wrote in his diary; "it is teaching people by demonstration." He continued, "The field directors carry out the work among the people. They tell the story of this disease in varied graphic forms and in terms simple enough that the common man, though he be illiterate, may see and understand." Education continued after diagnosis; each infected person received an envelope containing an appropriate dose of thymol and a card with printed directions for taking the medicine and preventing reinfection.

Science and culture intersected in the commission's efforts to raise public awareness about the treatment and prevention of hookworm disease. Of all the educational tools at the campaign's disposal, the microscope became one of the most important. "No exhibit is more effective," Rose wrote. "One person seeing these active larvae would go out and bring in friends. Persons coming in through curiosity, after seeing the exhibit would call for specimen containers for the whole family." Local culture took over the education work from there. "Some individuals and some whole families are holding out against treatment," Rose reported in 1911, "but they are being ostracized by their neighbors, and it is only a question of a short time when they must yield to the force of enlightened public sentiment." These grassroots features furthered the campaign's efforts beyond Rose's expectations.

People in the affected communities also needed to learn about proper sanitation. At the dispensaries, public health officials explained good sanitation in plain language. Community education programs resembled carnivals, with the organizers using refreshments and local children's choirs, public testimonials, and similar entertainments to encourage attendance. The campaign encouraged families and communities to install sanitary privies or "outhouses"—small toilet buildings erected away from the home—to prevent fecal contamination of the soil and thus break the hookworm transmission cycle. In keeping with Rose's pump-priming strategy, the Rockefeller Sanitary Commission offered to cover the costs of the educational campaigns if local governments paid for sanitation improvements.

Health exhibits with entertainment and a carnival-like atmosphere encouraged entire communities to come out and learn about hookworm. Exhibits like this one in Alabama encouraged attendees to not only be tested and seek treatment, but also to improve sanitation in an effort to ward off future infections. (Rockefeller Archive Center.)

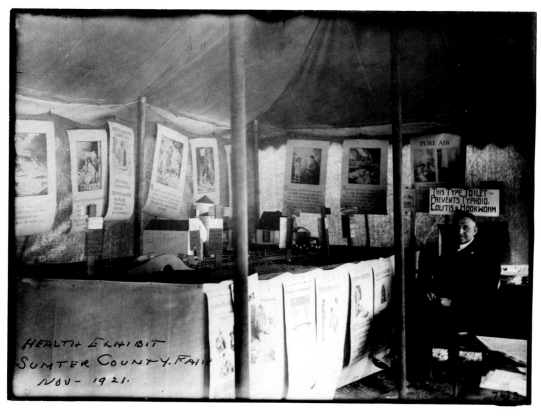

It was on the subject of privy construction, however, that Rose's wedge met its greatest resistance. Most homes in the South in the early twentieth century did not include indoor plumbing or toilets. Moreover, of the 250,680 homes inspected by the commission in 653 counties between 1911 and 1914, only half had a privy—nine out of ten of which were of the least sanitary kind, providing no protection from the transmission of hookworm and other diseases. Indeed, inadequate sanitation facilities were the norm in the South. The campaign therefore promoted a massive construction program across the Southern United States, and emphasized the enhancement of existing privies with a container that prevented soil contamination.

Charles Stiles promoted the LRS privy (named for its three inventors: L.L. Lumsden, Dr. N. Roberts, and Stiles), which the Rockefeller Sanitary Commission agreed was the most effective. But it was also the most expensive, and many communities resisted. Meanwhile other Southern towns passed ordinances specifying minimum health standards and used innovative advertising to promote the construction of privies. In front of one South Carolina courthouse, for example, stood a privy with its own public health message: "Build a privy now—use it always; It is cheaper than a coffin." Privy planning and implementation involved more than simple engineering techniques. Local leaders working with the Rockefeller Sanitary Commission realized that they had to take into account financial, social, cultural, and environmental factors. In other words, disease had to be understood as part of the whole social and environmental system.

Even when the commission was able to treat large numbers of people in a given community, reinfection as a result of poor sanitation eroded the overall effectiveness of the campaign. In 1913 leaders at the Rockefeller Foundation began to develop a far more comprehensive approach to hookworm aimed at total eradication. This approach became known as the "intensive method." The most important pilot study for the intensive method took place on Knotts Island, a small fishing community off the coast of North Carolina. Launched by G.F. Leonard, a physician with the Rockefeller Sanitary Commission, and C.L. Pridgen, with the North Carolina Board of Health Hookworm Commission, the project began with an intensive survey of the population. Fecal samples were collected from all but the seven residents who refused, and screened for the presence of parasites. Blood samples were also collected to test for malaria. Affected persons were targeted for treatment and

This sketch of a sanitary privy shows the use of containers to collect waste and prevent soil contamination. While this type of privy construction was ideal in halting the spread of hookworm, it was often too costly for individuals residing in one of the nation's poorest regions. (National Library of Medicine.)

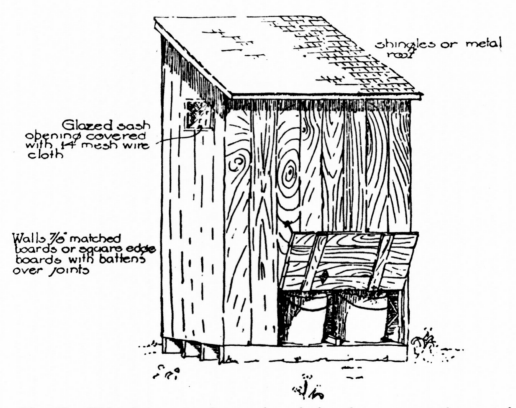

Fig. 17.—This shows a sanitary privy, designed to prevent the spread of disease. If a privy of this type were built on every farm and in every yard in villages, and if this privy were used by all persons, typhoid fever, hookworm disease, and various other maladies would almost or entirely disappear.

QUEEN MARGARET UNIVERSITY LRC

(To Be Tacked Inside of the Privy and NOT Torn Down.)

Sanitary Privies Are Cheaper Than Coffins

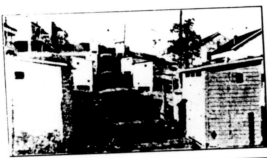

For Health's Sake let's keep this Privy CLEAN. Bad privies (and no privies at all) are our greatest cause of Disease. Clean people or families will help us keep this place clean. It should be kept as clean as the house because it spreads more diseases.

The User Must Keep It Clean Inside. Wash the Seat Occasionally

How to Keep a Safe Privy:

1. Have the back perfectly screened against flies and animals.
2. Have a hinged door over the seat and keep it CLOSED when not in use.
3. Have a bucket beneath to catch the Excreta.
4. VENTILATE THE VAULT.
5. See that the privy is kept clean inside and out, or take the blame on yourself if some member of your family dies of Typhoid Fever.

Some of the Diseases Spread by Filthy Privies:

Typhoid Fever, Bowel Troubles of Children, Dysenteries, Hockworms, Cholera, some Tuberculosis. The Flies that You See in the Privy Will Soon Be in the Dining Room.

Walker County Board of Health

follow-up. An innovative approach at the time, the intensive method was an immediate success: "All went as planned," Pridgen wrote. "I consider the hookworm work practically done."

The one remaining problem, however, was the need for sanitary privies to prevent reinfection. The prototype developed by Stiles was not appropriate for the island's sandy soil and water levels that fluctuated with rain and tide. Water pollution was a concern. Pridgen struggled to adapt the program to the local environment. "I have searched my brain," he wrote, "spent sleepless nights and made weeping appeals to all my friends in order to find a quick solution." There were economic obstacles as well. Pridgen lamented, "I feel that there is a simple solution somewhere but I can't get to it." Community support was the most pressing issue. "The greatest trouble is that we must figure against ignorance and carelessness," said Pridgen. On Knotts Island, the question of safe and affordable privy construction was not immediately

This poster from the Walker County Board of Health provides essential information on how to keep privies safe and sanitary, and warns that failing to keep a privy clean can lead to the death of a family member. (National Library of Medicine.)

solved. Neither was the question of how to continue to support the community's public health efforts once the privies were installed.

All in all, the comprehensive nature of the intensive method, which entailed a near total transformation of the community with regard to the spread of hookworm, still did not result in total eradication. As Leonard concluded, a long-term solution would have to come from sustained community education and sanitary improvements. In the great debate between seeking cures and transforming public health systems, represented by William Welch and Wickliffe Rose, the experiment with the intensive method seemed to favor public health.

The End of the Sanitary Commission's Work

Rose had hoped to extend the life of the Rockefeller Sanitary Commission beyond the five years originally outlined by Rockefeller and Gates. But by the end of 1914, the institutional structure for John D. Rockefeller's philanthropy was changing. In 1913 the Rockefeller Foundation had been chartered in the state of New York. Soon after the Foundation was created, the board established the International Health Commission as a subsidiary of the Foundation. Rose was chosen to lead this new organization, with a plan to attack hookworm in affected countries around the world. Under this new structure, the Rockefeller Sanitary Commission's work was absorbed into the Rockefeller Foundation at the end of 1914.

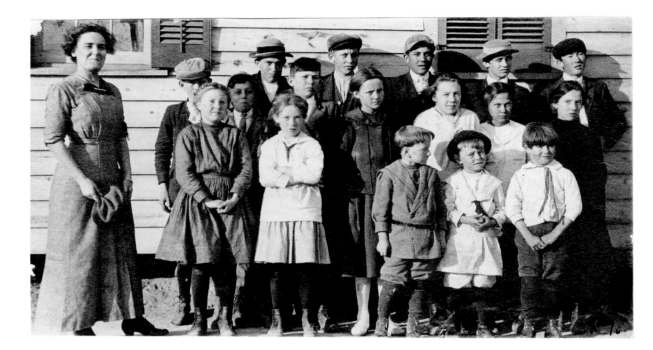

The hookworm campaign did not achieve Gates's goal of total eradication. Though the dispensary system convinced scores of people to be examined and treated for hookworm, fewer than 25 percent of estimated cases had been cured by mid-1914, and some of the most afflicted counties had not been visited. In areas that had been visited, additional clean-up campaigns to prevent reinfection and further spread of the disease had been effective, but costly.

Wickliffe Rose and others associated with the Rockefeller Foundation struggled to define the lessons learned from the campaign. The Foundation acknowledged that improving sanitation was a long and difficult process. Sanitary surveys proved to be both expensive and slow. As Rose remarked in 1914, it was "more difficult to get improvement in sanitation than to get people treated." Hygienic privy construction was taken up in some parts of the South, but it lagged behind other campaign projects. Finally, the initial hookworm program had excluded non-medical concerns such as economics, politics, and social norms. By the end of the campaign, Foundation leaders realized that, in choosing sanitation technology, they needed to consider socioeconomic, institutional, environmental, financial, and cultural factors.

In 1913 school children in Knotts Island, North Carolina, were tested and treated for hookworm as part of a comprehensive effort to free the island of the disease. However, finding suitable sanitation for the area and combating a local mindset resistant to change proved to be formidable challenges to eradication. Education and a public health system were required to achieve long-term goals. (Rockefeller Archive Center.)

Chapter One: A Wedge That Leads to Public Action

Despite these disappointments, the legacies of the Rockefeller Sanitary Commission were significant. With Rose at the helm, it had spent more than $680,000 ($15.8 million in 2013 dollars) on the largest and most complex community-wide health program carried out in the United States up to that time. Altogether, the commission and its network of county health agencies had examined more than a million people for hookworm infection and had treated more than 400,000. The commission had also promoted the development of health infrastructure so successfully that state appropriations for health work in the South had increased by 81 percent. And even after the Rockefeller Sanitary Commission was dissolved, hookworm eradication work continued in the South through 1917, with the continued financial cooperation of states in the American South.

> "Rose's vision of the campaign as a wedge to further the development of public health, which would in turn lead to social and economic development, proved highly successful."

Indeed, by the time the commission terminated its work, a network of state and local health units in 11 states was in place that would provide a model for the emerging field of public health for generations to come. Employing new operational methods and leadership styles to educate the public on matters of health and hygiene, the campaign had instilled in the general public an interest in scientific medicine and public health while encouraging programs for sanitation, health inspections, and school construction. This work led to increases in school enrollment and attendance as well as literacy. Overall, Rose's vision of the campaign as a wedge to further the development of public health, which would in turn lead to social and economic development, proved highly successful—so successful, in fact, that the leaders of the newly created Rockefeller Foundation believed that similar campaigns would help to substantially improve the lives of rural communities in developing nations around the world.

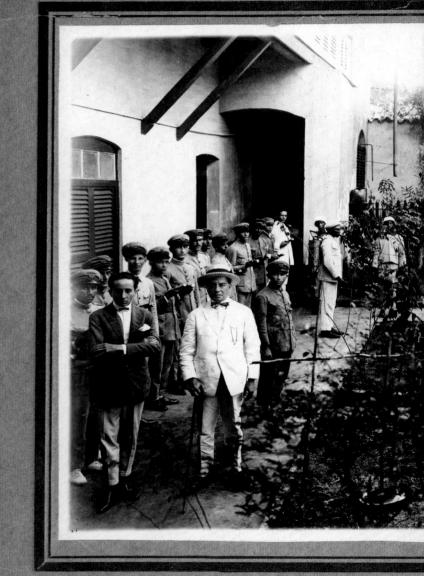

Kommissão da ...
— Missão R...

São Luiz - Ma...

Brazilian public health officials and the Rockefeller Foundation collaborated to launch a major campaign against yellow fever in the 1920s. From this work, the Foundation would learn lessons that would influence many of its future public health campaigns. (Rockefeller Archive Center.)

15056

e Amarella
efeller —

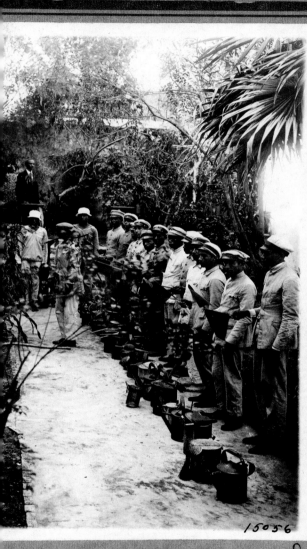

15056

nhão - Brasil. Florence M. Read.

A bxmª Snrta.

A. Ormandua

5.

THE FIRST
GLOBAL CAMPAIGNS

The International Health Commission, a subsidiary of the Rockefeller Foundation, was created in 1913 to champion the cause of preventive medicine throughout the world. "Its immediate object," explained the Foundation, was to carry the battle against hookworm to other nations and "to assist in the establishment of permanent agencies for promoting public sanitation and spreading the knowledge of scientific medicine." In keeping with Wickliffe Rose's idea of the entering wedge, the fight against hookworm would serve "as an excellent starting-point from which the various states and nations might develop and put into execution well-rounded, comprehensive programs for advancing the public health."

In many ways, hookworm represented the ideal disease for promoting Rose's wedge strategy. Diagnosis was relatively simple and also accessible to the layperson, who could see the worms in human feces or under a microscope. Treatment was usually effective. Prevention demanded specific strategies, such as building sanitary latrines and wearing shoes. And the social return on investment was very high.

The fight against hookworm also helped change attitudes about the overall benefits of investing in public health systems. Indeed, public education about hookworm in the American South had fostered both top-down and bottom-up strategies for promoting public health. Physicians and public officials recruited to the campaign played key roles as public leaders; meanwhile, individuals and families lobbied public officials to provide resources to maintain the campaign.

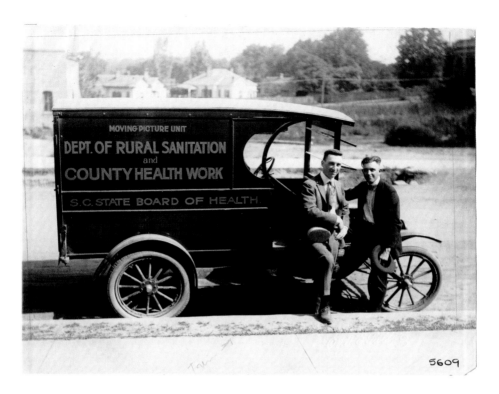

5609

Tactically, Rose hoped to apply all of these lessons learned in the American South to help developing nations around the world.

The first step in developing the Foundation's global campaign was to measure the extent of the problem. Rose dispatched experts to Asia and Latin America to conduct surveys, which revealed that hookworm infection was "an international problem of serious proportion," endemic in 54 countries. Prevalence ran as high as 90 percent in Puerto Rico and Colombia, and well above 50 percent in India and China. Hundreds of millions of people were infected worldwide.

Soon after these surveys were complete, the International Health Commission worked in concert with local officials to mount hookworm campaigns in several parts of the world. In every country, the commission began by conducting surveys to assess the prevalence of disease. Next, it used microscopic examination to confirm diagnosis and to monitor treatment of those infected. Finally, the commission employed sanitary measures to stop soil contamination and collaborated with local health professionals and public officials to develop public education campaigns.

Public health campaigns relied on a number of methods, including films, to teach people about disease and sanitation. Moving picture units, operated by doctors, traveled throughout a region to reach a wide audience with informative films meant to educate the public on communicable diseases. (Rockefeller Archive Center.)

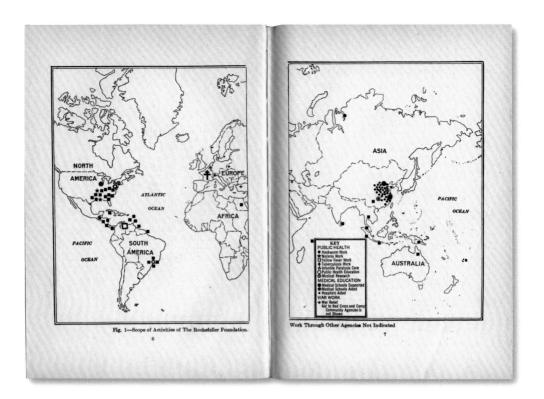

Fig. 1—Scope of Activities of The Rockefeller Foundation.

6

KEY
PUBLIC HEALTH
■ Hookworm Work
★ Malaria Work
□ Yellow Fever Work
▲ Tuberculosis Work
△ Infantile Paralysis Care
○ Public Health Education
◉ Medical Research
MEDICAL EDUCATION
● Medical Schools Supported
◐ Medical Schools Aided
■ Hospitals Aided
WAR WORK
✝ War Relief
   Aid to Red Cross and Camp
   Community Agencies is
   not Shown

Work Through Other Agencies Not Indicated

7

By the time it launched its international campaign in 1913, the Rockefeller Foundation understood that eradication was nearly impossible—except possibly in smaller communities like Knotts Island—so the global initiatives generally emphasized "relief and control." To further Rose's wedge strategy, the Foundation negotiated agreements that would integrate the campaign within the existing infrastructure for public health and provide for the gradual assumption of financial responsibility by the government.

Within five years of its founding the Rockefeller Foundation was firmly establishing itself as a global philanthropic organization. This map from 1917 shows the scope of the Foundation's work, including hookworm campaigns in South America and Southeast Asia, medical education in Asia, and war relief efforts throughout Europe. (Rockefeller Archive Center.)

In all, the commission established cooperative hookworm programs in 52 countries on six continents and in 29 island groups. Despite the overall uniformity in its approach, however, Rose and others at the Rockefeller Foundation soon realized that they had much to learn about working with other cultures and systems of government in a world still shaped by the global politics of imperialism. The lessons learned in this global campaign against hookworm—and in later campaigns against diseases like yellow fever and malaria—would have a profound impact on the Foundation's work in global health for decades.

The Rockefeller Foundation's global campaign against hookworm began with a dinner in London in August 1913. During his first trip across the Atlantic, Wickliffe Rose met with leaders of the British Colonial Administration at the sumptuous Marlborough Club, where he delivered a magic-lantern slide show on the work of the Rockefeller Sanitary Commission. Rose told his audience of the creation of the International Health Commission and offered to help fight hookworm throughout the British Empire. Lewis Harcourt, the British Colonial Secretary, pronounced the evening such a success that "I should not wonder if in the future we come to look back upon this evening and the gathering around this table as the beginning of a new day in the adminis- tration of our colonies and of a better civilization for all tropical countries."

In March 1914, with the consent of the British government, the International Health Commission began its first hookworm campaign abroad in British Guiana, a territory chosen for its relatively small size and proximity to the United States. In British Guiana,

The campaign to eradicate hookworm disease became truly global on April 16, 1913, when the International Health Commission administered its first dose of thymol to a patient in British Guiana. The patient, named Beni (number 5 below), later posed for this photograph surrounded by local and American officials. (Rockefeller Archive Center.)

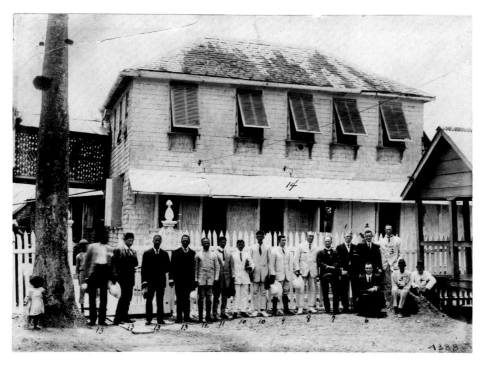

the commission adopted the intensive-method strategy, which was soon dubbed "the American method." Working with the families of generations of imported sugar plantation and rice farm laborers (the laborers themselves were treated by the planters) whose historical origins were in Africa, East India, China, and Portugal, the Foundation mapped the incidence of hookworm on the island and began treating people who were infected.

At first blush, working with colonial authorities was not much different than developing partnerships with county and state public health officials in the American South. Tensions emerged over treatment philosophies; the British generally preferred a lower, but more continuous, dose of thymol, while the Americans favored a stronger, but more purgative approach. Other conflicts developed over roles and strategies. Dr. A.T. Ozzard of the British Guianan Medical Service criticized the "Rockefeller Health Commission" for spending "vast sums of money" on surveys and treatment rather than building sanitary latrines. But these expenditures followed the Rose strategy. The officers of the International Health Commission believed that they were responsible for surveying, treating, and educating the public. "The subsequent introduction and maintenance of any sanitary measures to prevent reinfection," as historian John Farley explains, was the responsibility of local public health officials.

Ultimately, after five years of trying to resolve tensions and ambiguities in roles and responsibilities, the British chose in 1919 not to renew the hookworm campaign agreement in British Guiana. But by this time the commission—renamed the International Health Board (IHB) in 1916—had expanded its work into other countries and regions of Central and South America, where it faced other challenges and had to innovate and adapt to meet its goals.

RESPONDING TO LOCAL CULTURE

In Latin America and other parts of the world, the IHB frequently had to consider the role of local healers. This effort was not unlike the challenges that the Rockefeller Sanitary Commission had faced in the American South in its efforts to win allies within the local medical community. But epistemological differences between traditional healers and physicians trained in the scientific method could often lead to suspicion and conflict.

In Brazil, for example, during the hookworm eradication campaign in 1917, civil service employees were concerned that the IHB intended to displace self-taught native healers, known as *curanderos*, with practitioners who had been trained by medical schools in the urban centers. The power of curanderos

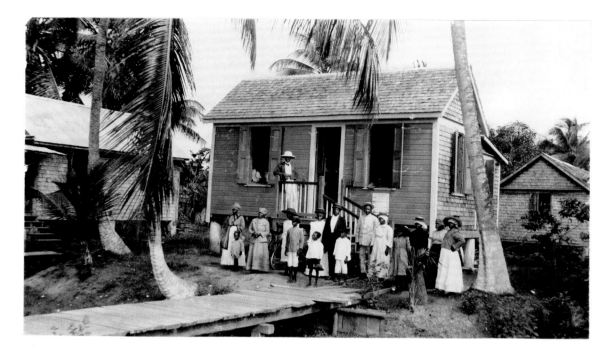

was based on a number of factors, including the curative effects of certain foods and plants as well as people's faith in the healers, in the healers' agents, or in supernatural beings. The conflict between curanderos and modern medical practitioners evidenced age-old divisions: modern versus traditional, urban versus rural, and the educated versus the self-taught.

Staff members of the International Health Board (IHB) attempted to balance respect for local cultures with the application of Western medicine. While their efforts often met with resistance, they also managed to treat the thousands of individuals who sought it, including these patients in Bagotville, British Guiana, who arrived at the IHB's local headquarters to receive treatment. (Rockefeller Archive Center.)

To address these tensions, the staff of the IHB in Brazil, Costa Rica, and other countries looked for ways to integrate native healers into public health campaigns. At the same time, some of the native healers would incorporate techniques learned from the IHB's staff into their work with local communities. Author Steven Palmer suggests that this produced a kind of medical pluralism that accounted for local cultural practices and helped to mitigate the impact of hookworm and other diseases.

IHB staff were also constantly challenged to understand and adjust to local conditions and cultures. In British Guiana, for example, the "East Indian wedding season," which lasted from February through the end of May, and the rhythms of rice cultivation had affected the availability of labor. Thus, IHB teams in the agricultural colony of British Guiana had only a few weeks each year during which they could do their work under optimal conditions.

In British Guiana and Colombia, some communities resisted providing the stool specimens required for microscopic examination because the methods and messages of the campaign ran counter to local beliefs and practices. Another issue involved the IHB's emphasis on the dissemination of an affordable sanitary privy, which local populations resisted for cultural as well as economic reasons. Over time, the IHB learned to work with these cultural differences as part of an ongoing process of adjusting to local conditions.

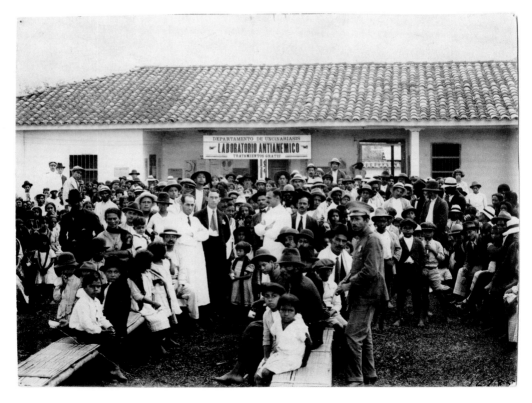

SETBACKS AND TENSIONS

The global hookworm campaign also faced challenges that played a key role not only in the overall development of the campaign, but also in the evolution of the field of public health. The most important of these issues related to the ethics of mass public health treatment programs.

In the American South, the drug thymol was the standard cure for hookworm disease, but it had uncomfortable side effects. Many patients refused to take it without a

By 1926 campaigns to eradicate hookworm had been initiated in 52 countries on six continents. In Cali, Colombia, patients gathered for treatment in front of a dispensary. (Rockefeller Archive Center.)

doctor's supervision, and researchers looked for an alternative medication. When World War One interrupted the supply of thymol, the IHB began administering oil of chenopodium to hookworm patients in Central America and the British Caribbean. Derived from a weed found throughout much of the United States, oil of chenopodium, or "wormseed oil," proved to be equally effective in ridding the body of worms. In fact, it was widely used by curanderos and other indigenous healers in Latin America and the United States.

But for some patients, especially children, this new treatment was very dangerous. From 1914 to 1934, 222 deaths occurred from oil of chenopodium poisoning. Eighty-seven percent of these victims were children aged 13 or younger. The IHB initially described some of these deaths as "tragic accidents," but as historian Steven Palmer has shown, they were, in fact, a product of the still-undefined ethical framework for medical innovation in the early decades of the twentieth century. For example, in the early years of the hookworm campaign, the Foundation "had no mechanism for effectively translating scientific evidence into safer field protocol," said Palmer. This deficiency was magnified by the "experimental" ethos of the hookworm campaign itself, which Palmer has described as the "first mass medication of international health."

According to Palmer, the Foundation's reaction to the fatalities from chenopodium treatments evolved over time. In the early years of the campaign, the IHB did not keep good records on fatalities. But as officials realized the importance of this information, data collection improved. The Foundation discussed fatalities in its annual reports as part of an overall evaluation of the safety and effectiveness of the hookworm campaign. And with greater information on the risks, the board adjusted dosages to find the right balance between safety and effectiveness. All of these efforts, as Palmer notes, "led to a gradual reduction in the incidence of fatal poisoning." They also helped contribute to the evolution of a stronger ethical framework for medical treatment, especially when poor and vulnerable populations were involved.

Tuberculosis in France

With the success of the hookworm campaign, at least in terms of its ability to encourage governments to invest in public health, the Rockefeller Foundation was increasingly willing to lend its expertise and resources to health crises in other parts of the world. The destruction wrought by World War One led to a serious decline in sanitary conditions in Europe and an increase in the level of disease. In France, particularly, tuberculosis reached epidemic proportions.

The Rockefeller Foundation became involved with this public health crisis through its efforts to help provide relief to war refugees. After a survey in January 1917 documented the extent of the disease, the Foundation created the Commission for the Prevention of Tuberculosis in France, operating under the auspices of the IHB. The commission concluded that its best avenue of attack was through a centralized national organization modeled after the National Tuberculosis Association in the United States. Under this system, all French agencies devoted to the prevention and treatment of tuberculosis were consolidated into "administrative machinery" directed by a central committee. The IHB intended to direct this system, but under the supervision of the French government.

The campaign against tuberculosis, however, tested the Rockefeller Foundation's ability to play a neutral role in a country's administrative political system. When rival departments within the French government competed for control of the central committee, Wickliffe Rose was persuaded that the Foundation had to act with some independence to avoid being seen as allied with one department over the other.

Another key strategy employed in France, which had already been tested by national tuberculosis campaigns in the United States, was a youth-focused traveling exhibit using lectures, slides, movies, posters, pamphlets, and press articles. American advertising techniques, such as the display of full-color posters on various social causes of the disease, had never been seen in France. For the tuberculosis campaign, they helped educate the public and represented a new tool in the array of strategies used for public health campaigns.

The Commission for the Prevention of Tuberculosis also adopted from the United States a special tuberculosis dispensary system. After the American method was demonstrated in two units—one in a rural community and one in a city—dispensaries were built throughout the country and staffed with *visiteuses d'hygiène*, who went out into the community to educate the sick about the disease, hygiene, and prevention. Whereas the commission wanted public health nurses to work in dispensaries and provide medical care, the French visiteuses d'hygiène did not dispense medications or medical advice; instead, they referred the ill to a physician. Up to that time, the French system had no public health nurses, and the role of the visiteuses d'hygiène was exclusively social and educational, not medical. To address this limitation, the commission supported ten-month training programs for visiteuses d'hygiène, as well as a two-year diploma program to train public health nurses throughout France. Training

While efforts were made to treat tubercular patients in France, great attention was also paid to preventive medicine in an effort to stop the spread of the disease before it overtook French cities. As part of this campaign, colorful posters advertised the services of visiteuses d'hygiène, women who visited infected areas and offered education on disease prevention. (Rockefeller Archive Center.)

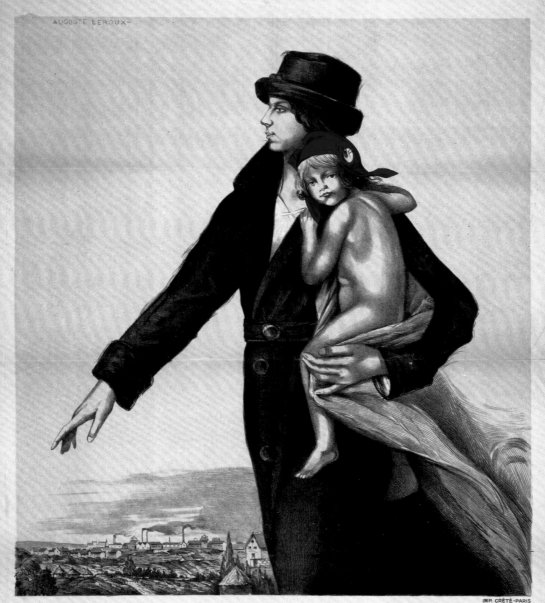

LA VISITEUSE D'HYGIÈNE EST L'AUXILIAIRE DU
MÉDECIN ET DES ŒUVRES SOCIALES DANS
LA CROISADE CONTRE LA TUBERCULOSE
ET LA MORTALITÉ INFANTILE.
SOUTENEZ-LA !

COMITÉ NATIONAL DE DÉFENSE CONTRE LA TUBERCULOSE, 66 BIS, RUE NOTRE-DAME DES CHAMPS, PARIS VI?
AVEC LE CONCOURS DE LA FONDATION ROCKEFELLER.

VILLE DE ROUEN

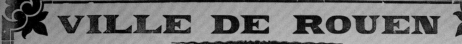

MISSION ROCKEFELLER

Commission Américaine de Préservation contre la TUBERCULOSE en France.

CIRQUE DE ROUEN

VENDREDI 12 DECEMBRE 1919, A 20 H. 30.

Sous la présidence de Son Eminence le cardinal DUBOIS, Archevêque de Rouen ;

GRANDE
CONFÉRENCE

SUR LA TUBERCULOSE

Par M. Ch. FUSTER

ET SUR

La Santé par l'Hygiène

Par Madame MARSAUX

LA MUSIQUE MUNICIPALE DE ROUEN

Sous la direction de M. SCHMIDT,

prétera son concours à cette conférence

qui sera suivie de

CINÉMA

ENTRÉE GRATUITE — DISTRIBUTION DE BROCHURES

Les ENFANTS non accompagnés ne seront pas admis.

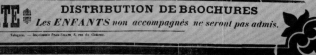

Valognes. — Imprimerie Paul-Simon, 8, rue du Château.

programs familiarized nurses with the scientific method, recordkeeping, and statistics, and taught them how to conduct public education campaigns as well as to structure home visits in infected areas.

The tuberculosis campaign in France was enormously expensive. By 1919 it accounted for 42 percent of the IHB's global expenditures. Foundation officials were never able to assess the overall effectiveness of the campaign. The mortality rate from tuberculosis in France declined, but some of this decline was undoubtedly a result of the general improvement in social conditions that followed the end of the war. For Wickliffe Rose, however, it was clear that the campaign had helped to cultivate what one public health official called "a widespread desire for improving the public health service."

Campaigns Against Other Diseases

As a result of its global hookworm eradication efforts and, later, the tuberculosis campaign in France, the Rockefeller Foundation realized that further research about prevention and treatment of tropical diseases was needed and that most countries had a shortage of health care workers trained for surveillance, treatment, and prevention of disease. These were among the concerns that the IHB addressed as it launched new campaigns against other diseases, including malaria in the U.S. South and Latin America, tuberculosis in France, and yellow fever in Brazil.

Building on the initial success on Knotts Island, for example, the Foundation in 1915 extended the intensive method for fighting hookworm to the battle against malaria, which was also endemic in the U.S. South and so virulent that it caused more sickness and death than all other diseases combined. Between 1912 and 1915, the U.S. Public Health Service had carried out a series of campaigns in mill towns in the American South to prevent malaria and treat victims. These campaigns led to a 66 percent reduction in the incidence of the disease, but the Public Health Service lacked the resources to build on these efforts. Wickliffe Rose and the other members of the IHB were impressed by the results and agreed to launch a series of experimental projects to determine whether the Foundation could develop an effective antimalarial campaign that local communities could afford to continue on their own.

Foundation officials began a trial of malaria eradication in Mississippi and Arkansas. Staff conducted surveys in which blood specimens were drawn and family histories were taken. Then an eight-week course

A 1919 poster advertised a public lecture in Rouen, France, where members of the Rockefeller Foundation-funded Commission for the Prevention of Tuberculosis in France discussed issues of the disease as well as hygiene. By 1922 the commission had suspended operations and its activities were administered by French authorities. (Rockefeller Archive Center.)

of quinine was distributed to people infected with malaria. This treatment was followed by an examination of new blood specimens. If infection remained, treatment started anew.

As with hookworm, public education played a critical role in these malaria campaigns. Foundation staff, working with local public health officials, encouraged the public to eliminate the breeding sites for mosquitoes. People in some counties were advised to drain the standing water around their homes, where mosquito larvae develop. In other communities, residents were counseled to add oil to containers of standing water to prevent larva development. The IHB also experimented with a larva-eating fish called the top-minnow in rural Mississippi in 1918, and subsequently in towns throughout Texas. Cheaper than the oil approach, this new technique led to a reduction in the incidence of malaria in Mississippi by 77 percent within the first year. Researchers quickly learned that these antilarval techniques were often more effective malaria prevention strategies than efforts to eliminate adult mosquitoes.

On the basis of the trials in Arkansas and Mississippi, the Foundation believed that malaria programs could be extended successfully to other tropical areas by combining a strategy of mosquito eradication in towns with screening and quinine distribution in rural areas where eradication seemed unfeasible. The first international malaria campaign modeled on the Foundation's efforts in the American South was launched in Nicaragua in 1921. The IHB then began a malaria program in Brazil. Soon, as former Rockefeller Foundation President Raymond Fosdick has written, the board had started projects "in a rapidly extending line that ran through practically every malarious region in the world, touching all the continents and many islands of the seas."

SAMPLE No. 2.

MOSQUITOES

Every Effort is Made to Keep Yazoo City Free of Mosquitoes.

Guests in this hotel are requested to notify the management if mosquitoes are found to be present.

The management is, in turn, requested to report mosquito nuisances to the Health Department, phone 249, who will examine into all complaints received and take the necessary steps to have such nuisances abated.

It is requested that this notice be conspicuously posted in each guest chamber, bath room and lavatory in your hotel.

W. E. NOBLIN, M. D.,
City and County Health Officer. 1923

BIRDSALL PRINTING CO., YAZOO CITY, MISS.

Anti-malaria campaigns in the United States required vigilance. In addition to health surveys and quinine treatment for infected persons, local officials, like these in Yazoo City, Mississippi, asked for the public's help in destroying mosquito breeding grounds and reporting areas of infestation. (Rockefeller Archive Center.)

Eradication of malaria-bearing mosquitoes proved difficult, however. The disease was transmitted by approximately 70 different species of *Anopheles* mosquito, and breeding habits among these species varied in different parts of the world. In the United States mosquitoes proliferated in areas where there were large quantities of standing water; in the Philippines *Anopheles* developed in rapidly flowing foothill streams. In Trinidad, meanwhile, mosquitoes bred in the water that collected on the broad leaves of certain trees. Even in focusing on one region, steps taken to limit the breeding sites of one type of mosquito might create new habitat for another malaria-carrying species of *Anopheles*. Eradication and prevention strategies, therefore, varied from region to region.

The IHB also struggled to measure the effectiveness of these campaigns. Although field officers were asked to generate data to be sent to New York, statistical accuracy was lacking until the board hired Persis Putnam in 1926. A former assistant director of educational work at the U.S. Public Health Service, she had earned a doctorate in statistics just prior to joining the Rockefeller Foundation. For the next 22 years, Putnam brought a new rigor to data analysis and epidemiology. She asserted the need for experimental controls and collecting comparative data to prove the efficacy of the Foundation's methods. Her work was particularly

Trying to rid the world of malaria-bearing mosquitoes proved a formidable task due to the variety of species and their unique breeding habits. These members of the International Health Board studied mosquito habitats in Puerto Rico in order to determine the best program for eradication in the territory. (Rockefeller Archive Center.)

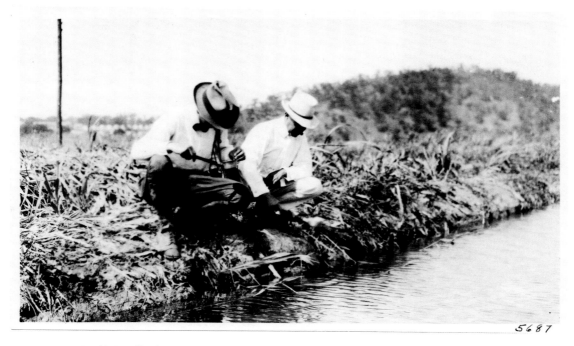

5687

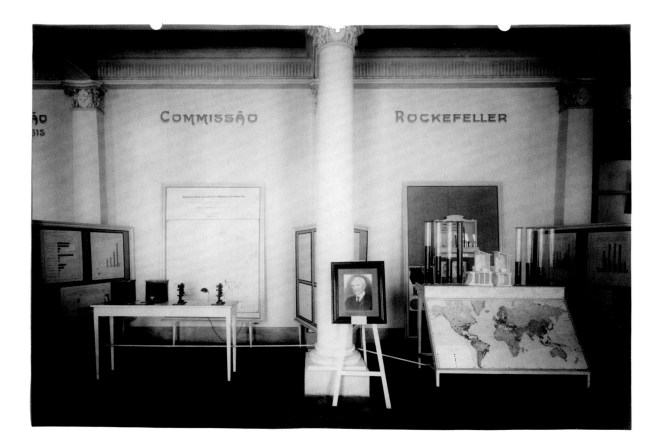

The International Health Board (IHB) presented an exhibit of its work in Brazil at the Independence Centenary International Exposition held in Rio de Janeiro in 1922. Throughout the 1920s the IHB was involved in Brazilian public health campaigns, including efforts to control yellow fever and hookworm disease. (Rockefeller Archive Center.)

valuable in Italy, where the IHB was challenged to prove the superiority of antilarval campaigns over the simple distribution of quinine to the population. Putnam's analysis of data compiled by Lewis Hackett and other field officers played a key role in convincing local officials to change their public health policies.

Along with improved data analysis, the Foundation also supported anti-malaria campaigns with research initiatives focused on the life cycle of the mosquito in different environments, the metabolism of the parasite injected by the mosquito, and the effects of various antimalarial drugs. Research, prevention, eradication, and public health campaigns organized by the Foundation between 1916 and 1939 played a significant role in reducing the impact of malaria in some parts of the world. But, as described in Chapter IV, real progress would be dependent on the development of a powerful new insecticide on the eve of World War Two.

In the fight against hookworm, tuberculosis, and other diseases, the Rockefeller Foundation learned to work with local health officials to minimize resistance to the Foundation's staff as "outsiders" and to maximize the transfer of knowledge and technology for improving community health. The Foundation gravitated to countries that had strong diplomatic ties with the United States and leaders or champions to help the cause. In 1916 Brazil fit the Foundation's criteria. Diplomatic relations were good, and Oswaldo Cruz, the director of public health in Rio de Janeiro, had done important work on yellow fever and bubonic plague that impressed the leaders of the Foundation. In addition, economic leaders in Brazil supported the idea of hookworm control in rural areas because they believed it would lead to greater productivity, particularly in the coffee industry. Between 1917 and 1922, funding for the hookworm campaign in Brazil grew from $12,000 a year to more than $2 million.

Brazil's geographic diversity and decentralized political authority presented complex challenges, however, as the IHB worked with local officials first to battle hookworm and later yellow fever. When yellow fever resurfaced in Brazil in the 1920s, after a period of absence, there was disagreement about the best way to address the problem. Local governments in key urban centers carried out short-term fumigation campaigns to destroy adult *Aedes aegypti* mosquitoes, the carriers of yellow fever. The Rockefeller Foundation, on the other hand, suggested preventing *Aedes aegypti* larvae from hatching in the first place by adding oil to containers of standing water or by releasing small, larva-eating fish into water containers—strategies that researchers had learned were effective against malaria in the U.S. South.

The antilarval measures were less expensive, more effective, and more efficient than fumigation, but they met with resistance in Brazil, where, in the absence of running water, households collected water in large storage containers and where people resented the intrusion of public health inspectors attempting to implement an antilarval strategy. Furthermore, politically attuned public health officials in the cities preferred the immediate results of fumigation to the apparently passive long-term outcomes of antilarval programs. Negotiations between the IHB and Brazilian officials led to the use of both antilarval strategies and fumigation in nationwide yellow fever campaigns in 1929. In a manner reminiscent of the display of public health posters in France, the IHB also funded educational films depicting antilarval methods that it hoped the public would use.

Disagreements also arose between government officials and IHB personnel over whether to target urban or rural populations. Believing that yellow fever was endemic only to urban centers with populations greater than 50,000, the IHB targeted those urban centers as well as coastal cities in the north, where the program was often effective. However, local public health officials argued that yellow fever was also widespread in rural areas, where the majority of Brazilians lived in the 1920s. Ultimately, the Brazilians were right. The Rockefeller Foundation embraced the idea that a "sylvan" or "jungle" form of yellow fever also posed a significant threat to more rural populations, and the Foundation worked with local officials to extend antilarval campaigns to smaller towns and rural communities.

The IHB also had to contend with Brazilians' perception that the health campaigns were merely an advance guard for imperialist domination, although these concerns were balanced somewhat by the positive perception that health campaigns would increase productivity among Brazil's workers. Yellow fever control became an issue of national pride in Brazil. As with the campaign against tuberculosis in France, politicians and scientists, as well as the public, clamored for the involvement of more Brazilians in the effort. Over the course of the campaign, the Rockefeller Foundation helped to strengthen and legitimize the role of the national government in an integrated approach to the control of yellow fever, which, beginning in 1931, was administered in Brazil under the auspices of the newly established Unified Yellow Fever Service.

Ultimately, as a consequence of successful mosquito control programs in Brazil, elimination of disease-carrying organisms became the basis of subsequent efforts to eradicate other diseases around the world. Thus, in Brazil there were both political and logistical victories for Rose's wedge.

MOVING FORWARD

Hookworm, tuberculosis, malaria, and yellow fever were not eradicated by the International Health Board in the 1910s and 1920s, nor was Western science transmitted directly and easily to countries outside the United States. Nonetheless, the IHB learned valuable lessons about how public health campaigns are mediated by the society, culture, and politics of host communities. Efforts to create systems to improve public health could be propelled or stymied by the hopes and fears of individuals at each of these levels—from an individual's embarrassment about being asked to provide a fecal sample, to a community's fear that it was being used as an "experiment," to a government official's hope for unending financial support.

During these early years, the Rockefeller Foundation had to repeatedly adjust its programs to accommodate local cultural concerns and environmental conditions as well as regional and national priorities, and it often collaborated with local people knowledgeable in these areas. The Foundation also had to work diplomatically with local bureaucrats who believed they already knew how to deal with a disease and simply needed funds from the Foundation's seemingly inexhaustible supply of money. Finally, experiences with hookworm, tuberculosis, malaria, yellow fever, and other diseases helped the Rockefeller Foundation and others in the emerging field of public health begin to define the ethical and intellectual framework for experiments and campaigns that aimed to perfect new ways of protecting the physical well-being of people around the world.

These campaigns led to the establishment and strengthening of public health services and health education in many countries. In Thailand, for example, with the support of Prince Mahidol Adulyadej, who studied public health and medicine at Harvard and was an heir to the royal throne, hookworm eradication became an opening wedge for building a public health system. In Brazil the IHB collaborated for six years in the creation of an institute of public health. But as Rose and others realized, these campaigns against disease and the development of public health systems were critically dependent on medical education and training for public health personnel. To strengthen these educational systems, the Foundation's leaders would need to overcome the resistance of entrenched interests. Philanthropic leaders like Wickliffe Rose and medical pioneers like Johns Hopkins University's William Welch would also need to reconcile their own competing visions of the future.

American and Brazilian directors of the Brazilian hookworm campaign posed together in 1921. From left to right: Drs. Mario Pernambuco, F.L. Soper, G.K. Strode, W.G. Smillie, L.W. Hackett, J.H. Janney, M.J. Faria, Alan Gregg, and Samuel Uchoa. (Rockefeller Archive Center.)

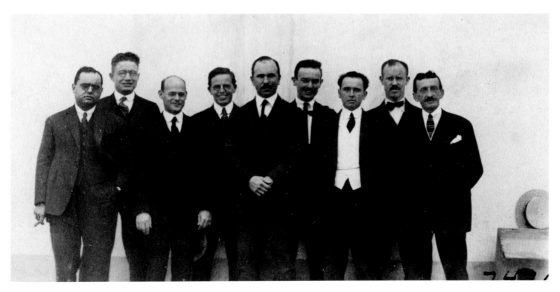

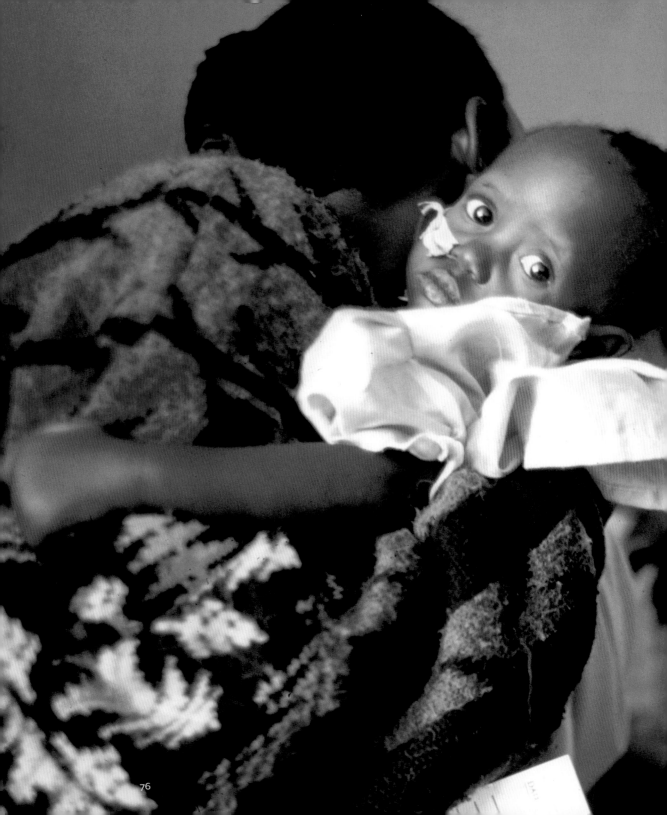

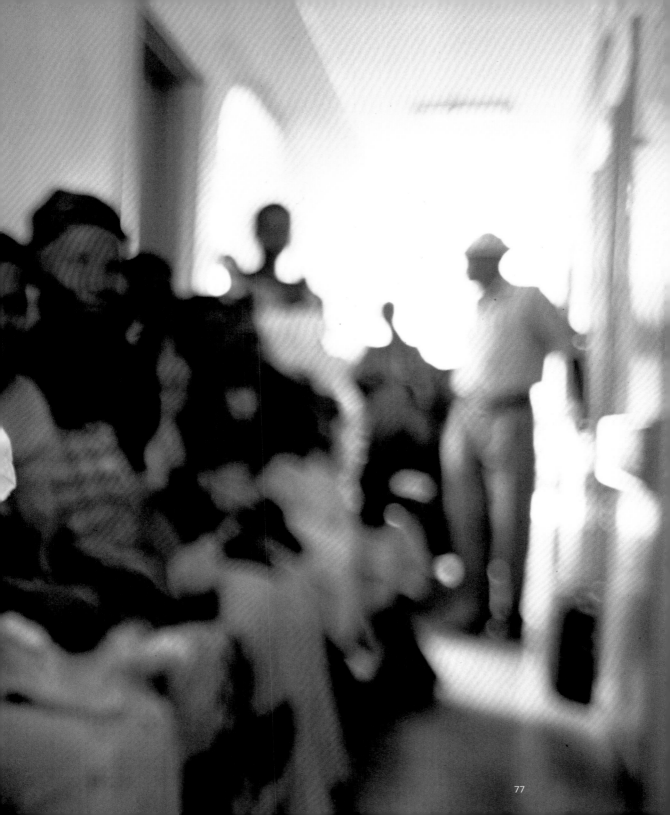

TRAINING THE CAREGIVERS

Wickliffe Rose had anticipated that the Rockefeller Foundation's campaigns to eradicate hookworm would be an "entering wedge" that would eventually lead host nations to consider "the whole question of medical education, the organizing of systems of public health, and the training of men for the public health service." Rose believed that there was a widespread disparity created by the need for physicians trained in public health and the failure of medical schools to meet the need. His assumptions were based, in part, on a report drafted in 1910 by Abraham Flexner, whose brother Simon Flexner was head of the Rockefeller Institute for Medical Research in New York and also a protégé of William Welch.

Abraham Flexner was an enigmatic man with big ideas about education reform. One of the first graduates of Johns Hopkins University, he had studied psychology at Harvard before writing a critique of higher education in the United States. Abraham was hired in 1908 by the Carnegie Foundation for the Advancement of Teaching to conduct a survey of North American medical schools

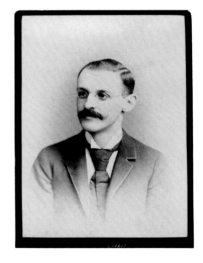

Abraham Flexner's *Medical Education in the United States and Canada* was a landmark critique of North American medical education. Among Flexner's chief concerns were the lack of scientific rigor in medical training and the abundance of for-profit medical schools that churned out unskilled doctors. (E. Klauber. Library of Congress)

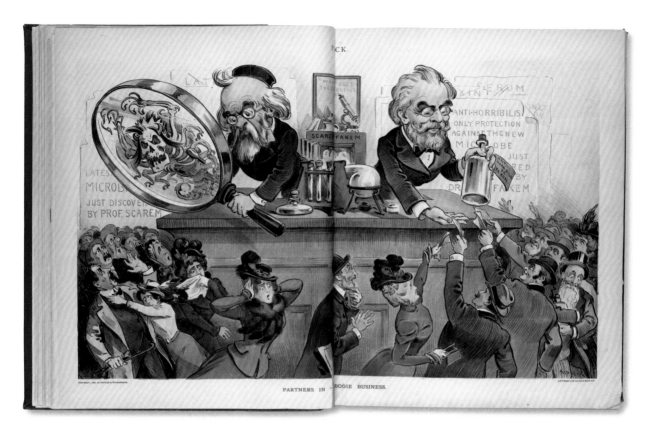

PARTNERS IN THE BOGIE BUSINESS.

for the purpose of making recommendations for their improvement. Flexner visited every medical school in the United States, and his report, widely publicized in 1910, showed that most for-profit, proprietary, degree-granting medical schools had mediocre instructors, curricula, and facilities. Many had such low admission standards that anyone with the ability to pay the tuition would be admitted.

Flexner reported that the United States had some of the best medical schools in the world, but also some of the worst. He recommended that the number of medical schools in the United States at that time be reduced from approximately 131 to 31, in order to ensure that the quality of medical education would keep pace with breakthroughs in medical science. Within these reformed schools, under Flexner's model, physician training would be founded on scientific principles, with clinical instruction provided by full-time professors who were also undertaking hospital-based research focused on improving patient care. Structural

Prior to the publication of the Flexner report and the reforms that followed, medical education and practice in the United States were not subject to significant regulation. As a result, nineteenth-century medicine was rife with scams, fakery, and unlicensed 'doctors' selling 'cures' to a gullible public. (Udo J. Keppler. Library of Congress.)

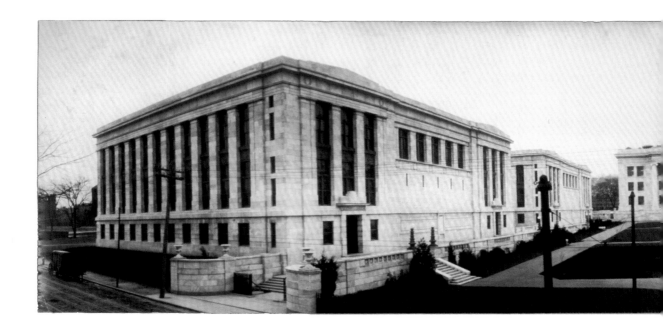

changes would include an emphasis on physics, chemistry, and biology; extensive hands-on clinical experience; and an expectation that professors would be engaged full-time in teaching and research so they would not be overburdened with the simultaneous demands of private practice or consultation.

The General Education Board allocated millions of dollars to improving medical education in the United States. Among the recipients was Harvard University, which received $1.4 million to improve its medical program. (S. Arakelyan. Library of Congress.)

Flexner's model was immediately attacked. Some accused him of muckraking. Others considered the model too dogmatic and largely insensitive to the needs of poor applicants, who would not be able to meet the higher standards for entry to medical school—increased to four years of premedical education in some states—or pay a higher cost for their education. Professors worried that being limited to full-time teaching would deny them income from private practice and paid consultations. Opposition also came from health practitioners who would suffer if the model became standardized, including traditional healers, some of them African American, and practitioners of alternative medicine.

At the same time, Flexner's report reinforced changes that were already underway in the field as the American Medical Association lobbied local and state governments to strengthen the licensing requirements for physicians. These tough requirements put economic pressure on many of the weaker, proprietary schools that believed additional investments in facilities and faculty would lead to increases in tuition and, eventually, a decline in

Chapter Three: Training the Caregivers

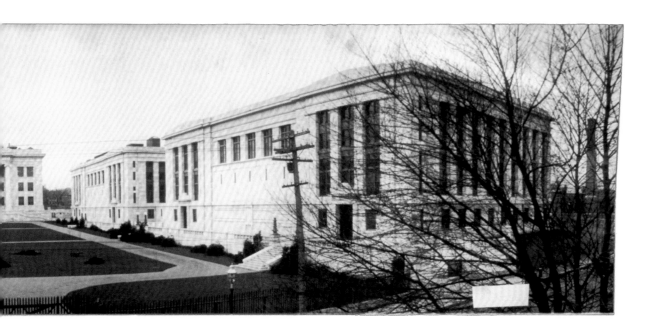

enrollments. Many chose to go out of business. Others affiliated or merged with a university. These changes set the stage for a major effort to strengthen the nation's remaining and most effective medical schools.

Investing in Medical Education

At the newly established Rockefeller Foundation, the Flexner Report was scrutinized and generally endorsed by Wickliffe Rose, William Welch, and other advisors and members of the board. As historian Paul Starr has written, it became the "manifesto" of a program that by 1936 would guide $91 million in funding from the Rockefeller Foundation and its sister institution, the General Education Board (GEB), to a select group of medical schools.

To lead this effort, Frederick Gates recruited Abraham Flexner, who was already a consultant to the GEB. In 1911, while the Rockefeller Foundation's charter was still pending before Congress, Gates asked Flexner, over lunch, "What would you do if you had a million dollars with which to make a start in the work of reorganizing medical education?" Flexner immediately suggested giving the money to Johns Hopkins to accelerate its development as a model institution for the rest of the country. Impressed by this conversation and by Flexner's work as a consultant to the GEB as well as the Carnegie Foundation for the Advancement of Teaching, Gates recommended that the GEB hire

Flexner as its assistant secretary, the second highest staff position. Elated, Flexner wrote to his brother Simon: "And so opens a new chapter!"

In his new position, Flexner moved quickly to encourage leading medical schools to adopt the "full-time plan" under which faculty received no outside income from clinical practice. He pushed through a major grant by the GEB to Johns Hopkins in October 1913 to help pay for full-time faculty, build and finance new laboratories, and expand enrollments. He also recommended major grants to Washington University in St. Louis and Yale University to help these institutions transition to full-time faculty.

The GEB provided funding during the early days of the medical education initiative, but its charter confined its grantmaking to the United States. After the Rockefeller Foundation had been established to work throughout the world, and as Flexner and other Rockefeller advisors oversaw the expansion of the program internationally, the Foundation provided the grants, ultimately establishing a separate Division of Medical Education in 1919.

In the United States, Rockefeller philanthropy played a critical role in the transformation of medical education. By endowing these leading schools, the Foundation essentially condemned proprietary medical-training institutions— those with only one or two instructors, whose main income included private practice and consultation—and helped accelerate the consolidation of medical education in the United States. From a high of 165 institutions in 1906, the number of medical schools in the United States fell to 70 by the late 1920s.

The Rockefeller Foundation also rewarded the University of Chicago for adopting the Flexner model, pledging one million dollars ($21.5 million in 2013 dollars) for the creation of what became an integral component of medical education: the modern teaching hospital. By 1917 all additional monies needed by the university had been raised, with an aggregate value of more than $14 million.

These efforts to provide financial incentives for the reform of medical education were driven by deep-seated beliefs that commercialism in medicine was not a good thing. Gates, Flexner, and others within the Rockefeller philanthropies were suspicious of poorly trained doctors as well as of pharmaceutical companies, many of which were not far removed from patent medicine makers who promised to cure every known human ailment with a few swallows of their amazing elixirs. For good reasons, these Rockefeller insiders hoped to strengthen public-sector prevention, even as they worked to improve medical education. To promote public health, however, they would need to train a new generation of experts attuned to the circumstances that affected the well-being of whole populations.

The need to educate practitioners went hand in hand with the emergence of a new era in the history of public health. In the nineteenth century, the sanitary reform movement had sought to improve public health by improving sewer systems in urban areas. The discovery of bacteria and the development of the germ theory of disease in the 1870s led to improvements in water systems and medical treatment. Both revolutions led to better health and longer lives. They also prompted institutional reforms, including the first local health departments and the creation of the diagnostic laboratory as the scientific arm of the health department.

All of these initiatives and debates were ongoing when the General Education Board gathered in New York on May 27, 1915. When Wickliffe Rose arrived—as described in the Introduction—he expected William Welch to provide the plan that the two of them had developed for a model "School of Public Health" with an emphasis on the development of a national training system in the field. Instead, the document Welch shared with Rose only hours before the meeting was dramatically different.

The new "Welch-Rose Report" contained very little of Rose's draft. Rather than create a "School of Public Health," the plan called for the establishment of an "Institute of Hygiene." As historian Elizabeth Fee has noted, the change in title alone signaled a shift in emphasis from teaching to research, and from practice to science. Welch's version of the report "essentially ignored Rose's proposed system of state schools, practical demonstrations, and extension courses." Plans to train public health nurses and inspectors had also disappeared, along with the development of public health as "a distinct profession" separate from medicine. Instead, Welch envisioned an institution that would focus heavily on research and cultivate and advance the science of hygiene rather than meet the institutional needs of the public health service for trained personnel. It would cater to the interests and needs of physicians, rather than a broader audience of public administrators.

Rose agreed to Welch's revisions; he never explained his decision. In 1915, deeply immersed in his work for the International Health Commission and war relief, he may have decided that Welch's plan represented a good start. He was also inclined to be deferential to Welch, who was a highly regarded scientist and physician.

Rose, Flexner, and Rockefeller Foundation Executive Secretary Jerome Greene were appointed as a committee of three to choose a home for the first institute of public hygiene. Their choice narrowed quickly to either Harvard or Johns Hopkins. Rose favored Johns Hopkins, argues historian Elizabeth

"The Institute of Hygiene," also known as the "Welch-Rose Report," proposed a plan for public health education. While Wickliffe Rose envisioned a program that taught practical skills to nurses, engineers, and others outside the medical profession, William Welch drew up a plan that was directed at the medical community and emphasized scientific research as an inroad to public health. (Rockefeller Archive Center.)

Fee, because the full-time faculty was more independent from the influence of the medical profession, whom Rose saw as major opponents of the expansion of public health. Flexner agreed, and Jerome Greene bowed to the majority.

The selection committee's recommendation was ratified by the Executive Committee of the Rockefeller Foundation in 1916, when the Foundation appropriated $267,000 ($5.73 million in 2013 dollars) to launch the Johns Hopkins School of Hygiene and Public Health. With an organization, building plan, budget, and curriculum designed primarily by Rose and Welch, the school opened to students in 1918, and Welch served as its first director. Endowed with $6 million, the research-oriented school supported nearly 40 faculty members by 1922 and emphasized bacteriology and the germ theory of disease, fields of knowledge considered essential for future public health personnel working in local and state health departments.

Over the next few decades, the Johns Hopkins School of Hygiene and Public Health became a leader in the fields of public health education and research. To some extent the competing visions of both Rose and Welch were frustrated. Rose's concept of a national system of public health agencies developed all too slowly. By 1929 only 467 of the nation's approximately 2,500 counties had public health agencies. That represented a 40 percent increase over 1920, but it was still far short of addressing the needs of the American people. Meanwhile Welch's optimism that physicians would be drawn to the field of public health proved unfounded. As Fee notes, cultural and economic forces—shaped by exciting innovations in diagnosis, therapeutics, and surgery—proved far more attractive to most doctors, while public health struggled to overcome its image as the poor stepchild of medicine.

Despite these disappointments, over the long run the Hopkins model would play a major role in the development of public health. In 1922, with a Rockefeller Foundation endowment and following the model developed at Hopkins, Harvard University established its School of Public Health beside the Harvard Medical School. Before the end of the decade, with support from the Foundation, several other major universities in the United States established or reorganized their public health programs as well, including Yale, Columbia, and the University of Michigan. The Hopkins model would also influence the development of public health education and research abroad, especially in China, where the Rockefeller Foundation would make the largest single investment in its history.

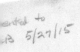

° 200L
Institute of Hygiene ?files

...rted to
...B 5/27/15

INSTITUTE OF HYGIENE

...ng a Report by Dr. William H. Welch
...and Wickliffe Rose to the General
...Education Board, submitted in 1915

...rence * on training for public health service held at
...eneral Education Board in New York on October 16, 1914,
...o develop substantial agreement on the following points:
...tal need in the public health service in this country at
...s of men adequately trained for the work; (2) that a dis-
... toward meeting this need could be made by establishing
... place a school of public health of high standard; (3)
...itution, while maintaining its separate identity, should in
...n of economy and of efficiency be closely affiliated with a
...ts medical school; (4) that the nucleus of this school of
...hould be an institute of hygiene.

...Rose and Dr. Welch were asked to formulate a plan for such an
...ygiene and in compliance with this request offer the following
...is designed to set forth the scope and general character of
...of the institute and the service which it should render in train-
...ne, preventive medicine and public health and in the advancement
...jects. If desired, the report can be supplemented by a detailed
...f organization, plan of building, budget and courses of instruc-

- - - -

... Abbott, Dr. Herman M. Biggs, Dr. Simon Flexner, Mr. Jerome D.
...Dr. Victor G. Heiser, Dr. Edwin O. Jordan, Mr. Starr J. Murphy,
...H. Park, Dr. Wickliffe Rose, Dr. M. J. Rosenau, Dr. Theobald
...Dr. George C. Whipple, Dr. C.E.A. Winslow, Dr. Wm. H. Welch, Prof.
...ackson, Dr. F. Cleveland, Dr. Wallace Buttrick, Dr. E. C. Sage and
...raham Flexner.

2

...IN ENGLAND AND IN GERMANY.

...ealth movement and of the culti-
...may be found especially in the
...n 1848 and in the establishment
...kofer in Munich in 1865. The
...from the discoveries relating
...ctious diseases and the con-
...diseases. It is instructive
...conceptions and directions of
...In Germany every university
...ucted by a professor and
...ented broadly in all its
...laboratory courses and field
...n England on the other hand,
...stly governmental or inde-
...ublic health administra-
...d. Those desiring to
...he diploma in public
...least nine months of
...d medical officer of
...t seems obvious that
...e English systems, and
...scientific and the practi-

...HE NEEDS IN AMERICA.

...cking both in laborato
...public health work.
...s, but none is comple
... schools attempt some
...s all inadequate and

...es is at present the
...th work, and is recog.
...alth officials, socia
...istration, national,
...ained leaders and tre
...apidly growing appre
...omising careers of u
...bility, character an
...ents and physicians
...es of hygiene and
...owledge in this
...he great needs of
...of hygiene.

...ss of persons
...se who expect
...ese will aim
...red in some

Political and economic turmoil in China had paved the way for U.S. Secretary of State John Hay's Open Door Policy and the advancement of American interests in the early years of the twentieth century. Frederick Gates and John D. Rockefeller's other philanthropic advisors saw an opportunity to contribute to the improvement of education in China by establishing a great university along the lines of the University of Chicago.

To explore this idea, Rockefeller funded the Oriental Education Commission in 1908 to survey China's educational institutions. The commission concluded that there was a need for a great university in China, but it noted that Chinese officials were wary of secular reforms.

At the same time, many American and European missionaries were hostile to the idea of a Rockefeller-backed university that might rival their influence, and provincial politicians would demand that their appointees control any such institution. From this report Frederick Gates concluded that development of a major Rockefeller-funded university was not feasible.

Students and faculty of the class of 1922 in medical zoology at the Johns Hopkins School of Hygiene and Public Health. The interdisciplinary curriculum had offered students the opportunity to engage in public health research while receiving practical training for future work in the field. (Rockefeller Archive Center.)

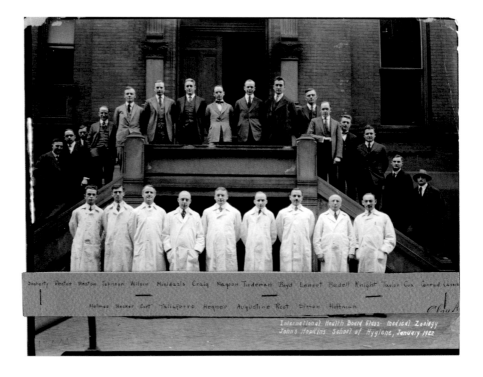

Chapter Three: Training the Caregivers

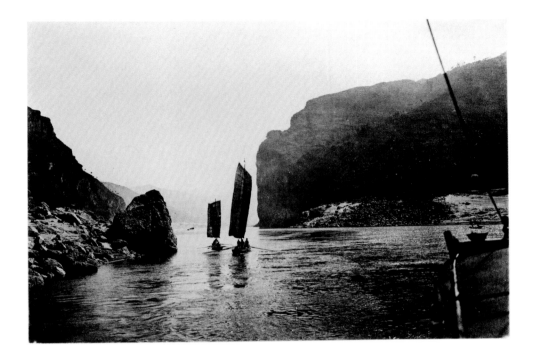

As the global hookworm campaign continued, meanwhile, stimulating Rockefeller interest in foreign medical and public health education reform, China once again rose to the top of the list of potential projects. Medical education seemed far less controversial or politically challenging. In January 1914 the Foundation's board of directors convened a conference composed of officers from Christian missionary boards, medical missionaries who had deployed to China, and Chinese dignitaries who were visiting New York. The purpose of the conference was to discuss how the Foundation could best stimulate the creation of a modern medical system in China, including a movement for public and personal hygiene to prevent disease. As a result of this conference, the Foundation's board of directors voted to send a three-person commission to survey medical education and public health needs.

China was particularly attractive to the Rockefeller Foundation because of its history in medicine and health. Frederick Gates, for example, believed that "no land, whether in America or Europe, has any system of medicine at all comparable in efficiency or promise" to that of China, although he did not think it was rooted in scientific ideas. He had long been in communication with medical missionaries as well as with those who were compiling the history of the missions. And prior to the creation of the survey commission,

China was a long-time interest of the Rockefeller family. John D. Rockefeller Sr. and John D. Rockefeller Jr. had both faithfully supported Baptist missionary causes in Asia prior to the creation of the Rockefeller Foundation. (Rockefeller Archive Center.)

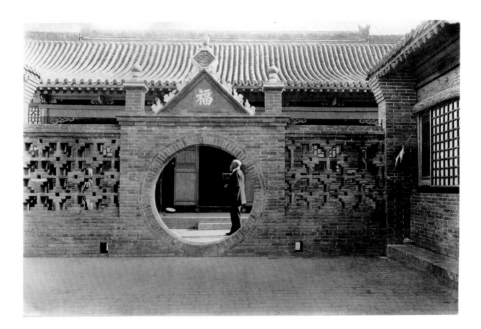

Gates had laid out a four-step plan for the gradual and orderly development of a comprehensive system of medicine in China. The commission would explore whether Gates's plan was realistic.

The commission members visited 17 medical schools and 97 hospitals in 11 of China's 18 provinces. They also consulted with government officials and regional missionaries who were responsible for more than 300 clinics throughout the country. Generally, they found that Western medicine had not yet noticeably affected the Chinese health care system. Nor was the practice of medicine subject to government regulation in China, where most health care was delivered by practitioners of traditional medicine who had usually inherited both the healer's role and secret medicinal recipes. Chinese medicine relied on traditional treatment methods such as acupuncture, and surgery was nearly unknown. Because dissection of human cadavers was contrary to traditional beliefs and viewed with particular horror, knowledge of internal human anatomy was limited. Western science, including physics and chemistry, was not taught in the Chinese equivalent of high school, while most of the medical schools visited by the commission were small and run by either individual doctors or missionaries. Aside from a few provincial institutions, there were only two government-funded medical schools—Peking Medical Special College and Peiyang Military Medical College. The Beijing school had only 70 students and 10 professors at the time.

In 1908 the Rockefeller-funded Oriental Education Commission traveled to China to survey China's educational institutions. The commissioners documented their travels in photographs and reports, and at Taiyuan, Shanxi, they found the "best inn at which the party stopped." (Rockefeller Archive Center.)

The survey commission's report, submitted in October 1914, played a major role in shaping the Foundation's strategy. To assure high standards, the commission recommended a large-scale, long-term initiative to build and develop a few major institutions at key locations. To integrate Chinese medicine with the development of the scientific community in the West, instruction should be in English and the Foundation should award fellowships for Chinese students to study abroad.

The Foundation's board of trustees established the China Medical Board a month later. John D. Rockefeller Jr. was appointed chair and Roger Greene was appointed resident director in China. With Greene's assistance, the Foundation purchased the campus of the Peking Union Medical College (PUMC) from the London Missionary Society in 1915 and embarked on a multi-year effort to expand and upgrade the school's faculty and facilities. By 1917 China had become "the most important foreign recipient of Rockefeller philanthropy."

If China's health care system was to be modernized, such efforts were critical. In 1921 discrepancies between the Chinese and American medical education systems were enormous. There was only one medical student for every 175,000 people in China, and one physician for every 120,000. In the United States the numbers were one student for every 8,000 and one physician for every 720. The United States had five times as many medical students as China and 37 times as many physicians, for a population roughly a quarter the size.

At the Peking Union Medical College dedication ceremony in September 1921, John D. Rockefeller Jr. noted, "The purpose of the China Medical Board was to develop a medical school and hospital of a standard comparable with that of the leading institutions known to western civilization." In other words, it was "the Johns Hopkins of China." PUMC consisted of laboratories, a pathology building, a 250-bed hospital with approximately 30 private rooms, and a large outpatient department. The hospital administration unit included quarters for resident physicians and interns. There was a dormitory for nurses as well as industrial plants to supply water and electricity. By 1930 the hospital had 346 beds and had treated 5,071 inpatients along with 134,312 outpatients.

From the start, the goal was to train China's future medical leaders. Standards and curricula were designed to produce physicians, professors, scientists, and public health administrators. Following the Flexner model and the Johns Hopkins example, laboratory experience and clinical demonstrations in hospital wards were emphasized. Most graduates competed at the highest level internationally, and many went on to receive advanced degrees from American institutions.

But this single medical college was not designed to solve the health services problem in China. "The China Medical Board recognized from the outset," John D. Rockefeller Sr. noted, "that only the Chinese nation itself could cope with a task so colossal as the establishment of modern scientific medical education throughout the Republic and all that Western civilization could do would be to point the way."

The China Medical Board's work also went hand in hand with efforts by the International Health Board (IHB) to strengthen medical education in other parts of Asia. Led by Wickliffe Rose, staff surveyed medical schools in the Philippines and Siam (now Thailand) to learn how doctors were trained and how the education system could be improved. These surveys revealed that training in public health was lacking or nonexistent and that little was being done for public hygiene. The IHB also investigated medical education in India in 1915, and additional surveys were commissioned there in 1921 and 1928. Researchers estimated that no more than one percent of the population of India had access to well-trained physicians. The Foundation responded in many cases, when the surveys were complete, by offering grants and loaning physicians as well as other experts to help bolster medical and nursing training programs in these nations.

President Xu Shichang of China (left) talks with John D. Rockefeller Jr. at the Presidential Palace in the Imperial City in 1921. Rockefeller had traveled to China to dedicate the newly opened Peking Union Medical College. (Rockefeller Archive Center.)

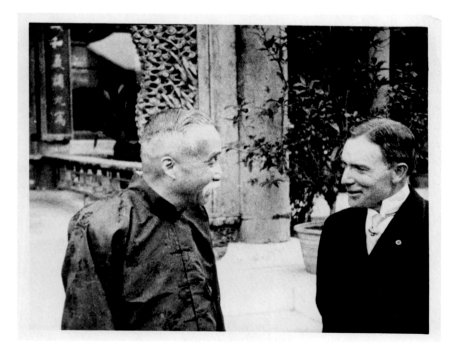

Chapter Three: Training the Caregivers

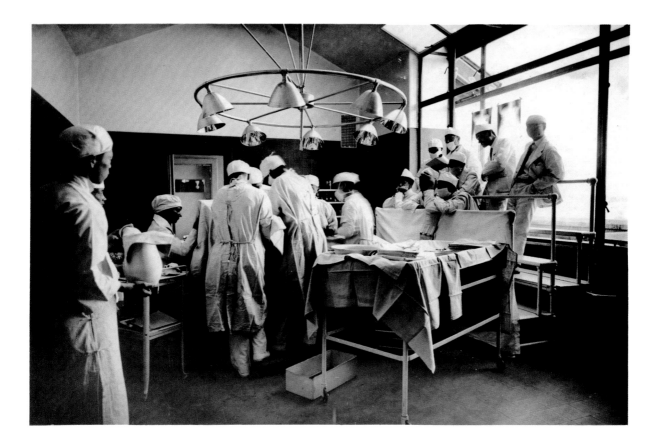

In Thailand the IHB, working closely with Prince Mahidol, assisted in the building of a first-rate medical school at Siriraj Hospital in Bangkok. In addition, Foundation officers negotiated with the Thai government for the development of a medical school at Chulalongkorn University in 1923. The Foundation agreed in the meantime to support the training of several Thai professors and to provide first-rate instructors. Although this project, like many IHB endeavors, had developed when a lack of trained personnel was discovered during the hookworm campaign, public health work and preventive medicine had a relatively low priority in the IHB's development of a medical education system in Thailand. Eventually, course work in public health and rural health problems was offered in a health district adjacent to the medical school. (See *Innovative Partners: The Rockefeller Foundation and Thailand* for more on this history.)

Students at Peking Union Medical College (PUMC) watch as a surgery is performed. Prior to the opening of PUMC, Western medical techniques, including surgery, remained largely unknown in China. (Rockefeller Archive Center.)

As the Foundation worked to propagate the Flexner model in countries around the world, the officers discovered problems with medical and public health education almost everywhere they surveyed. These problems were not limited to the developing world; even the great powers struggled with hookworm, tuberculosis, and malaria. In many places, health care systems were underfunded. Patterns also began to emerge. The farther away one traveled from metropolitan centers, the smaller the number of clinicians and the lower the quality of their training. At the outskirts of society, medical care, if it was available at all, was rudimentary, supplied by medical missionaries or traditional healers. For some, medical care could not be found within several days' walk. Around the globe, health demands outpaced the ability of education systems to supply high-quality medical personnel.

Realizing that it could not remedy all of these shortcomings even with its vast resources, the Foundation chose a combination of approaches to do the most good under the circumstances. It built up a centralized training and education system

Thai medical students conduct experiments in a physiology lab. In addition to opening a medical school in Chulalongkorn University, the Rockefeller Foundation supported Thai professors and medical students through international fellowships meant to offer practical training and exposure to methods of Western medicine. (Rockefeller Archive Center.)

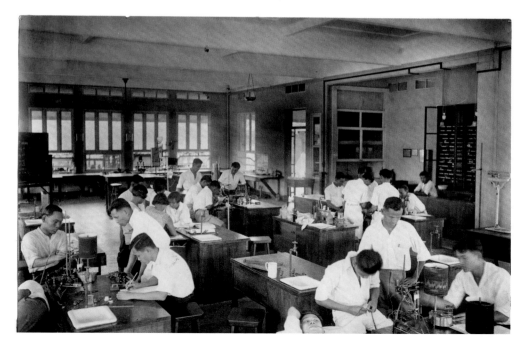

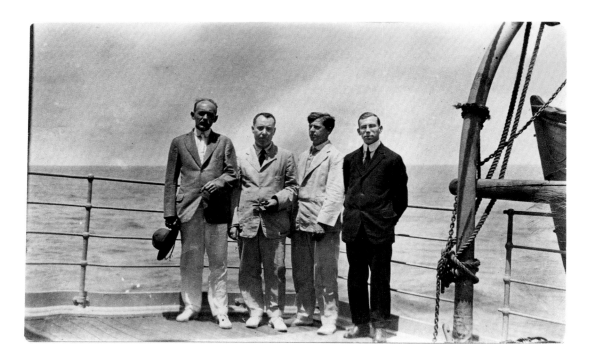

in each country consisting of a few prestigious schools that would attract the best and brightest students. It strengthened any existing colleges and universities that had substantial international influence, or had that potential. And it developed fellowship programs to ensure that students would have postgraduate opportunities, allowing the system to perpetuate itself for years to come.

Although China received the majority of Foundation funds invested in educational institutions abroad, other areas also benefited. The IHB commissioned 15 surveys in Latin America between 1916 and 1929. Richard Pearce, chair of research medicine at the University of Pennsylvania and, from 1919, director of the Foundation's Division of Medical Education, evaluated medical and public health systems in Brazil and later surveyed Chile and Paraguay. Alan Gregg, associate director of the Division of Medical Education, surveyed Mexico and Colombia.

In Brazil a Foundation survey led the government to establish a department of ankylostomiasis to fight hookworm disease. The IHB also agreed to assist the University of São Paulo in establishing a department of hygiene, and to help the Belo Horizonte Medical School create a department of pathology.

In 1916 officers from the International Health Commission (IHC) set sail for Brazil to survey medical education and public health systems. From left to right: Bailey Ashford researched the feasibility of portable field clinics to treat hookworm patients; Richard Pearce led the team; John Ferrell was associate director of the IHC; and William Garvey served as secretary. (Rockefeller Archive Center.)

The first school of hygiene and nursing in Rio de Janeiro was endowed in 1926; a department of hygiene was opened in connection with the Faculdade de Medicina e Cirurgia at São Paulo; and a department of pathology was introduced at the Oswaldo Cruz Institute in Rio de Janiero.

LONDON SCHOOL OF HYGIENE AND TROPICAL MEDICINE

In Europe, Rose and Welch admired England for its proficiency in teaching public health administration and Germany for its scientific approach to hygiene, but, they wrote, "the ideal plan will give due weight to both." In London Rose embarked on a remarkable effort to persuade authorities to establish a school of hygiene to strengthen public health in Britain and its colonies.

Rose and Rockefeller Foundation President George Vincent traveled to London in 1919, shortly after the end of World War One, to meet with officials in the Colonial Office. Vincent made it clear that the Foundation was interested in supporting a school of public health on par with Johns Hopkins. The British were keenly interested in the plan, but it was not until May 1922 that the IHB

The London School of Hygiene and Tropical Medicine was one of the largest international recipients of Rockefeller Foundation funding for medical education. Foundation officials believed that public health education in London had the potential to impact many of the poorer regions of the world that were part of Britain's colonial empire. (Rockefeller Archive Center.)

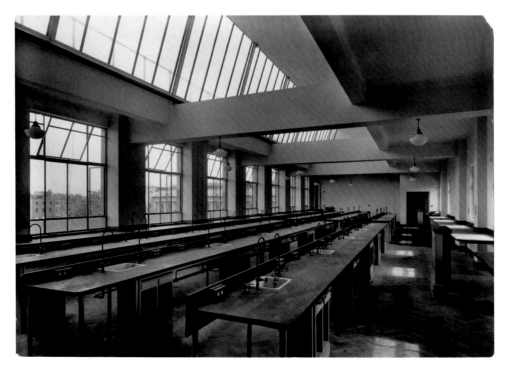

approved the site for the new campus. According to historian John Farley, Foundation officials and British authorities agreed that the new school would provide training and incorporate facilities for research.

As the negotiations were taking place, however, leaders at the London School of Tropical Medicine, which had been established in 1899, grew concerned that the new school would diminish their institution. They successfully lobbied to combine their institution with the school of public health to create the London School of Hygiene and Tropical Medicine. The combination of the two schools created an institution that would support the training of public health officials in many of the British colonies and pave the way for improvements in the health and well-being of some of the world's poorest citizens.

The Foundation's efforts in London represented only one part of an overall initiative to strengthen medical education in Europe. In 1917 surveys had revealed that the public health education system was at least partially inadequate in many countries. To overcome these deficiencies, the Foundation provided support to developing medical schools and programs for public health. In 1920, for example, the newly formed Czechoslovakia was the first country in Central Europe to receive Rockefeller support for the creation of a state institute of hygiene. The Foundation later continued to support public health, nursing, and social work in Central and Eastern Europe. It also assisted demonstration projects in rural and urban sanitation, in public health, and in popular health education. Moreover, the Foundation provided fellowships to train people who came to occupy positions of leadership in these fields. All of these efforts worked to build capacity within each country, but the Foundation also endeavored to promote an international exchange of ideas and a global scientific conversation in the fields of medicine and public health.

International Students in U.S. Medical Schools

Once new universities had been established and medical education had been strengthened in the United States, the Rockefeller Foundation, from 1920 to 1930, provided postgraduate opportunities for 4,400 fellows, students, public health officers, and professors from 48 countries to travel to the United States to conduct research or training in medicine, nursing, public health, and hygiene. In 1921 the IHB had also set up an apprentice training program in sanitary engineering with the agreement that, after completing their training, these new professionals would have secure employment at the federal, state, or county level in their home countries.

Be a Trained Nurse

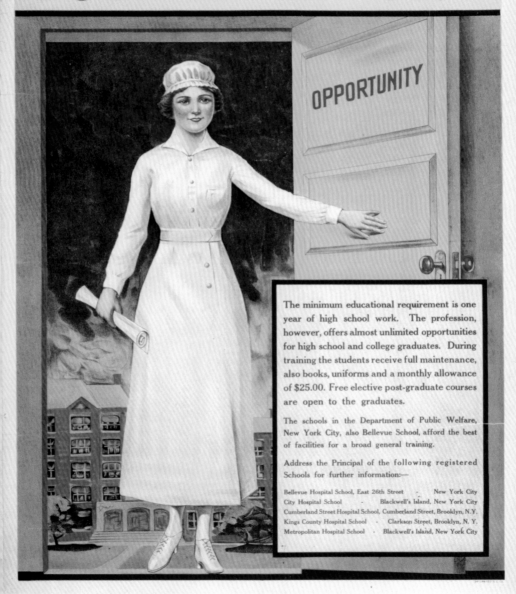

Another focus during the 1920s was the training of future leaders in science, which became a chief concern of Foundation officials. It was a time of extraordinary optimism, driven by the belief that conditions could be improved with the application of scientific knowledge and the use of the scientific method. "This is an age of science," Wickliffe Rose wrote in 1923. "All important fields of activity, from the breeding of bees to the administration of an empire, call for an understanding of the technique of modern science." Indeed, Rose held to the view that a nation's ascendancy was directly linked to the degree to which it supported science: "The nations that do not cultivate the sciences cannot hope to hold their own."

Founded in 1923 under Rose's leadership, the Foundation's International Education Board directed its resources to the physical sciences. It provided grants for the rehabilitation of European research centers along with travel fellowships to American institutions for chemists, physicists, and mathematicians. The fellowships, which typically granted funds for one year, played a significant role in the internationalization of science in the 1920s, a process that contributed to the development of medical education and research.

Training Nurses

Wickliffe Rose and Rockefeller adviser Frederick Gates believed that good health depended on a functioning system for the prevention and cure of disease. In his gentlemanly debates with William Welch, however, Rose had conceived of a system with many types of well-trained players, including nurses. In 1918 the Foundation had sponsored a conference to discuss public health nursing education, which led to the creation of the Committee for the Study of Public Health Nursing. In typical fashion, the committee began its work with a survey of the field, including hospital nursing. Josephine Goldmark, a prolific writer and activist who had campaigned for child labor laws and the rights of workers, served as the executive secretary of the committee and wrote the report. She recommended that nurses be trained in a university, and that public health and hospital nurses should complement academic studies in science with work in practical clinics in a hospital setting. In the way that Abraham Flexner's report on medical education had provided the blueprint for reform, Goldmark's book, *Nursing and Nursing Education in the United States* (1923), led to dramatic changes in nursing education.

Throughout the nineteenth and early twentieth centuries, nursing provided one of the few professional opportunities open to women. Recruitment posters during World War One highlighted the important role of nurses, but despite this importance, nursing education only began to receive serious attention in the 1920s. (Library of Congress.)

The Rockefeller Foundation would play a key role in implementing the recommendations of the Goldmark Report. In the United States, the Foundation provided a grant to the Yale School of Nursing to improve the education of public health nurses based on the Goldmark proposals. In Canada the Foundation made a pivotal grant to the University of Toronto's nursing school to help it become a model for nursing training.

The Foundation had also commissioned an extensive survey of nursing education in Europe, conducted by Frances Elisabeth Crowell. In 1922 and 1923 she visited Austria, Bulgaria, Czechoslovakia, England, Hungary, Italy, Poland, Romania, and Yugoslavia. Her report, issued the same year as Goldmark's, echoed Goldmark's observations in a number of ways. As a profession, nursing was perceived as lower-class work or as a vocation for members of a religious order. Nurses tended to have little formal education and were often poorly treated. Unlike Goldmark, however, Crowell tended toward Rose's point of view that an army of nurses—rather than an elite cadre of professionals—was needed to serve public health needs. Crowell's recommendations sparked controversy among many of the leaders and advisors of the nursing program at the Rockefeller Foundation, who believed that professionalizing nursing was a high priority.

As with the movement to foster a broad-based public health training initiative, Crowell's vision could not overcome the institutional impulse to advance the frontiers of science as opposed to promoting the application of existing knowledge through institutions designed to meet the needs of the masses. Given the background of the Foundation's leaders and their deep investment in basic science in the 1920s, this direction was not surprising. In some sense it reflected the underlying strategy for the Foundation's philanthropy, which was focused on root causes and using its resources to bring other institutions to the process of making permanent change.

ADJUSTING TO LOCAL NEEDS

As the Foundation pursued medical education based on the Flexner model, it encountered some resistance to various aspects of its programs. In China, immediately after the opening of Peking Union Medical College, Chinese specialists called for modifications to the Western-style curriculum. For example, they demanded research focused on the country's primary medical problems, including parasitic diseases and trachoma of the eye. Investigations into the complementary use of the nation's historic pharmacopeia were also urged. PUMC's leaders listened to these concerns, but the institution's policies were primarily shaped by the priorities of Western medical education. In addition, because the funds used for buildings, equipment, and training for leaders in research, teaching, and administration came primarily from the Foundation, it sought to maintain control over the institution. But Chinese influence grew over the years. While Westerners initially comprised a majority of the faculty, the number of Chinese members increased substantially after 1928. By 1940 the faculty included 109 Chinese and 10 Westerners.

The Foundation never intended its support for medical education to help countries meet their immediate health needs. Rather, the trustees envisioned stimulating national support for public health by eradicating a disease while modeling the best in medical education. With its philosophy of "raising the peaks," the Foundation was generally committed to the idea of training an elite corps of physicians who would provide leadership and supporting institutions that would serve as a model for other funders, including private donors and governments. But the Foundation's work often raised local expectations. In Thailand, for example, the IHB's development of a medical education system placed a relatively low priority on public health work and preventive medicine. Local health officials criticized this strategy, concerned that the new medical school graduated only a small number of physicians per year. Similarly, medical students in Latin America in the 1920s clamored for higher enrollment numbers and lower fees.

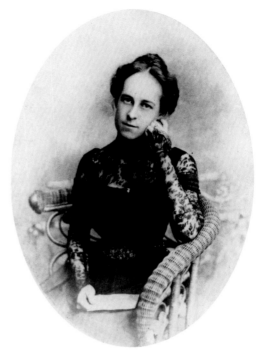

Frances Elisabeth Crowell joined the Rockefeller Foundation in 1917 as part of the Commission for the Prevention of Tuberculosis in France. Following the war, Crowell remained in Europe to conduct an extensive survey of nursing on behalf of the Rockefeller Foundation. In her findings, Crowell advocated for more public health nurses, rather than an elite cadre of university-educated nurses. Her recommendations went largely unheeded by the Foundation. (Rockefeller Archive Center.)

Around the world, the Rockefeller Foundation also had to adjust to different levels of government involvement in the field of medical education. In countries where the government played a major role in the administration of medical education, changes were born of governmental decree, not experimentation or competition. This was in sharp contrast to the U.S. system, where a medical school's curriculum was largely independent of government.

All of these variations in local institutions and culture forced the Rockefeller Foundation to be flexible in its effort to promote reforms in medical education while still following the basic outline of the Flexner model. In attempting to overcome resistance on the part of some citizens, politicians, religious leaders, or medical professionals, the Foundation often had to experiment with new approaches. For example, while physician John Grant was department head and associate professor of hygiene and public health at PUMC from 1921 to 1935, he approached public health differently from other Rockefeller officers. Responsible for training public health workers, Grant focused on introducing preventive medicine into the curriculum and strengthening the capacity to develop a national health care system. He came to be known as "the spirit of public health" in China.

Born into a Canadian missionary family in Ningbo, China, in 1890, Grant was not a typical Rockefeller field officer. Following in the footsteps of his father, medical practitioner James Skiffington Grant, he earned an undergraduate degree from Acadia, a liberal-minded Baptist college in Nova Scotia, followed by a medical degree from the University of Michigan in 1917. Joining the IHB after graduation, Grant was part of its hookworm campaign in North Carolina, spent a short time in China, and oversaw a hookworm and malaria survey in Puerto Rico. He then returned to the Rockefeller Foundation-created Johns Hopkins School of Public Health, where he earned his master's degree in 1921.

Grant was sensitive to Chinese society and culture, and had a strong aversion to the Western assumption of superiority. Unlike many of his Western peers, he socialized with and befriended Chinese people. In the early 1920s he established urban demonstration units in Beijing, providing medical services for its first ward, an area close to PUMC with a population of approximately 100,000 people. The program served as a training ground for public health specialists. Students devoted four weeks to working at a public health station—a time equal to their rotations in medicine, obstetrics, and surgery—a major innovation later duplicated by large American universities like Johns Hopkins and Harvard.

Grant went on to develop a rural health demonstration unit in Ting Hsien (known today as Dingxian) in the late 1920s. It consisted of a district health center with administrative offices, a 50-bed hospital, a laboratory, classrooms for training, and seven subordinate stations that served more than 75 villages. PUMC graduates, whom Grant had inspired to enter public health, directed the program. In 1934 the Rockefeller Foundation extended the project to other

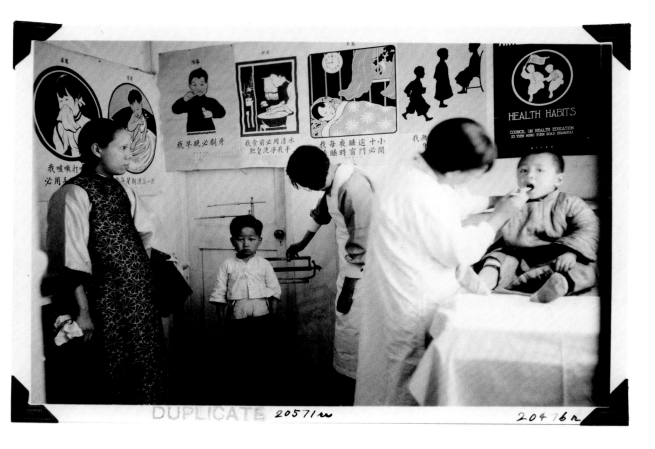

DUPLICATE 20571✧

health districts. Care at the subordinate substations was provided by a health officer, one or more public health nurses, and an attendant, whose technical competency was overseen by the district health center. The program served as the model for the famous "barefoot doctors" that emerged decades later—local doctors selected by villagers who carried out simple health care measures.

In the 1930s, Grant worked closely with Selskar M. Gunn, the Rockefeller Foundation's vice president. Gunn was a graduate of the Massachusetts Institute of Technology who had worked in public health before joining the Rockefeller Foundation. He had served as the associate director of the Commission for the Prevention of Tuberculosis in France and then directed the Foundation's European programs in the late 1920s. After a trip to China in 1931 that included travels with Grant, Gunn drafted a report for the Foundation's trustees that envisioned a highly innovative program to address the needs of the rural poor.

Public health nurses examine children at a preschool clinic in China. Small clinics like these were promoted by Rockefeller Foundation officer John Grant as a way to serve China's large population while providing practical training to China's public health students. (Rockefeller Archive Center.)

Gunn wanted to "dispel [the] impression that Foundation interests in China were largely medical." Along with Chinese health officials, he grew concerned that PUMC was not addressing problems of immediate priority. By the 1930s the International Health Division (IHD)—known as the International Health Board before 1927—had begun to support holistic programs of community development in China. This led to a new line of thinking about the interrelationships between public health and social, economic, and political conditions. In Gunn's view, public health required medical expertise and social science knowledge. Gunn's ideas were as unconventional as Grant's, shaped by an emerging idea of social medicine that he had encountered during his work in Europe.

Gunn's interdisciplinary program in Northern China was designed to promote "rural reconstruction" and "the correlation of the Foundation's existing medical program [that of PUMC] with public health work." It involved PUMC's Department of Preventive Medicine (which

Selskar Gunn joined the Rockefeller Foundation as associate director for the Commission for the Prevention of Tuberculosis in France. Following the commission's disbandment, Gunn remained in Europe to direct operations in health and the social sciences. Influenced by programs in European social medicine, Gunn later became the architect of the Foundation's China Program—a multidisciplinary approach to modernization through health, education, and agricultural reforms. (Rockefeller Archive Center.)

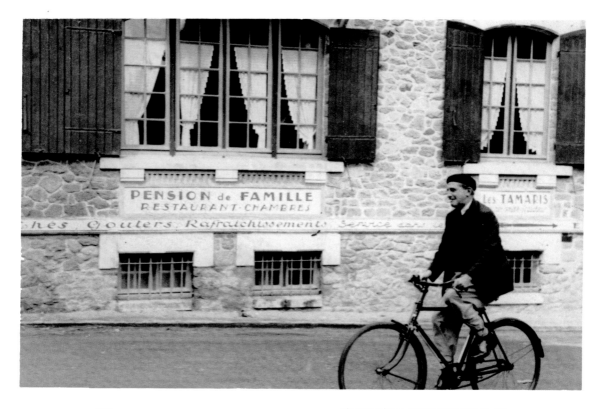

Chapter Three: Training the Caregivers

Grant had founded) and several other universities and institutes. Gunn asked for more than one million dollars ($17.1 million in 2013 dollars) on a three-year trial basis, and the IHD gave its approval in 1935. Gunn headed the effort, developing educational, social, and economic programs in rural China. Local fellowships were also awarded.

Extending beyond rural health and social problems, in April 1936, John Grant—who had become Gunn's assistant in China—formed the North China Council for Rural Reconstruction (NCCRR), which represented a number of leading Chinese universities that formed the institutional core of the program. Under the auspices of the IHD, the NCCRR created departments of economics, public works, social work, and civic administration, bringing together research, training of personnel, and political administration. Funds supported applied research as well as field projects for composting, developing modern farm implements, controlling gastrointestinal diseases, and breeding plants and animals. Social programs included birth control, school integration, adult education, and financial advice.

Japanese military expansion in China soon altered the trajectory of the NCCRR collaboration. Japanese forces seized and occupied Beijing in July 1937, and Japanese bombers and ground troops destroyed Nankai University, which had received millions of dollars in Rockefeller Foundation grants. According to historian Mary Brown Bullock, many staff and students were able to flee and join with others from Qinghua and Peking University to form what became Lianda University in Kunming. The NCCRR relocated its work to Guizhou Province in southwest China, and was renamed the China Council for Rural Reconstruction. Meanwhile in Beijing, PUMC continued to operate independently for several years, but with the attack on Pearl Harbor in Hawaii, the Japanese seized PUMC and closed the medical college, although the hospital was allowed to remain open. The nursing faculty escaped and, remarkably, moved their operations to Chengdu, where they reopened their school in 1942. But several American members of the China Medical Board were imprisoned until the end of the war.

Despite war and revolution, the legacy of the Rockefeller Foundation's work in China would carry forward for decades. John Grant and Selskar Gunn believed that human health is affected by social and economic forces. Their view was not shared by all at the Rockefeller Foundation, where some leaders in medical education and medical science preferred to focus on the pathology of specific diseases, but the initiatives launched during the first half of the twentieth century by Grant, Gunn, and the Foundation—in China and elsewhere around the world—would influence the fields of public health and medical education in the postwar years.

Between 1913 and the start of World War Two, the Foundation was able to promote a transformation of medical education in China and many other parts of the world, based on the Flexner model. Throughout these years, the Foundation learned by doing. As the Foundation's Alan Gregg concluded in 1933: "Failures were most commonly associated with incompetent recipients, premature hopes on our part of progress in fields where no advance has taken place, and over-confidence in the social, economic, and cultural matrix in certain countries." The Foundation recognized that it needed to develop a better understanding of the capacity of grant recipients; to provide funding in fields that had shown advances; and to better assess whether a country's infrastructure and culture might support or impede the reformation, modernization, and Westernization of medical education.

Nevertheless, in roughly three decades the Foundation had contributed to the rise of "the expert" in medical education, characterized by high standards, superlative credentials, and specialized skills. Along the way it had paid for the building, organization, or reorganization of many university medical colleges where caregiver education would include research and education as well as practice in labs, hospitals, and elsewhere. Indeed, funding from the General Education Board and the Rockefeller Foundation had helped to create a worldwide network of high-quality schools and institutes of medicine, nursing, and public health, each related to the others through key centers at Johns Hopkins, Harvard, Beijing, London, Brussels, and Toronto. This network included institutions in ten Western European locations, 16 in China, six others in Asia and the Pacific, and an additional six in the United States, Canada, and Latin America.

Equipment to be used by a station physician at a vaccination unit in China. Health education in rural China required finding unique ways, like these posters, to communicate with a largely illiterate population. (Rockefeller Archive Center.)

To further the development of this network, the Foundation sent its officers and field staff to train health workers in foreign lands. It awarded fellowships to students from across the world to be educated in leading medical schools. It purchased medical and scientific journals for medical schools worldwide. All of these initiatives, which aimed to promote an international culture of science in the field of medicine, were increasingly supported by the Foundation's investments in scientific research and endeavored to push forward the frontiers of knowledge.

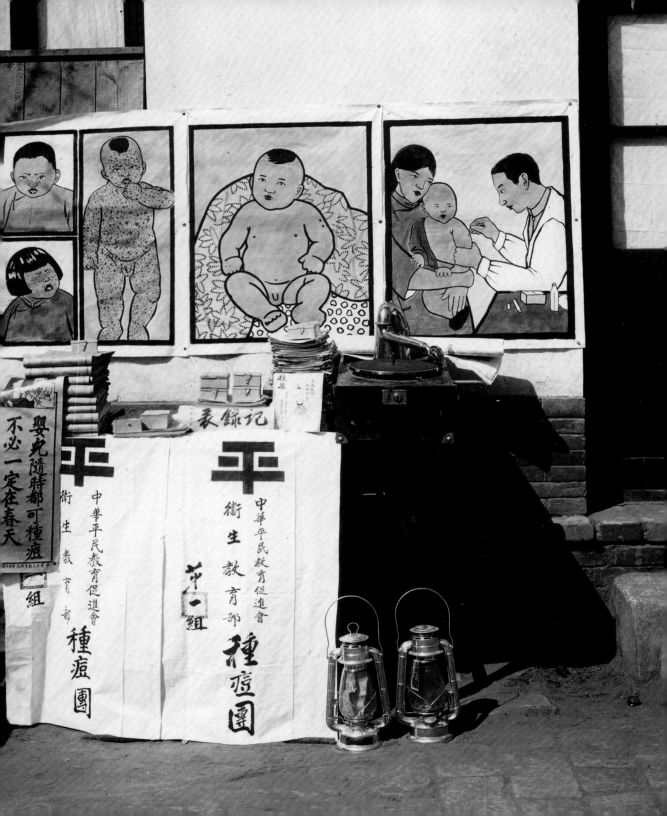

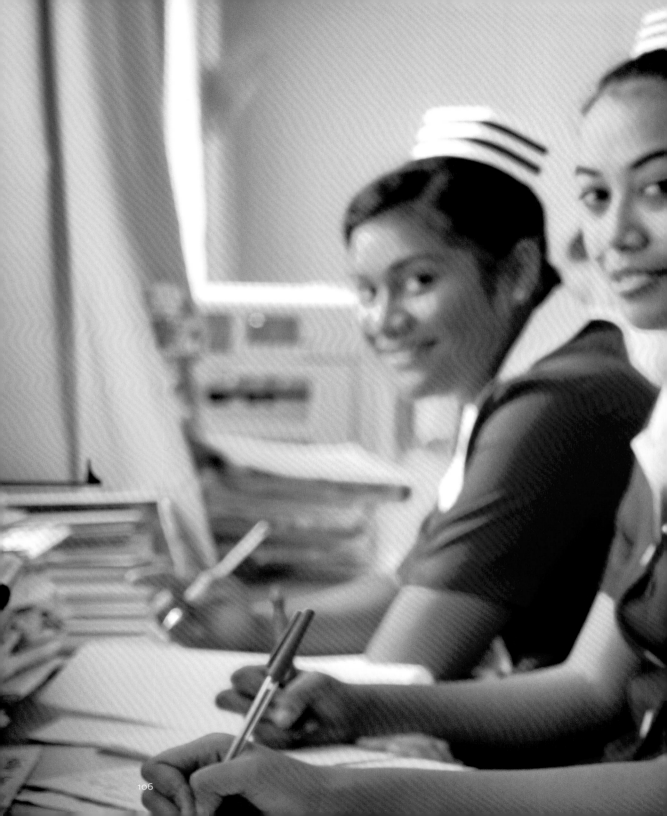

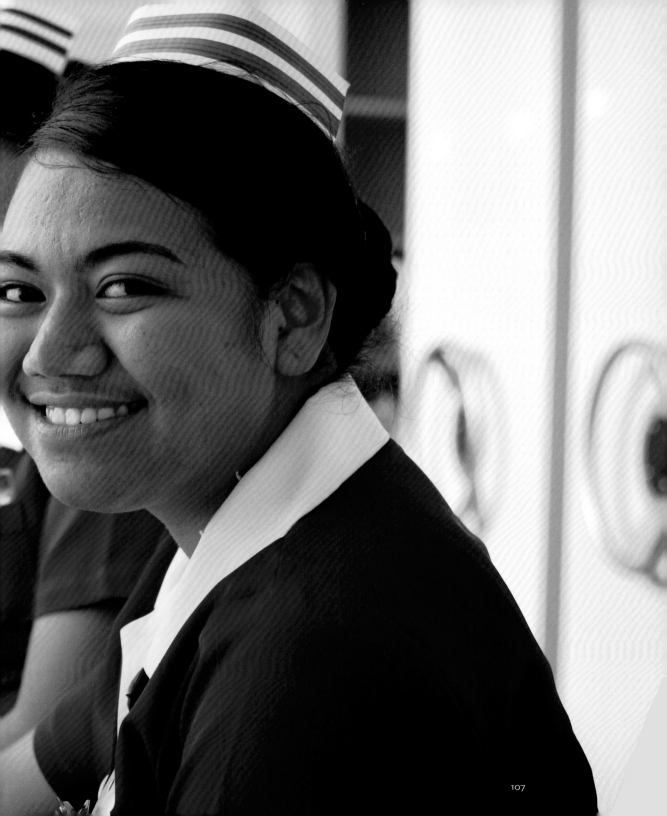

FINDING CURES

Summering in 1897 at Lake Liberty, New York, Baptist minister Frederick Taylor Gates had chosen an unlikely book for his vacation reading: the second edition of William Osler's 1,050-page tome, *The Principles and Practice of Medicine*. Originally published in 1892, while Osler was physician-in-chief at the newly established Johns Hopkins Hospital in Baltimore, *Principles* summarized the preceding 70 years of clinical pathology and was in fact the last work by a single author that attempted to address humankind's every illness or injury. The book was considered so important that it was translated into French, German, Spanish, and Chinese, and remained a seminal work for decades.

Osler's *Principles*, while it might seem odd summer reading for a man of the cloth, was not that unusual a choice for Gates. From personal experience he had long been skeptical of the medical profession. Although he came from a line of physicians, he had lost several family members to illness and had nearly died himself of an undiagnosed malady. As a minister, Gates had also counseled numerous physician-parishioners who had confessed to him varying degrees of medical deception. Osler, a renowned "medicinal nihilist," confirmed Gates's skepticism; the majority of treatments recommended at the time had no real basis in science and were largely ineffective, if not harmful. In fact, medicine at the end of the nineteenth century could "cure" only a handful of diseases—including rabies, diphtheria, hookworm, and malaria—and many of these cures would not prevent reinfection or relapse.

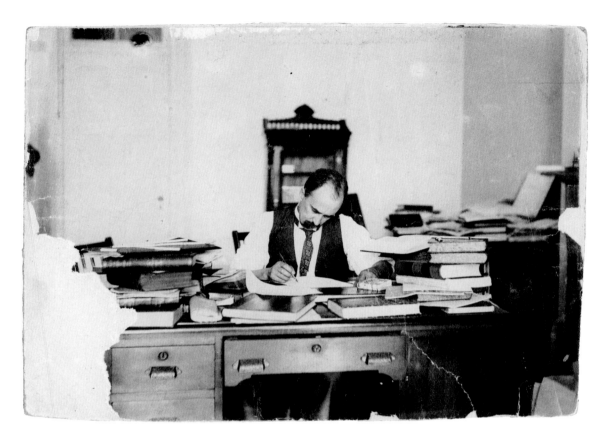

Gates understood why the scientific study of medicine had been woefully neglected. Having worked with John D. Rockefeller in planning the University of Chicago, he knew most researchers lacked the basic equipment of scientific investigation. Important theories of disease, such as Pasteur's germ theory, had not been fully disseminated. And proprietary medical colleges, without endowments, could not afford to do research. Instructors interested in scientific research had to fund their work from private-practice revenues.

William Osler, a leading physician of his era, was the author of the landmark medical textbook *The Principles and Practice of Medicine*. His career included positions as a professor of medicine at McGill University in Montreal, physician-in-chief and a founding father of Johns Hopkins Medical School, and chair of the Department of Medicine at Oxford University. (National Library of Medicine.)

After he finished reading *Principles*, Gates wrote, "The only thing I saw was the overwhelming need and the infinite promise, worldwide, universal, eternal." Compelled, "possessed" even, to address the situation, in 1897 Gates began urging Rockefeller to direct his philanthropic efforts toward the fundamental reform of medical education and the development of a medical research infrastructure. He believed that Rockefeller's support for scientific research could lead to cures for disease.

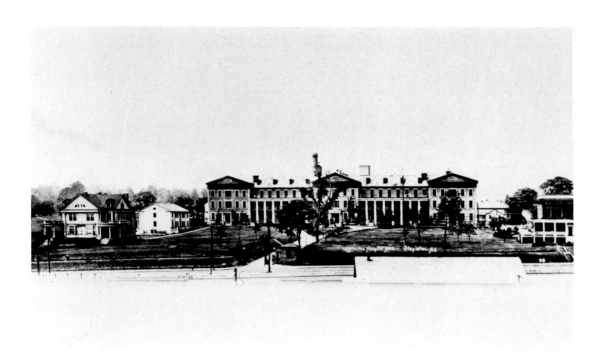

Central to Gates's vision was the creation of an institute for the scientific study of medicine. He wrote repeatedly to Rockefeller and others in positions of power, urging them to support this new direction. Some of his letters envisioned a grand legacy for the institution, like the Pasteur Institute in Paris. Other memoranda addressed important potential breakthroughs, such as the discovery of new disease-causing germs, and the worldwide suffering that would be alleviated through the development of cures. Gates predicted that Rockefeller's leadership would prompt other benefactors to establish similar institutes. He also enlisted John D. Rockefeller Jr. in the effort to persuade his father to establish a scientific research institution. Persistence paid off. In 1899 Rockefeller Sr. hired attorney Starr J. Murphy to investigate the best aspects of such a potential research institute.

The U.S. Marine Hospital Service at Stapleton, Staten Island, New York, was the sole institution conducting government-funded medical research in the late nineteenth and early twentieth centuries. The opening of the Rockefeller Institute for Medical Research in 1901 modernized American science by providing the necessary funding and environment for unfettered research into health and disease. (National Library of Medicine.)

Efforts to solidify the ideal institute languished, however, until January 1901, when Rockefeller's first grandson died of scarlet fever at age three. Although a cure existed—a serum derived from horse blood—the boy's physicians reportedly said there was nothing they could do. Within six months, on June 14, 1901, the Rockefeller Institute was incorporated, four years after Gates read Osler's *Principles*.

Chapter Four: Finding Cures

The Rockefeller Institute was modeled after the Koch and Pasteur Institutes in Germany and France, which had opened in 1880 and 1888, respectively. Its mission was to "conduct, assist and encourage investigations in the sciences and arts of hygiene, medicine and surgery, and allied subjects, in the nature and causes of disease and the methods of its prevention and treatment and to make knowledge relating to these various subjects available for the protection of the health of the public and the improved treatment of disease and injury."

At the turn of the twentieth century, this kind of scientific patronage was in its infancy in the United States. The federal government funded only limited medical research at the Hygienic Laboratory of the Marine Hospital Service at Stapleton, Staten Island, New York. The laboratory was a precursor of the Public Health Service. Established in 1887, its federally funded research was limited by congressional mandate to "infectious" and "contagious" diseases and matters of immediate public health thought to be due to immigrants. Government scientists were prohibited from pursuing their own research interests or engaging in expensive and open-ended basic science projects.

According to historian Victoria Harden, this limitation on government participation in science was due, in part, to "deeply ingrained American opposition to the establishment of government patronage for any special group," including scientists working for the public good. For their part, scientists feared government control over research priorities. As late as 1928, one scientist said, "We [Americans] naturally question governmental participation in scientific matters because we feel that anything having a political flavor cannot be above suspicion." In contrast, Germany, France, and England all supported their premier research institutes with public funds. In the end, the impetus for privately funded institutes, such as the Rockefeller Institute, came from scientists who believed that basic research was the key to medical advances in the twentieth century and that private philanthropy was the appropriate source of support.

With its private endowment, the new Rockefeller Institute was free from federal restrictions and could support any basic research project. Prior to the federalization of science in the 1930s—with the passing of the Ransdell Act, which established the National Institutes of Health—the Rockefeller Institute was America's only major biomedical research facility. As such, it would play a key role in the transformation of medical education and medical science envisioned by Gates. And it provided a missing piece in the emerging medical and health system in the United States.

Over the following decades, the institute developed in parallel with other Rockefeller initiatives, notably the General Education Board, the Rockefeller

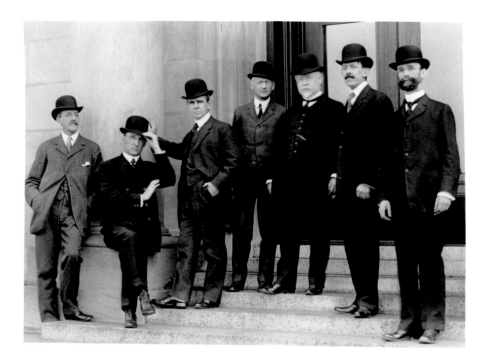

Sanitary Commission, and the Rockefeller Foundation (and its subordinate International Health Board). As these different Rockefeller-supported institutions came into being, officers and staff found themselves working across organizational boundaries, sometimes struggling to reconcile interwoven but competing priorities. The success of these organizations in achieving their mandates is therefore the story of how Rockefeller personnel learned through trial and error to balance finding cures through scientific research with the exigencies of improving health within communities—all the while training medical professionals capable of treating the whole patient.

The first Board of Scientific Directors of the Rockefeller Institute for Medical Research stood together for a picture in 1909. From left to right: T. Mitchell Prudden, Christian A. Herter, L. Emmett Holt, Simon Flexner, William H. Welch, Hermann M. Biggs, and Theobald Smith. (Rockefeller Archive Center.)

SCIENCE IN THE SERVICE OF HEALTH

In its early years, the Rockefeller Institute developed its research focus through a series of organizational experiments. Initially it supported researchers across the United States through fellowships. But in 1903 a steering committee proposed that a research center be built to accomplish more through consolidated efforts. Simon Flexner, a renowned pathologist and member of the committee, was elected the institute's director in 1903. He accepted after resigning his faculty position at the University of Pennsylvania.

Everything about Flexner's background made him seem destined for his new role. Driven by childhood memories of the U.S. financial panic of 1873 and the death of his father, Flexner was focused on achieving a career in either pharmacy or medicine, or both. An avid reader, raised among argumentative siblings, Flexner displayed a high intelligence distinguished by strong logical thinking. He excelled in his studies, and received his medical degree from the University of Louisville at age 26. Flexner's interest and skill in pathology, coupled with the fact that he was one of the few physicians to own a microscope, led him to be consulted by many local physicians. In his view, an accurate diagnosis was best found through examination of physical samples. He came to believe wholeheartedly that the laboratory could help the sick. His younger brother Abraham, having recently graduated from Johns Hopkins, urged Simon to go there to further his studies in pathology. Working alongside Osler and William Welch at the Johns Hopkins Hospital, Flexner learned to mentor research scientists.

By training and inclination, Flexner was the right person to direct the design of the new institute. After a trip abroad to Europe to study the latest developments in medicine and laboratory science, he returned to open the institute's first laboratory, the Division of Pathology, Bacteriology and Experimental Surgery, in 1906. A year later he established the Divisions of Physiology, of Pharmacology, and of Chemistry. Units for cancer research, biophysics, and animal and plant pathology were added over the years.

Just as the Koch and Pasteur Institutes had affiliated hospitals, the Rockefeller Institute added its own hospital in 1910, under the directorship of the clinician Rufus Cole, to study poliomyelitis, pneumonia, syphilis, heart disease, and other pathologies. In contrast to existing American and European teaching hospitals, the staff at the Rockefeller Institute's hospital was engaged full-time in clinical work, treating patients free of charge, and engaging in independent, original clinical research in their own laboratories physically separated from the rest of the institute. Approaching patient care as research, resident staff had full control of a ward, where they could study patients of interest from admission to discharge. All aspects of a disease were explored, from its fundamental chemistry and biology to the bedside treatment of the afflicted.

The laboratory and hospital facilities were fully endowed and well equipped. The institute soon developed a culture of privilege, in which senior scientists were encouraged to take a long view, pursuing a line of fundamental research to its conclusion, a tradition that lasts to the present. Given this environment, it is not surprising that the novelist Sinclair Lewis used a fictionalized Rockefeller Institute as the setting for much of his 1925 Pulitzer Prize-winning novel *Arrowsmith*, about the culture of medicine and related research.

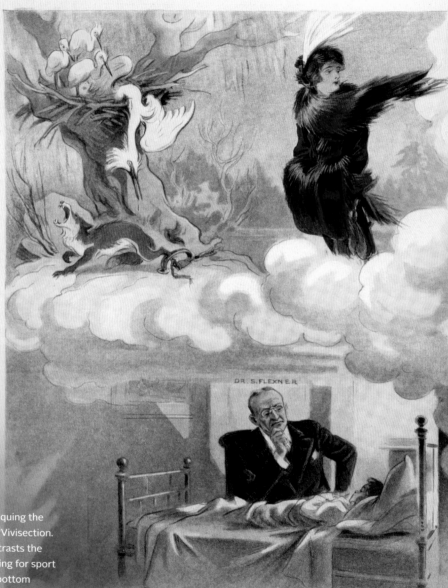

DR. S. FLEXNER

THE PUCK PRESS

on from *Puck*, critiquing the
ovement, is titled "Vivisection.
criticized." It contrasts the
science with hunting for sport
or fashion. In the bottom
rrel and Jacques Loeb
n a laboratory, while Simon
t the bedside of a sick child.
e prominent scientists at the
te for Medical Research.

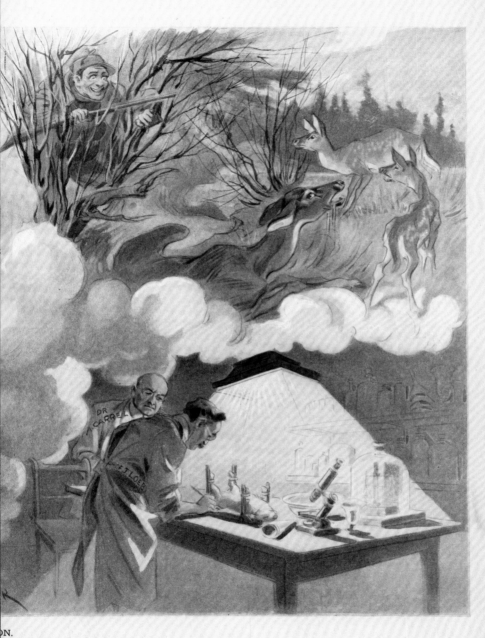

ON.

CRITICIZED.

After his initial contribution of one million dollars in 1901, John D. Rockefeller Sr. continued to support the institute; its endowment grew to $23 million dollars by 1920 and $65 million dollars by 1928 ($884 million in 2013 dollars). In addition, the Rockefeller Foundation provided occasional grants to the Institute to support research. The institute quickly attracted and employed many outstanding scientists. Through 1940 numerous advances at the hospital in the biochemical field covered a variety of subjects, such as the chemical activities and interactions of proteins, carbohydrates, fats, hormones, vitamins, mineral elements, and water in living things.

Early on the institute drew a diverse group of biochemical researchers whose discoveries would have a profound impact on scientific knowledge, including Oswald T. Avery, who characterized the *pneumococcus* and its virulence, laying the groundwork for new treatments of pneumonia, which was serious and widespread, particularly in wintertime. The immunologist Karl Landsteiner identified and classified the human blood groups (A, B, AB, and O)—a feat that won him the Nobel Prize in Physiology or Medicine in 1930. Wendell Stanley became world-famous in the 1930s for the crystallization of the tobacco-mosaic virus—a big step in demystifying the underlying structure of living things. By 1940 the Rockefeller Institute had become one of the most important centers for virus research in the United States. Virus researchers there and elsewhere were no longer preoccupied with the effects of viral infection but with the structure and composition of the viruses themselves.

ROCKEFELLER INSTITUTE AND ROCKEFELLER FOUNDATION

In 1913, as Oswald Avery began his investigation of pneumococcal pneumonia at the Rockefeller Institute, the Rockefeller Foundation received its charter from the state of New York. Expanding on the success of the Rockefeller Sanitary Commission, the Foundation launched the International Health Commission to "follow up the treatment and cure of [hookworm] disease with the establishment of agencies for the promotion of public sanitation and the spread of the knowledge of scientific medicine." In 1916 the commission became the International Health Board, which in 1927 was made a division—the International Health Division (IHD)—within the Foundation.

From its inception in 1913 to its termination in 1951, the IHD conducted field and basic laboratory research primarily on hookworm, yellow fever, and malaria. It also investigated influenza, rabies, syphilis, tuberculosis, anemia, schistosomiasis, undulant fever, and yaws, a skin and bone disease spread through human-to-human contact. As laboratory-based virus and vaccine research increased, the IHD set up and operated its own research laboratories in New York, Brazil, and West Africa that primarily addressed yellow fever. But it also supported laboratories across the world in Managua, Beijing, Bogotá, Beirut, Bangkok, and Munich, among other cities, and on the island of Penang in Malaysia, to address diseases that were endemic there. In this way scientific advances in epidemiology and biology were disseminated immediately to improve disease control in the field.

At his desk at the Rockefeller Institute for Medical Research, Oswald T. Avery analyzes the results from his research. Avery's work led to improvements in diagnosing and treating pneumonia, and also laid the groundwork for efforts to understand DNA and for modern genetic research. (National Library of Medicine.)

Overall, the type of laboratory research conducted by IHD staff differed from that of the Rockefeller Institute in that it was intimately tied to investigations in the field, whereas the institute pursued basic research that might not have any immediate impact on public health. However, this distinction was not always clear. Over the years, different IHD directors brought differing perspectives to their charge. Wickliffe Rose, for example, believed strict laboratory investigation was "unpredictable." As his earlier debates with William Welch suggested, Rose wanted knowledge to be disseminated, not just discovered, and under his direction the IHD's efforts were geared to that end. Frederick Russell, on the other hand, after succeeding Rose in 1923, put a greater emphasis on the discovery of new knowledge. At times a compromise of sorts was reached between the Rockefeller Institute's work in basic science and the IHD's research in support of fieldwork, with institute scientists joining IHD personnel in the field. Simon Flexner readily encouraged cross-fertilization among scientific staff inside as well as outside the walls of the Rockefeller Institute.

Russell was by inclination and training a laboratory scientist. As a physician in the U.S. Army Medical Corps, he had risen through its ranks over 22 years to become a one-star general directing the Army's entire Laboratory Service during World War One. Building on the success of IHD field labs in Brazil and Nigeria, he soon called for more basic laboratory research and began to position the IHD to set up its own lab in New York. With Flexner's support, the IHD opened its Yellow Fever Laboratory in 1928 in space provided at the institute. This increasing focus on laboratory research signaled the IHD's shift away from public health fieldwork, which would occur in the 1930s and continue after Wilbur Sawyer, the head of the IHD's laboratory service, succeeded Russell as director in 1935.

The IHD and Yellow Fever

The Rockefeller Foundation's efforts to fight yellow fever reflected the IHD's growing emphasis on research as the primary path to public health, and evidenced the cross-fertilization that took place among Rockefeller Institute and IHD personnel. As the IHD worked with various governments in Latin America to organize and sustain campaigns to control the population of yellow fever-carrying mosquitoes (see Chapter II), scientists at the Rockefeller Institute worked to gain a better understanding of the disease and search for a possible vaccine. The brilliant and accomplished scientist Hideyo Noguchi was an early pioneer in this effort. Born in the Fukushima prefecture of Japan in 1876, Noguchi survived a horrible burn accident as a child that left

The International Health Division set up its first yellow fever research laboratory in Africa in 1929. Headquartered in Lagos, Nigeria, the West Africa Yellow Fever Commission eventually included staff doctors, field directors, and lab assistants throughout West Africa, including A. Maurice Wakeman, pictured here with his assistants in Accra, Ghana. (Rockefeller Archive Center.)

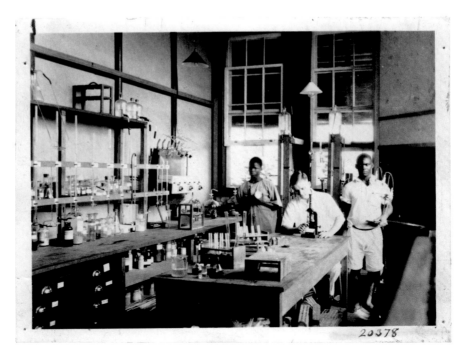

Chapter Four: Finding Cures

him with only partial mobility in his left hand. The care and treatment he received fueled his interest in medicine as an adult. After graduating from medical school, Noguchi moved to the United States in 1900 and soon joined the staff of the Rockefeller Institute. In 1913 he isolated the spirochete bacteria in the brain that could lead to paralysis in patients with syphilis. He was nominated for the Nobel Prize for this work. Noguchi participated in a Rockefeller Foundation commission to Ecuador, and in 1918 he began to work on the cultivation of yellow fever in cell-free tissue and to experiment with vaccine development.

Unfortunately, Noguchi mistakenly identified the causative agent for yellow fever as another spirochete, which he believed was closely related to the bacteria that caused infectious jaundice or Weil's disease. Noguchi created a yellow fever vaccine at the Rockefeller Institute that was tested with remarkable success, and IHD staff inoculated more than 20,000 people in Latin America by 1925. In Mexico and Peru, eradication efforts in the early 1920s that used Noguchi's vaccine—in combination with other public health strategies—seemed to successfully control yellow fever, and the leaders of both the Rockefeller Institute and the IHD believed that a cure for yellow fever was at hand.

After the Rockefeller Foundation sent its second Yellow Fever Commission to Africa in 1925, however, and the IHD opened a laboratory in Lagos, Nigeria, new research began to cast doubts on Noguchi's work. In June 1927, a 28-year-old man named Asibi came to the lab suffering from yellow fever. One of the IHD's scientists, Adrian Stokes, took some of Asibi's blood and injected it into a rhesus monkey, which developed a fever. This "Asibi" strain helped researchers prove that a virus, and not Noguchi's spirochete, was the active agent. But Stokes died after he became infected while working in the laboratory.

Embarrassed by what appeared to be a serious error on his part, Noguchi sailed for Africa in October 1927 in an effort to redeem his findings. He worked furiously over the next several months, but his research was poorly organized and even "chaotic" according to one fellow scientist. Then Noguchi himself contracted yellow fever, and died on May 21, 1928. In the meantime, an experiment using blood from patients in South America who had survived yellow fever, and developed an immunity, proved effective in protecting monkeys in Lagos. The tests conclusively undermined Noguchi's theory.

After three more IHD staff died from yellow fever, a "well-equipped and well-organized" lab was seen to be essential. It was obvious that the IHD field labs in South America were overburdened and unable to maintain the level of control needed to safely develop a vaccine. It was decided by the IHD that while field labs would continue efforts to determine which mosquitoes

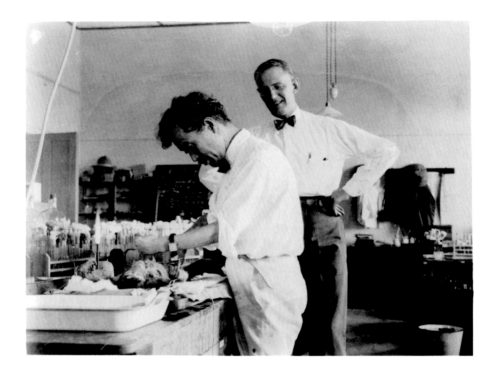

carried the disease, how the viruses developed within them, and whether or not seasonal fluctuations made a difference, a safer, more controlled environment would be needed to identify the virus and develop a vaccine.

By October 1928, Frederick Russell had secured approval to use two rooms at the Rockefeller Institute for the Yellow Fever Laboratory mentioned earlier. One room was reserved for monkeys infected with the Asibi strain of the virus. To guard against accidentally infecting the staff, everyone who entered this room wore white trousers, a long white coat, rubber gloves, and a rubber apron. The garments were sanitized after each use. Despite these precautions, seven of the lab's personnel came down with yellow fever, including the lab's director Wilbur Sawyer. Fortunately, no one died.

A number of major inventions emerged from the IHD laboratory in its pursuit of a yellow fever vaccine, including the ultracentrifuge and the viscerotome, which was a device that enabled liver biopsies without a full autopsy. It made determination of a cause of death from yellow fever a simple matter, and furthered epidemiological surveys. The ultracentrifuge, capable of 30,000 to 60,000 revolutions per minute and generating a force up to 260,000

Hideyo Noguchi, pictured here with Johannes Bauer in a field lab in Ghana, conducted extensive research in the quest for a yellow fever vaccine. While Noguchi believed he had found success in 1925, later research by members of the West Africa Yellow Fever Commission showed that Noguchi had misidentified the causal agent of the disease. (Rockefeller Archive Center.)

Chapter Four: Finding Cures

times gravity, was key to isolating the yellow fever virus, which is smaller than a single protein. These innovations paved the way for the ultimate development of an effective vaccine.

In 1926, while he was a teaching fellow at Harvard, a young research scientist named Max Theiler had also uncovered Noguchi's error. The son of Swiss immigrant Arnold Theiler, "the father of veterinary science" in South Africa, Theiler had studied medicine at the University of Cape Town, St. Thomas' Hospital in England, and the London School of Tropical Medicine. He received a Diploma of Tropical Medicine and Hygiene in 1922. Socially reticent but intellectually curious, he became more interested in research than the practice of medicine and joined the staff of the Harvard Medical School in 1922. In the summer of 1929 he began experimenting with the development of a vaccine for yellow fever. When Wilbur Sawyer, the director of the IHD's yellow fever lab, heard about this work, he recruited Theiler to join the IHD to help develop a vaccine that would protect the lab's staff.

Soon after he arrived in New York, Theiler was able to infect, as well as inoculate, mice. His experiments showed that long-lasting immunity could be conferred by injecting them with serum from humans who had been infected 30 to 70 years earlier. The ease of using mice instead of monkeys in epidemiological studies prompted renewed interest in finding and testing vaccines. Meanwhile Wilbur Sawyer and another researcher, Wray Lloyd, worked on a yellow fever blood test for humans, and from 1931 to 1936 the IHD conducted a worldwide survey of yellow fever immunity in humans.

Meanwhile Theiler continued to incubate the yellow fever virus in a series of tissues of different types—a process called "serial passage"—in an effort to attenuate the virus, or reduce its potency, even though it was still alive, allowing it to confer immunity against the original or parent form. In 1931 he developed the first yellow fever vaccine by serial passage through mouse brain tissue. This version of the vaccine, when added to fresh but sterile human immune serum globulin, produced no cases of yellow fever. The vaccine worked with the lab's staff, but the large amount of serum required for inoculation made it impractical for mass application.

Theiler's next step was to pass the virus through mouse embryonic tissue. The result was reduced virulence, which required less human immune serum, but it could still only be used on a small scale. Researchers eventually discovered that if the virus was passed through embryonic tissue devoid of brain or spinal cord components, it became even less virulent.

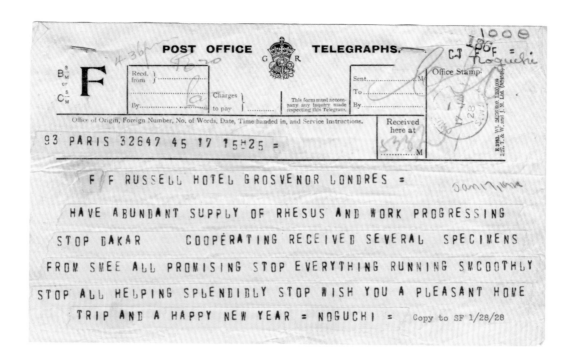

POST OFFICE TELEGRAPHS. G R

93 PARIS 32647 45 17 15 25 =

F F RUSSELL HOTEL GROSVENOR LONDRES =

HAVE ABUNDANT SUPPLY OF RHESUS AND WORK PROGRESSING
STOP DAKAR   COOPÉRATING RECEIVED SEVERAL   SPECIMENS
FROM SWEE ALL PROMISING STOP EVERYTHING RUNNING SWCOOTHLY
STOP ALL HELPING SPLENDIBLY STOP WISH YOU A PLEASANT HOME
TRIP AND A HAPPY NEW YEAR = NOGUCHI =   Copy to SF 1/28/28

By 1937, after more than 100 such passages, Theiler isolated an attenuated yellow fever virus—known as 17D—suitable for use as a preventive vaccine that did not require fresh human immune serum globulin for vaccination. By 1938 more than 40,000 people had been inoculated against yellow fever using 17D, with some 90 percent being fully or partially immunized. For his discovery of the vaccine, Theiler received the 1951 Nobel Prize in Physiology or Medicine.

In a telegram to International Health Division Director Frederick Russell, Hideyo Noguchi wrote that he had an abundant supply of rhesus monkeys and that his research was progressing smoothly. Sadly, Noguchi died just over four months later after contracting yellow fever in Africa. (Rockefeller Archive Center.)

A Problem with the Vaccine

Theiler's 17D may not have required fresh human immune serum globulin for vaccination, but it did require such serum for production, which led to problems. A significant portion of the people who were vaccinated became jaundiced. The IHD tried to fix this problem by using a new strain of the virus and by heating the human serum to 56 degrees centigrade to kill the jaundice-causing agent, but the problem soon reappeared.

After the outbreak of World War Two, as the United States prepared its forces for fighting, the U.S. War Department decided to vaccinate tens of thousands of soldiers headed for tropical environments. The Rockefeller

Foundation promised to manufacture these doses. More than six million doses were produced for American and British troops, but the reports of jaundice continued. Given the revised protocol in preparing the vaccine, the IHD insisted initially that the vaccine was not causing the jaundice. They suspected outbreaks of hepatitis. But as they monitored a group of 817 soldiers in California, the evidence pointed to the vaccine. At a press conference in July, Secretary of War Henry Stimson reported that 28,585 people who had been vaccinated had experienced jaundice, and 62 had died. Scientists at the IHD raced to discover the source of the contamination.

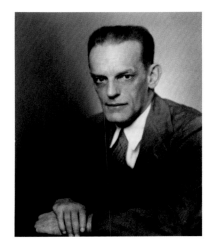

Max Theiler is credited with the discovery of 17D, the vaccine used to inoculate against the yellow fever virus. The vaccine, created in 1937, still remains in use today. In recognition of his efforts, Theiler received the Nobel Prize in Physiology or Medicine in 1951. (Pach Brothers, New York. Rockefeller Archive Center.)

Researchers tracked down more than 1,500 of the nearly 2,000 donors who had provided serum for the vaccine. It was eventually determined that a small percentage of donors who had been presumed to be healthy were in fact suffering from liver problems, and their blood had contaminated the 17D vaccine. In fact, the Rockefeller Foundation's statistician Persis Putnam was ultimately able to tie 86 percent of the jaundice cases to six particular lots of vaccine. As historian John Farley has written, "The evidence indicated that there was nothing fundamentally wrong with the Rockefeller vaccine."

But the risk of contamination had to be eliminated from the manufacturing process. Vaccinations were halted while the IHD scrambled to develop a safer method. The new procedure used chicken embryo pulp rather than human serum. By the time Secretary Stimson held his press conference, the Rockefeller Foundation had already converted to this new system. The jaundice problems did not reappear, and the U.S. military had reported no cases of yellow fever among the troops in the meantime.

The IHD's Virus Laboratory, Typhus, and DDT

Yellow fever was not the only disease that threatened troops during World War Two. Research into typhus prevention and control also became urgent. Throughout history, wartime conditions had led to outbreaks of this deadly disease, which was caused by lice that tucked themselves into the folds of their victims' clothing. The afflicted soldiers developed fever and red spots on their arms, back, and chest, which progressed to gangrenous sores while the victims suffered delirium. Napoleon's men had succumbed to this dread disease by the thousands during the army's retreat from Moscow in 1812.

Under Wilbur Sawyer's leadership, the IHD had begun working with the U.S. military on typhus prevention in 1939. Shortly thereafter, IHD scientists initiated experiments to develop a typhus vaccine or an insecticide that would kill the louse that carried the disease. Working closely with Harvard bacteriologist Hans Zinsser, the IHD was responsible for laboratory research on the typhus-spreading louse as well as field experiments to assess whether Zinsser's findings could be replicated in the field. Over the next several years, the Foundation field-tested a number of insecticides with volunteers in a camp for conscientious objectors in New Hampshire and in villages in Mexico. The insecticides proved very effective in killing the lice, but one chemical seemed particularly effective.

Men of the U.S. Army Signal Corps line up at Fort Jay on Governors Island, New York, to be vaccinated against yellow fever. In 1942 reports of vaccine-related deaths led researchers to discover that a small portion of the vaccines had been derived from individuals with liver problems. The deaths ultimately led to a vaccine that did not use human serum. (U.S. Army Signal Corps. Rockefeller Archive Center.)

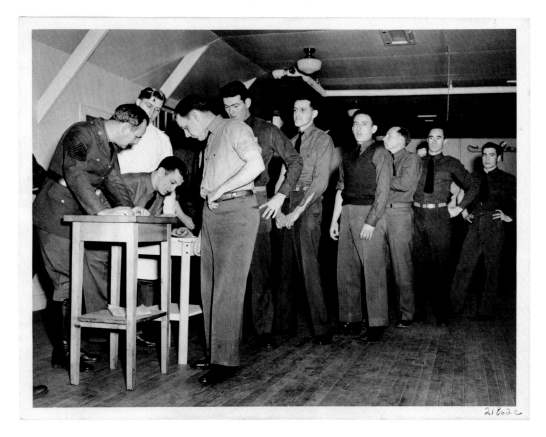

Chapter Four: Finding Cures

In 1939 Paul Müller, a Swiss chemist employed by J.R. Geigy A.G., rediscovered a chemical formula that had been synthesized 65 years earlier by a graduate student at the University of Strasbourg named Othmar Zeidler. Müller tried using this formula, known today as DDT, as an insecticide and found that it was remarkably effective. Tests also showed that it seemed harmless on humans. Geigy soon began using DDT in a louse powder called Neocid and a general insecticide called Gesarol. In 1942 a sample of DDT was sent to the U.S. Bureau of Entomology and Plant Quarantine in Orlando, Florida, for testing, and the Orlando team shared these results and some of this new insecticide with the IHD's louse researchers in New York.

Fred Soper, an epidemiologist with the IHD, soon carried DDT to Europe to battle lice and mosquitoes. Later dubbed "the Mosquito Killer" by writer Malcolm Gladwell, Soper had grown up in Kansas and earned a doctorate at the Johns Hopkins School of Public Health before joining the Rockefeller Foundation. He then followed in the footsteps of William Gorgas, killing mosquitoes in Latin America in the 1930s to prevent malaria and yellow fever. Efforts under Soper's direction between 1939 and 1941 led to the eradication of the mosquito known as *Anopheles gambiae*, the carrier of malaria, from Brazil. He also oversaw the annihilation of the same species from the lower Nile region in the 1940s. Soper applied a regimented approach to mosquito eradication, deploying a veritable army of sprayers, larvae collectors, and supervisors. This authoritarian strategy became known as "malaria discipline" in the public health lexicon, and would be softened, if not repudiated, by later generations of IHD and Rockefeller Foundation leaders. But at the time, Soper was praised for his effectiveness.

Soper was appointed to the United States of America Typhus Commission in 1943, which had been established by President Franklin Roosevelt to develop a way to limit the impact of typhus on the military and civilian populations. Under the aegis of the IHD and the commission, Soper traveled to the Mediterranean that year to aid in the fight against malaria and typhus. The Typhus Commission asked the IHD to oversee military anti-lousing experiments in Cairo, Egypt. But bureaucratic infighting between the IHD and the military and logistical difficulties led to disappointing results. Meanwhile epidemics raged in Algeria that summer.

The Rockefeller typhus team, under the auspices of the Red Cross and the Pasteur Institute, shifted its focus to Algeria, testing insecticides and application methods on human populations. Charles Wheeler, an IHD scientist under Soper, developed a new technique of applying insecticide with a compressed air gun, which reduced application time by 90 percent and did not require disrobing. Soper and his team also used DDT for the first time in

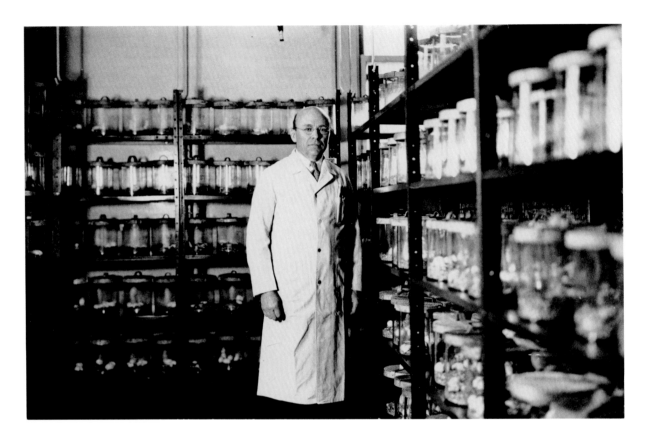

In 1935 Wilbur A. Sawyer took over the leadership of the International Health Division. While Sawyer maintained the research-focused mandate initiated by Frederick Russell, he was also forced to deal with a particular set of health emergencies brought on by World War Two. (Thomas P. Hughes. National Library of Medicine.)

Algeria and were impressed with its long-lasting effects. Ultimately, the treatments were enormously successful.

Having demonstrated the efficacy of the new DDT-based louse powder and application in North Africa, the IHD aided delousing efforts in Naples, Italy, from December 1943 through January 1944. More than 1.3 million people were treated in a single month. As Raymond Fosdick, a historian, biographer, and former president of the Rockefeller Foundation, has written, "The epidemic which might have taken thousands of lives collapsed with astonishing rapidity."

DDT was also quickly brought into the wartime effort to fight malaria. After the Allied invasion of Sicily in July 1943, an estimated 200,000 troops were infected. Infection rates soared to near 192 in every 1,000 soldiers. U.S. Colonel Paul Russell, a former member of the IHD staff, launched a campaign to stop these infections. In March 1944, at the request of the U.S. Army, the IHD introduced methods for controlling mosquito populations using DDT. Infection rates plummeted.

Chapter Four: Finding Cures

The IHD's work with yellow fever, typhus, and malaria reflected Frederick Russell's decision to expand research efforts in 1927. Like most research laboratories focused on developing new pharmaceuticals or treatments, however, the Foundation experienced more failure than success, and at times these setbacks were frustrating. For example, IHD researchers began looking at a variety of diseases including influenza and the common cold. Three separate research teams collected nasal samples from subjects before, during, and after a flu season in an attempt to identify a causative bacteria, but none was found. Then Alphonse Dochez, a Belgian-American physician, received a three-year grant from the IHD in 1931. His research led to the realization that the common cold and influenza are caused by a "multiplicity of viral strains," which provided the health community with important insight, but no cure.

Likewise, the IHD's Virus Laboratory began to study influenza in the mid-1930s, and in 1939 began work on a vaccine. The vaccine was administered and tested during the winter of 1940-1941 in the United States and provided to Allied troops, but it met with limited success. IHD director Wilbur Sawyer also allocated funds for rabies research in 1936 after Leslie Webster developed a way to test for the disease using mice. The IHD helped fund a unique rabies laboratory in Birmingham, Alabama, where rabies was particularly virulent in the local dog population. But researchers were ultimately unable to produce an effective vaccine, and the IHD abandoned this work.

In 1927 the Foundation had made tuberculosis a research focus. At the time, there was a global hunt for an effective vaccine. In February 1928 IHD Director Frederick Russell arranged for Eugene Opie, then director of the Henry Phipps Institute at the University of Pennsylvania, to go to Jamaica for two weeks to investigate the prevalence of tuberculosis on the island. Opie's detailed family graphs of tuberculosis patients and their relatives revealed that 78 percent of people who had migrated to Jamaica as adults died within one year of infection. Opie suggested that Russell establish a survey clinic like that at Phipps. Rufus Cole, a scientific director at the Health Division, encouraged Russell to offer support for this research and to make him an associate director of the IHD. Russell agreed to both suggestions.

Opie accepted both the offer of support for the clinic and the IHD associate directorship. Over the next decade he developed a vaccine that he asserted lessened the severity of TB. In 1940 it was given to 7,739 Kingston residents, but no outcome data was ever collected. In the end, this research proved disappointing as well.

If the pattern of medical research often leads to failure, success is almost always a product of layers of discovery by various individuals and teams. The story of penicillin reflects both a succession of discoveries and at least two instances where Rockefeller philanthropy played a critical role in development.

In 1928 British scientist Alexander Fleming discovered a mold growing on a culture plate of staphylococcus bacteria. The mold seemed capable of killing the bacteria around it. Fleming isolated the substance and named it "penicillin," studying it for a short time before reporting his discovery in the *British Journal of Experimental Pathology*. Fleming was unimpressed with his discovery, in part

A worker on the Italian island of Sardinia uses a hand-flint gun to spray mosquito breeding grounds with DDT. The use of DDT led to dramatic decreases in the incidence of malaria among Sardinia's population. (Rockefeller Archive Center.)

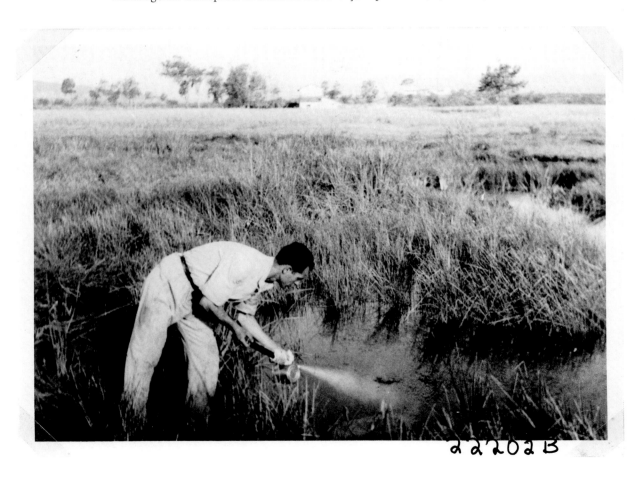

because he had seen too many others prematurely celebrate germ-killing substances as miracle cures and also because it proved difficult to concentrate the active ingredient.

Fleming's paper later came to the attention of Ernst Chain, a biochemist who had fled Nazi Germany in 1933 and was working with pathologist Howard W. Florey at Oxford University. Florey was doing research related to bacteria-killing enzymes when, in 1936, he wrote to the Rockefeller Foundation asking for £250 (about $24,000 in 2013 dollars) to purchase laboratory equipment. The application eventually found its way to Warren Weaver, the director of the Foundation's Division of Natural Sciences, who approved the grant. With this money, Florey and Chain were able to continue their work.

Fleming's paper seemed like a key that could unlock Florey and Chain's work, but the men were still strapped for funding. The British government provided some support, but research funds were in short supply after the outbreak of World War Two. In February 1940, the Foundation approved an additional $5,000 grant ($83,300 in 2013 dollars), which allowed Florey and Chain to purify penicillin and prove its effectiveness against bacteria. The Foundation then provided funds for Florey to come to the United States and meet with pharmaceutical companies in order to rush this new antibiotic into production. Penicillin saved millions of lives during the war and afterward. For their discovery, Florey and Chain, along with Fleming, were awarded the Nobel Prize in Physiology or Medicine in 1945.

Pointing to the Future

As the officers and staff at the IHD were applying their skills and knowledge to defeating yellow fever and similar diseases, new scientific fields were emerging. In 1933 the Foundation pioneered new research on "experimental biology," which was later named "molecular biology" by Warren Weaver, the director of the Foundation's Natural Sciences Division. Linking biology to physics and chemistry, this "new" biology focused on fundamental physiochemical explanations, microorganisms, and submicroscopic processes, although its links to vaccine development were indirect.

This new program supported scientific research from the 1930s through the 1950s at universities in the United States and elsewhere. The field of molecular biology is associated with the elucidation of the structure of DNA by J.D. Watson and F.H.C. Crick in 1953, and the detection of the proteins myoglobin and hemoglobin in 1958 and 1959. In the dozen years

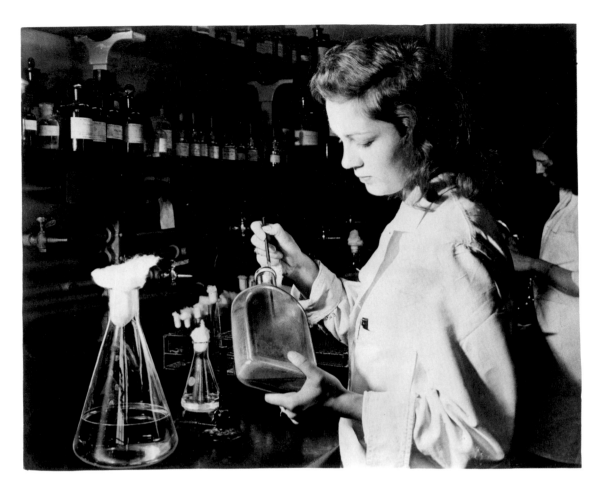

following Watson and Crick's discovery, Nobel Prizes were awarded to 18 scientists for their research into the molecular biology of the gene, many of whom had been funded by the Rockefeller Foundation.

In fact, Frederick Gates's vision of what medical education could be had led to the creation of the Rockefeller Institute for Medical Research, America's first biomedical institute, and to the formation of what would become the International Health Division of the Rockefeller Foundation. Ample funding allowed scientists to develop a longer timeline for their investigations, sometimes stretching over decades. Thanks to John D. Rockefeller's endowments, researchers were liberated to move beyond the treatment of disease, delving deeper into the very

While the discovery of penicillin can be traced to Alexander Fleming's detection in 1928, the research leading to its isolation, proven effectiveness, and production can be credited to Ernst Chain and Howard W. Florey, who were able to pursue their efforts due in part to funding from the Rockefeller Foundation. With Chain and Florey's discovery, lab technicians at Merck & Co., Inc. in 1944 began manufacturing penicillin for patients. (Merck & Co., Inc. Rockefeller Archive Center.)

Chapter Four: Finding Cures

structure and function of viruses and their hosts. This freedom produced noted Nobel Prize winners such as Max Theiler, Karl Landsteiner, Ernst Chain, and Howard W. Florey.

The Rockefeller Institute and the Rockefeller Foundation's IHD had initiated scores of projects that were not addressed by any other agency or institution at the time, researching and battling diseases that were affecting millions across the globe. The IHD was the vanguard of infectious disease detection. It not only had the staff in the field, but researchers who used state-of-the-art techniques and technology to objectively identify changing patterns in the emergence and spread of infectious diseases. Perhaps more important than any specific research project conducted by the Foundation was its overall approach. As historian David Kinkela puts it, the work was "multi-tiered, combining lab research with fieldwork, scientific knowledge deployed with dispassionate efficiency, and an unquestioned belief in technological solutions to complex ecological problems."

"The IHD was the vanguard of infectious disease detection. It not only had the staff in the field, but researchers who used state-of-the-art techniques and technology to objectively identify changing patterns in the emergence and spread of infectious diseases."

In the laboratory and working often at the cellular level, this dispassionate, scientific approach was a tremendous innovation. Failure, more often than not, was a given. Rare successes—with yellow fever or penicillin—seemed almost miraculous in terms of their benefit to humanity. Around the world, people celebrated these accomplishments. Unfortunately, as World War One proved to a generation of survivors, humanity's tendency toward violence and its destructive capacity kept pace with its ability to prevent, treat, and cure the afflicted. For some of the leaders of the Rockefeller Foundation this dark side of human behavior brought the deepest grief imaginable.

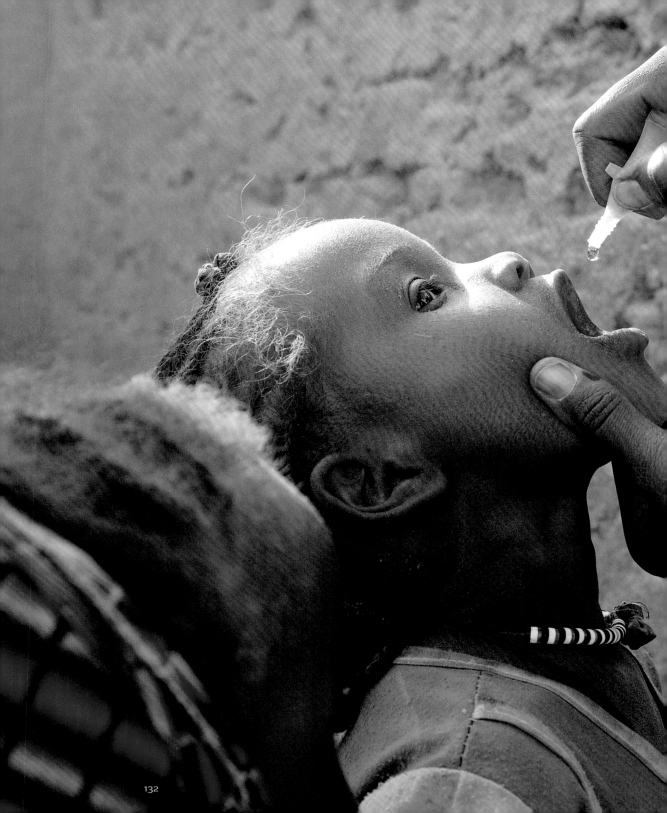

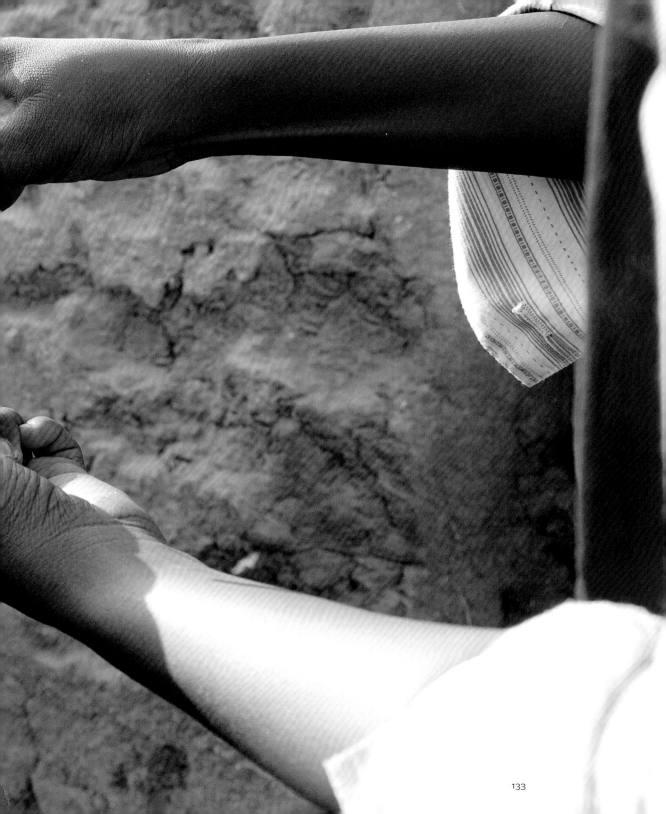

THE LIFE OF THE MIND

On the morning of April 4, 1932, Rockefeller Trustee Raymond Fosdick awoke to a quiet house. It was nearly nine o'clock. He had slept late on this Monday, no doubt because for the first time in months his family was together under one roof. These days, he and his wife Winifred—Win to her friends—and their two children were too often apart. He traveled frequently in his role as a member of the executive committee of the Rockefeller philanthropies, for his law firm, or to promote peace and international cooperation, a carryover from his involvement with the League of Nations after World War One.

Win and their ten-year-old son, Raymond Blaine Fosdick Jr., were normally in Lake Placid, New York, where the boy attended a private school. Their daughter, Susan, 16 years old, was usually away at Bryn Mawr College outside Philadelphia. For much of the year, the family's home in Montclair, New Jersey, was closed—opened only when the family gathered for holidays, as they had this Easter.

After 22 years of marriage, the tension between Raymond and Win sometimes infused family gatherings. According to one family friend, Win was "unable to meet life as normal people do," and when attempting to socialize she was "tight as a string," so nervous that she could not eat. After the birth of their son, she developed bipolar disorder (then known as manic depression), the most disturbing symptom of which was paranoia. Fosdick had tried to get her help. Win went to Europe for the winter of 1928 and apparently sought psychiatric treatment, but her condition had persisted after her return.

Fosdick was concerned about his wife, but he delighted in his children. This weekend, his obvious affection for them had ignited in Win a simmering, jealous rage. As the family slept, Win carefully paid her bills, typed the minutes from a women's group meeting, left money for the servants, wrote a will, and drafted a note explaining what she was about to do. Holding the .38 caliber Colt revolver her husband had purchased for a hunting trip, she slipped into the room where her daughter slept and fired a bullet into her head, killing her instantly. She then went to Blaine's room and killed him. She had planned to murder her husband, but for some reason changed her mind. Pressing the muzzle against her heart, she pulled the trigger and fell dead beside her son's bed.

Raymond Fosdick slept through the gunshots. The next morning, he dressed and went down to breakfast. Surprised that no one else was awake, he went back upstairs to investigate. Entering his son's room first, he found the boy bloodied and still, and Win on the floor with the revolver beside her. Horrified, he rushed to Susan's room only to find her lifeless body. Distraught, he called Win's doctor. After confirming the obvious, that all three were dead, the doctor called the police and Fosdick's brother, the minister Harry Emerson Fosdick, who came immediately. When John D. Rockefeller Jr. heard the news, he too went straight to Montclair to support his longtime colleague and friend.

For weeks after the funerals, Raymond Fosdick lay in bed in his brother's apartment, unable to sleep or eat. At one point he was hospitalized for a nervous condition. Over and over, he searched for something he might have done differently. "The numbness goes," he wrote many years later in his autobiography, "but the ache remains; and one lives with the eternal question, unanswered and unanswerable: Why? Why?"

Fosdick was not the only Rockefeller Foundation leader to suffer the loss of loved ones to mental illness. At the time of the Fosdick deaths, Max Mason served as the Foundation's president. A distinguished mathematical physicist,

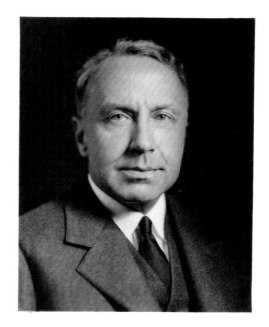

Raymond Fosdick presided over the Rockefeller Foundation during one of its most influential periods. From 1936 to 1948, the Foundation conducted extensive research on yellow fever and malaria, assisted China in its efforts to modernize, contributed to impressive advancements in the natural sciences, and initiated a program in agriculture in an effort to stave off global hunger. (Rockefeller Archive Center.)

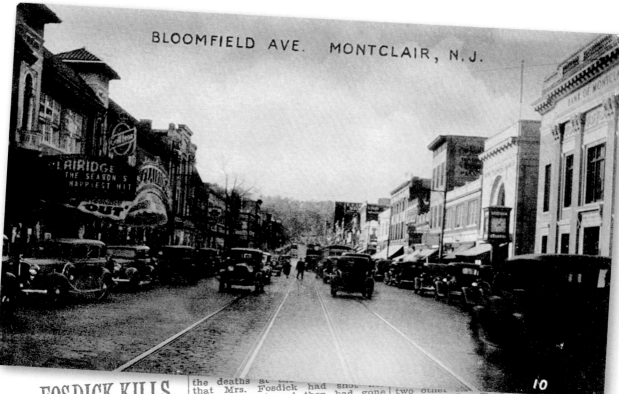

BLOOMFIELD AVE. MONTCLAIR, N.J.

FOSDICK KILLS AND 2 CHILDREN

Continued from Page One.

elope marked "The will of
d Fosdick" and a letter to
band's law partner, Chauncey
, of 61 Broadway, New York,
she had named executor of
ate.

artland declined to discuss
tents of the will, saying that
other documents had been
over to the police for return
amily.

etter contained personal re-
he indicated, adding, "A pos-
otive for her act was shown
etter. Due to her psychosis,
apparently a little jealous of
band's affection for their chil-
his was due entirely to her
al mental state."
artland said that her malady
manic depressive psychosis.
lepressions are subject to vio-
ictuations of mood, ranging
lation to deep melancholy.
are usually victims of this
is.

ifts of Money for Servants.

Fosdick had prepared for her
vith great care and had left
irs in perfect order. Besides
she left a sheaf of checks to
—ications. She left pres-

the deaths at ___ ___ ___
that Mrs. Fosdick had shot ___
daughter first and then had gone
immediately to her son's room,
killed him and then herself. Only
three shots had been fired. The
bullet with which she killed herself
had sped on upward and lodged in
the wall six feet above the floor.

Mr. Fosdick telephoned Dr. Victor
B. Seidler of 16 Plymouth Street,
Montclair, who had been treating
Mrs. Fosdick. Dr. Seidler hurried
to the house and after determining
at a glance that the mother and
children were dead telephoned the
police. Chief Edward F. Reilly assigned Captain Thomas Claren and
Detective Sergeant Fred Gallagher
to investigate the deaths and noti-
fied the Medical Examiner's office.

Other members of the family, including Dr. Fosdick, were summoned
to the home. A police guard was
placed at the house to prevent intrusion.

Both the Medical Examiner and
the police quickly pronounced the
case one of double homicide and
suicide, but made the usual investigation.

Husband Bought the Pistol.

The revolver was one which
Fosdick had bought some years ___
for a hunting trip in the Northwes
He kept it in a bureau drawer ___
the third floor and, according to
police, did not know that Mr. ___
dick knew of its existence. ___
loaded and additional cartrid
were locked in a desk in Mr.
dick's study on the first floor

The bodies were taken to Kin___
morgue in Orange. Autopsies were
performed there by Dr. Martland
and Dr. Brien and the bodies were
then removed to the Home for Ser-

two other ___ ___ ___
lano and Mrs. Fred Hewlet___
brother, George D. Finlay Jr., all
Montclair.

She was married to Mr. Fosdick
Dec. 2, 1910, in the home of ___
parents here. Dr. Fosdick, then
young clergyman in the First B___
tist Church here, his first pastora
performed the ceremony. John P
roy Mitchel, afterward Mayor
New York, was among the guests

Mr. Fosdick already has had a
reer of unusual distinction and is
present engaged in many public
tivities. He was graduated fr
Princeton in 1905, taking a mast
degree there also in 1906. After tra
ing for the law he entered practic

In the early twentieth century Montclair, New
Jersey, was a growing town with excellent
schools, influential churches, and a thriving arts
community, which attracted prominent New York
City businessmen who wanted easy access to
the city and a small-town environment for their
families. Among Montclair's notable residents
were a number of key Rockefeller Foundation
officials, including Raymond Fosdick, Frederick
Gates, and Starr Murphy. The deaths of Win
Fosdick and her two children shocked this
otherwise stable community. (Photo: Montclair
Historical Society. Article: New York Times.)

Mason had been the president of the University of Chicago before coming to the Foundation in July 1928. His first wife, Mary Louise, had been institutionalized, and she died of pneumonia shortly before Mason left Chicago for New York. John D. Rockefeller Jr. had suffered a mental breakdown in his early twenties, and his sister Edith was first a patient of, and later a therapist trained by, the Swiss psychiatrist Carl Jung. Even John D. Rockefeller Sr. had suffered bouts of depression. These personal experiences would play an important part in shaping what became a major initiative of the Rockefeller Foundation in the 1930s—the search for scientific explanations for human behavior and physiological treatments for mental illness.

Psychiatry, Mental Hygiene, and Social Control

Mental illness had baffled physicians and victimized families for generations. Those who suffered from it were ostracized by society and frequently confined at home or in institutions where they received little treatment. Insanity was often associated with evil spirits or moral corruption. In the late eighteenth century, one emerging group of physicians and scientists began to look for biological explanations, while therapists sought explanations in the personal and social experience of the patient. These twin paths for the development of neuroscience and psychiatry would define the development of the field in the twentieth century and often lead to controversy.

Psychiatry evolved without clear breakthroughs in treatment on either path, but there were tantalizing insights in both arenas. German researchers developed a basic functional map of the cerebral cortex in the 1880s, and discovered that the brain responded to electrical stimulation. A neurohistologist named Alois Alzheimer found a biological explanation for the dementia that affected many older patients. In 1917 Viennese psychiatry professor Julius Wagner-Jauregg seemed to discover that a malaria-induced fever could cure the psychoses of patients who had been infected with syphilis and contracted neurosyphilitic disease. His work led to the development of a malaria-induced "fever cure" for psychosis (see Chapter IV). All of these insights appeared to strengthen the idea that mental illness had biological roots that could eventually be discerned and treated.

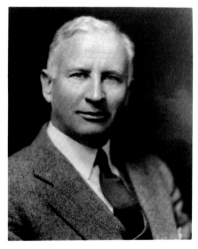

Max Mason had directed the Natural Sciences Division of the Rockefeller Foundation for only three years before he was promoted to Foundation president in 1929. Mason's personal interest in understanding human behavior led to increased funding for psychiatric research during his tenure. (Rockefeller Archive Center.)

On a path that paralleled this physiological research, the field of psychotherapy flourished under the influence of Sigmund Freud, Carl Jung, and others who focused on the influence of the unconscious mind and the lasting effects of childhood experiences and social interactions on the personality. As these ideas were popularized, they influenced the theories of social scientists, especially those working in sociology and anthropology, and offered a countervailing framework for understanding human behavior that was often at odds with the traditional moral framework provided by more conservative religious leaders. This maelstrom of ideas, new and old, often made the Rockefeller Foundation's efforts to develop the science of human behavior controversial.

To the Victorian generation, which included Frederick Gates and John D. Rockefeller Sr., social problems like prostitution, alcoholism, gambling, rape, robbery, and murder were often framed in strictly moral or religious terms. But with the rise of Progressivism, younger board members increasingly viewed these issues as problems in "social control." While the term may sound nefarious today, when early leaders of the Rockefeller Foundation used these words they were primarily concerned about human welfare.

For John D. Rockefeller Jr., the need for social control became clear when he served as foreman of a grand jury convened to investigate prostitution in New York City. At the time, prostitution was flourishing across the United States. "Vice commissions" set up in major cities revealed that the men of New York, Chicago, and Pittsburg spent more than $100 million ($2.1 billion in 2013 dollars) on prostitution, nearly three-quarters of the amount given to charity in those cities. This was at a time when one percent of the nation was solely dependent on religious donations and another 10 to 15 percent was living at or below the poverty line. The dangers of prostitution were also measured in health statistics: one man in 20 was infected with venereal disease, and approximately one in five hospital admissions was for paralysis related to syphilis.

Over the course of the investigation in New York, John D. Rockefeller Jr. interviewed experts from every religious and community support organization in the city. With his own money, he also hired 14 investigators who interviewed hundreds of witnesses: prostitutes, their patrons, and their "owners." Overall, the investigation revealed that there was no organized "white slave trade" in New York. The prostitutes and their pimps were not members of any syndicate or mafia family. Each pimp was independent, but they knew one another in such a way that few women could escape.

Recognizing that women were victimized by prostitution, Rockefeller recommended that the pimps, and not the prostitutes, be the focus of

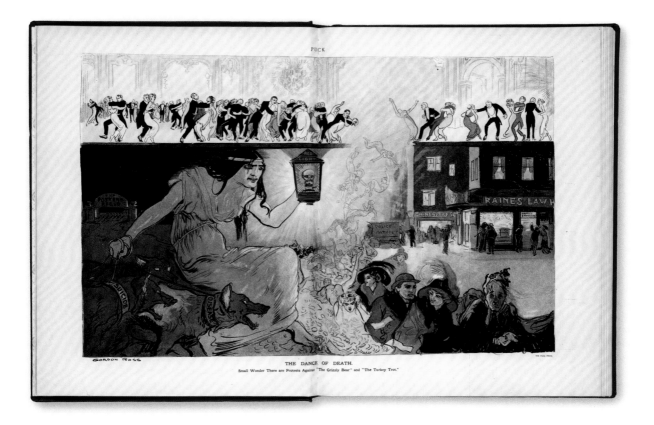

THE DANCE OF DEATH.

Small Wonder There are Protests Against "The Grizzly Bear" and "The Turkey Trot."

future police sweeps. Furthermore, he advised that sex education training be set up in schools. But more important, he argued for a special commission to further study the entire cycle of prostitution in order to make policy changes.

Rockefeller's investigation also dispelled the myth that prostitution was a matter of immorality among the throng of foreigners entering the country. Between 1910 and 1915, more than 35 investigations at the city and state level revealed that the enterprise was run primarily by and for men. Prostitutes were just as likely to be second- or third-generation U.S. citizens as immigrants. The cycle of prostitution was one of dependency and coercion, born out of economic desperation.

Rockefeller realized that the city government was unlikely to do much about the problem. As the grand jury was ending its work, he searched for some way to promote continued research and action. It was during this period that he met Raymond Fosdick, still a young lawyer at the time, who

In this 1912 illustration titled "The Dance of Death," couples are pictured dancing just above an image of a prostitute holding back the dogs of "disease," "insanity," and "suicide." The cartoon vividly expresses early twentieth-century anxieties in the United States about moral order, changing sexual relations, and societal ills. (Library of Congress.)

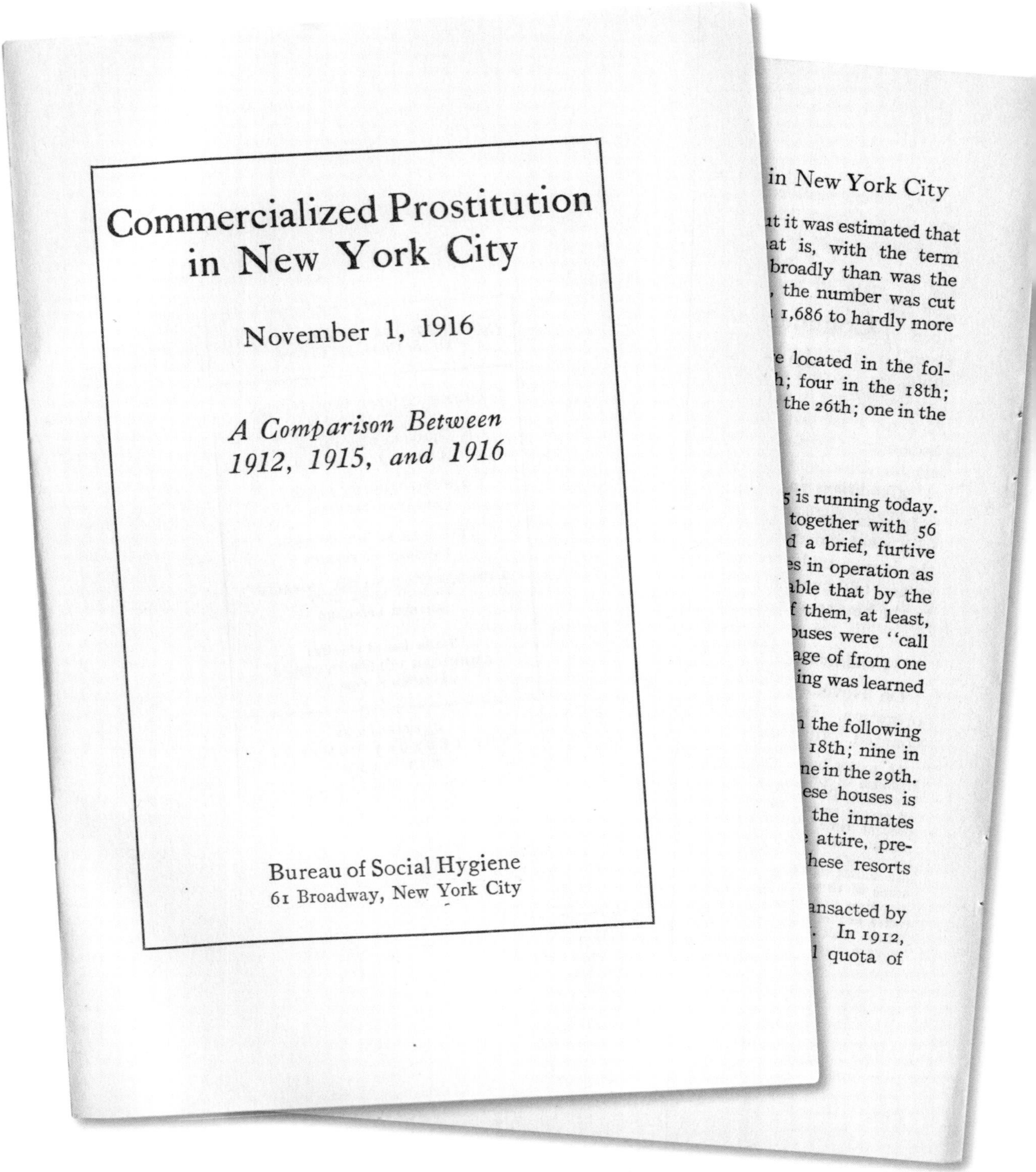

Commercialized Prostitution in New York City

November 1, 1916

A Comparison Between 1912, 1915, and 1916

Bureau of Social Hygiene
61 Broadway, New York City

it it was estimated that
at is, with the term
broadly than was the
, the number was cut
1,686 to hardly more

e located in the fol-
h; four in the 18th;
the 26th; one in the

5 is running today.
together with 56
d a brief, furtive
es in operation as
able that by the
f them, at least,
ouses were ''call
age of from one
ing was learned

the following
18th; nine in
ne in the 29th.
ese houses is
the inmates
attire, pre-
hese resorts

ansacted by
. In 1912,
quota of

was working for the mayor. A Princeton graduate who had worked in a settlement house in New York before coming to city government, Fosdick, like Rockefeller, was a Progressive who believed in the scientific method and the role of experts in solving social problems. The two men had much in common, and this initial meeting would eventually lead to a deep and lifelong friendship.

Soon after, in 1913, Rockefeller organized and financed the American Social Hygiene Association, with its research arm, the Bureau of Social Hygiene, to carry forward the work of the grand jury. Rockefeller endowed a hygiene laboratory at the New York State Reformatory for Women and established a municipal diagnostic clinic for venereal disease—one of the first in the country. At the lab, researchers and diagnosticians began to recognize that many of the women confined to the reformatory were suffering from mental illness.

Following his service as foreman on a grand jury investigating prostitution in New York City, John D. Rockefeller Jr. launched the Bureau of Social Hygiene to conduct studies and formulate public policy related to a number of societal ills, including prostitution and juvenile delinquency. (Rockefeller Archive Center.)

Through the Bureau of Social Hygiene, Rockefeller also financed studies of addiction and juvenile delinquency, as well as major scholarly studies of prostitution by George Kneeland and Abraham Flexner. When Raymond Fosdick quit his job with the City of New York, Rockefeller recruited him to the Bureau to undertake studies of police systems in Europe and the United States. This work led to campaigns against red-light districts, public service messages that promoted prophylactic use, and education about sexually transmitted diseases. All of these initiatives deepened Rockefeller's interest in the relationship between social conditions and the mind of the individual.

Mental Hygiene

In 1900 Clifford W. Beers tried to commit suicide by throwing himself from the upper window of his parents' home in Connecticut. Beers had grown up in New Haven, attended Yale University's Sheffield Scientific School, and graduated in 1897. But after working as a clerk in New York City he had become increasingly depressed. After recovering from his injuries in 1900, Beers was confined in a series of mental institutions, where he suffered degrading treatment and physical abuse. When he was finally released in 1904, he resolved to write a book about his experiences. Psychiatrist Adolf Meyer, from Johns Hopkins University, offered to help.

Beers's book, *A Mind that Found Itself*, revealed much about the hidden world of the asylum in the U.S. In 1906 mentally ill patients occupied more hospital beds in the United States than all other patients combined. Approximately one in every 300 people was institutionalized for being insane. Historians have struggled to explain the tremendous rise in asylum populations at the end of the nineteenth century. Some argue that the proliferation of asylums reflected the larger pattern of institution-building in Western culture in this era, a pattern that gave rise to new universities, government agencies, and hospitals that absorbed social functions that had once been taken care of in the home, church, or community. Other historians, however, suggest that many asylum inmates were not mentally ill, but nonconformists or social misfits who were committed for their failure to follow social mores. In any case, most asylums became little more than warehouses for the afflicted.

Widely read, Beers's book sparked a social movement that led him across the nation and around the world, advocating on behalf of the mentally ill. With Adolf Meyer, William Welch, and philosopher William James, Beers founded the Connecticut Society for Mental Hygiene in 1908 to improve care and treatment of the mentally ill. The following year, the National Committee for Mental Hygiene (NCMH) was created and dedicated to improving asylums, educating physicians in psychiatric clinics, providing support to discharged patients, and preventing mental illness.

This movement on behalf of the mentally ill and mental hygiene was at its height when the Rockefeller Foundation was established in 1913. The board of trustees recognized the importance of mental hygiene research and set out to "contribute to the discovery of needed facts and to the diffusion of the most reliable information by which this important field of public health is to be governed." Acting on the recommendation of William Welch, the Foundation hired psychiatrist Thomas Salmon in 1914 to develop a strategy and program in this arena.

Salmon had worked as a bacteriologist in state psychiatric hospitals in New York before turning to psychiatric research and patient advocacy. After moving to the U.S. Public Health Service, he was assigned to Ellis Island, where he evaluated immigrants. Appalled by the treatment of immigrants awaiting deportation, many of whom showed symptoms of mental illness, he sought to improve their care. In 1912 he had become the NCMH's

In 1908 Clifford Beers published *A Mind That Found Itself*, an autobiographical account of his time in a mental institution after suffering bouts of paranoia and attempting suicide. Beers's book focused attention on the treatment of the mentally ill and led to a reform movement that sought to educate doctors and improve patient care. (H. Schervee. Alan Mason Chesney Medical Archives, Johns Hopkins University.)

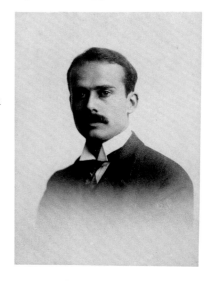

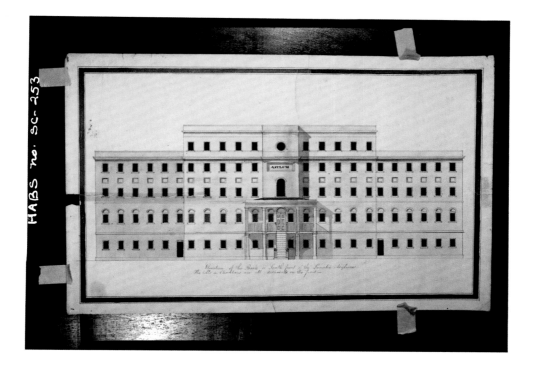

HABS no. SC-253

first medical director. During his tenure, he initiated a series of surveys of the mentally ill using a system of standardized records and statistical analyses that were in line with emerging social science methods.

The Rockefeller Foundation funded these surveys because it believed that related fields such as mental hygiene, heredity, alcoholism, and venereal disease "should be approached as one broad problem." As with many Rockefeller projects, the Foundation's first step was a series of surveys of mental institutions in each of several states, beginning with South Carolina and then expanding to 12 more states, hoping that the results of these surveys would lead to changes in the diagnosis, commitment, and care of the mentally ill.

Salmon's surveys revealed that many communities isolated the mentally ill in charity houses, where they remained secluded and received little if any care. The surveys also revealed an extensive unmet need for mental health services. For every person under psychiatric care, another person needed but did not receive it. This was true for both outpatient care and inpatient hospitalization. These results prompted state legislators to allocate significant new funding for mental hygiene reform.

At the "lunatic asylum" in Columbia, South Carolina, and at other asylums around the United States, mentally ill patients were often neglected or abused. Calls for deinstitutionalization, improved care, and psychiatric research gradually led to new investment in the science of the brain and the treatment of America's mentally ill. (Library of Congress.)

Salmon's studies revolutionized the organization and administration of mental institutions in the United States. They also suggested that many convicted criminals were suffering from mental illness. In 1916 the Foundation granted $10,000 ($200,000 in 2013 dollars) to the NCMH to establish a new medical facility at Sing Sing prison in upstate New York that emphasized psychiatric diagnosis and treatment. It was the first mental hygiene center of its kind in a penal institution in the United States. In making the grant, the Foundation underscored its concern for the relationship between "mental abnormalities or disease" and criminal behavior, and endorsed the appropriate humane treatment of individual prisoners. As the Foundation noted in its 1917 annual report, "The public attitude toward mental maladies is still affected by superstition and ignorance," and the Foundation hoped to dispel these beliefs.

Salmon found that 59 percent of criminals had psychiatric conditions but were not "insane" by the standards of the day, meaning that they did not require inpatient hospitalization. He also found a high recidivism rate among parolees. The Rockefeller-funded studies revealed that the penal system failed on two counts: it did not identify inmates that might benefit from mental hygiene, and it did not rehabilitate many criminals,

Soldiers diagnosed with neurosis, nervous diseases, or "shell shock" recovered by fishing and swimming at the U.S. American National Red Cross Hospital in Blois, France, during World War One. Treatments for shell shock, which was poorly understood at the time, ranged from electroshock therapy to rest cures in tranquil locations. (National Library of Medicine.)

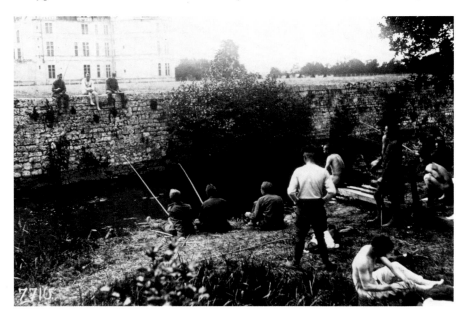

perhaps because of a lack of psychiatric intervention. Salmon advocated that the accused be given mental examinations before trial and incarceration. These initiatives marked the beginning of a much larger effort in forensic psychiatry in the United States.

World War One redirected the Foundation's mental hygiene initiative as the NCMH worked with the U.S. Surgeon General to address mental health issues in the military. The Foundation funded Salmon's visit to Europe in 1917 to study the nature and treatment of nervous diseases (then known as "shell shock") in military hospitals. This work helped shape the development of U.S. Army policy on mental health. All draftees and volunteers would be screened to exclude individuals who were "mentally or nervously unfit for military service," and during later military engagements, psychiatrists were positioned as far forward as was safe, to support infantry personnel.

ROCKEFELLER FOUNDATION DIVISION OF MENTAL HYGIENE

After the war, in 1919, Salmon proposed that the Foundation establish a Division of Mental Hygiene. He suggested that its functions should be "(1) the study of psychiatric school clinics and other opportunities for mental hygiene work in childhood, (2) consideration of the present status of psychiatric studies in delinquency and crime, (3) a study of the facilities for undergraduate and postgraduate training in psychiatry and mental hygiene, and a study of the function, development and administration of university psychiatric hospitals." The trustees demurred, however, fearing that postwar relief efforts would overwhelm the Foundation's ability to fund other programs. Frustrated, Salmon left the Foundation in 1921 to become a professor of psychiatry at Columbia University. Despite his departure, the Foundation continued through 1929 to fund NCMH efforts to address "problems of defects and delinquency in children and criminality in adults, with nervous and mental disorders, with the classification, treatment, and custodial care of the feeble-minded and insane, and related questions." Altogether, Foundation expenditures in mental hygiene from 1914 to 1929 totaled $805,709.11 ($10.3 million in 2013 dollars).

The Rockefeller Foundation also funded several mental hygiene investigations that examined the impact of alcohol and drug use. Before the 1919 Volstead Act, which prohibited the sale of alcohol, the per capita use of alcohol in America was three times as high as it is today, on par with each person drinking one to two bottles of 80-proof liquor per week—about 90 bottles each year. Seventeen times more money was spent on alcohol than was given to charity.

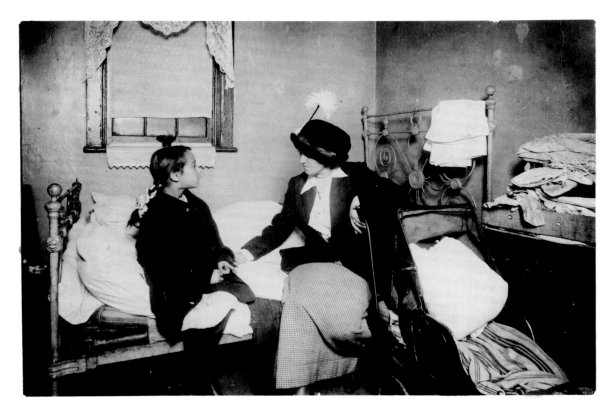

Many psychiatrists of the day believed that alcohol caused mental disorders. Other people suggested that it indicated a "degenerate" constitution and was "nature's way of weeding out the unfit." This idea of "degeneracy" reflected an increasingly popular notion that mental illness was hereditary and worsened or degenerated with each generation. Progressives did not subscribe to this view. Rather, they asserted that people stressed by factory work and urban living resorted to alcohol and other drugs as a solace, which provided only temporary relief and ultimately left the person wanting more.

A public health nurse, working with the Department of Public Charities in New York City in 1913, speaks with eight-year-old Ida List, the daughter of an alcoholic. In the early twentieth century doctors and reformers debated whether alcoholism was inherited or a reaction to the stress of modern urban life. (Library of Congress.)

John D. Rockefeller Jr., a third-generation teetotaler, backed one of the greatest social experiments in American history: Prohibition. He supported the Anti-Saloon League (ASL), matching ten percent of all its donations. But in 1926, after the ASL supported a measure that imprisoned Volstead Act violators, Rockefeller withdrew his monetary support. And in 1932 he abandoned the dry movement altogether, acknowledging that it had led to the "colossal scale" of criminal activity related to Prohibition.

Chapter Five: The Life of the Mind

Rockefeller funded the Liquor Study Committee, composed of his trusted advisor Raymond Fosdick and several researchers, to examine the social effects of legislation regarding the production, distribution, and sale of alcohol in other countries. The results of the study were published to widespread acclaim in 1933 in *Toward Liquor Control*, which encouraged two strategies for states: to control all sales of liquor so as to remove the profit motive, or to strictly regulate the sale of alcohol through the issuance of licenses. Additional Foundation funding led to the two-year follow-up study *After Repeal*, which examined the effects in the 15 states that had adopted monopoly control and the 25 that utilized central licensing. Overall, the study suggested things were "going well."

REORGANIZATION AND THE RISE OF PSYCHIATRY

By 1927 Raymond Fosdick had become a close advisor to John D. Rockefeller Jr., who was serving as the chairman of the Rockefeller Foundation. Fosdick had been a trustee since 1921 and was on the boards of the Rockefeller Institute for Medical Research, the Laura Spelman Rockefeller Memorial, the China Medical Board, and the International Health Division. He had also become a trustee of two other Rockefeller philanthropies, the General Education Board and the International Education Board. When Rockefeller became concerned about the lack of coordination between all of these entities, Fosdick orchestrated a major reorganization that consolidated authority and funding within the Foundation.

For some, the reorganization marked the end of an era. Wickliffe Rose retired, as did Abraham Flexner, who protested the diminution in authority of the General Education Board he headed. President George Vincent stepped down shortly after the reorganization and was soon succeeded by Max Mason from the University of Chicago. Frederick Gates, who had already stepped down from the Foundation's board, died in 1929. The reorganization led to a redefined program for the Rockefeller Foundation. While promoting the well-being of mankind remained the core mission, the trustees embraced a new goal—the advancement of knowledge.

As these transitions in leadership and program were taking place, the Foundation commissioned a report from trustee David L. Edsall, the dean of the Harvard Medical School. Edsall presented his memorandum to the trustees in 1930 during a meeting in Princeton, as they were contemplating major changes in the Foundation's program. He encouraged the Foundation to deepen its involvement in the field of psychiatry, noting that psychiatry had been "distinctly separated from general medical interests" and describing the need for a greater understanding of diseases of the mind. His recommendations built upon the work of the Foundation and other Rockefeller philanthropies in mental and social hygiene, as well as in medical research and education.

Alan Gregg listened to Edsall's presentation with enthusiasm. His appointment to succeed Richard Pearce as head of the division of Medical Sciences was confirmed at the Princeton meeting, which meant he would be responsible for implementing a new program focused on psychiatry. A Harvard-trained physician who had served on the front in World War One, Gregg had joined the International Health Board in 1919 and worked for several years in Brazil. While he was still in medical school, he had been mentored by James Jackson Putnam, the chief of the department of Neurology and one of the earliest proponents of psychoanalysis in the United States. Gregg had met Sigmund Freud and Carl Jung in 1909, when Freud made a celebrated trip to America to deliver a series of lectures. Gregg later described these experiences as a "turning point" in his life, shaping his fascination with psychiatry.

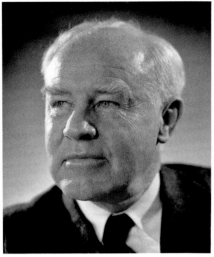

As director of the division of Medical Sciences of the Rockefeller Foundation, Alan Gregg focused on building the field of psychiatry. Gregg directed funding that helped to standardize psychiatry as part of medical school curricula and to support individual researchers working in the field. (Rockefeller Archive Center.)

Over the next 18 months, Gregg began to develop Edsall's recommendations into a program. He visited psychiatric research facilities in the United Kingdom, Canada, and the United States. He was undoubtedly encouraged by trustee Raymond Fosdick, who was by this time the effective leader of the Rockefeller Foundation's board of trustees, working closely with chairman John D. Rockefeller Jr.

Then in April 1932 came the murder of Fosdick's children and the suicide of his wife. For three weeks, Fosdick's own mental state was so fragile that he was hospitalized with "neuritis." After he left the hospital, he could not work for months. Rockefeller invited him to Warm Springs, Virginia, and the following summer Fosdick retreated to the coast of Maine. He returned to work in New York in the fall, believing it would provide a path back to mental stability. He tired easily, but gradually he resumed his pivotal role on the board.

In April 1933, almost exactly a year after the death of Fosdick's wife and children, Alan Gregg presented his multi-phased plan to make psychiatry and neurology the major focus of the division of Medical Sciences to the Rockefeller Foundation's board of trustees. Because these disciplines were so poorly developed in 1933, Gregg suggested that the Foundation would have to build these fields. It would start with education and training, expanding the personnel and the institutions that would sustain future research and development. Grants-in-aid would follow to support the most promising investigators and research scientists. Eventually, as leaders emerged in each field, more substantial grants and endowments would follow to sustain these institutions over the long run. Ultimately, advancements in research and the professionalization of psychiatry would lead to better care and transformations in the social, legal, and educational systems that would account for the realities of mental illness.

With Rockefeller chairing the board meeting and Max Mason leading as president of the Foundation, the policy options that Gregg presented had deeply personal overtones. Months later, in the Foundation's annual report, President Mason made it clear that this new strategy represented more than a decision to devote substantial resources to the development of psychiatry and neurology. Across the board, the Foundation had decided to focus on advancing knowledge in "subfields which contribute more directly to the general problem of human behavior, with the aim of control through understanding." Over the next two decades, motivated by the desire to advance the scientific understanding of the mind and human behavior, and by the private longing of Fosdick and others for answers to questions that seemed unanswerable, the Foundation supported pioneering research in arenas that others were unwilling or unable to explore.

SEXUALITY

Human sexuality was probably the most controversial topic for Foundation-sponsored research. John D. Rockefeller Jr.'s work with the Bureau of Social Hygiene had raised his awareness of the exploitation and health issues related to sexual behavior, and the Rockefeller Foundation was a pioneer in promoting scientific research on human sexuality from 1914 to 1954. Initially the Foundation provided funds to the Bureau of Social Hygiene to conduct sex research, with an emphasis on factors that led to prostitution as well as on its reform. After Katherine Bement Davis became general secretary of the Bureau, she argued that prostitution could not be reduced or controlled without deeper understanding of human sexuality.

Davis's efforts led to the creation of a partnership between the Bureau of Social Hygiene and the National Research Council and the formation in 1921 of the council's Committee for Research in Problems of Sex. With

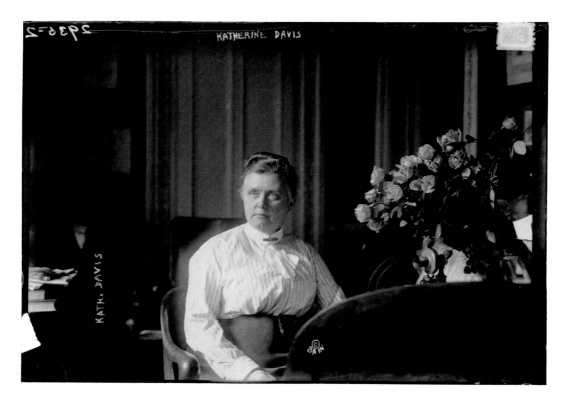

funds provided by Foundation trustees, the committee worked to promote "systematic comprehensive research in sex in its individual and social manifestations." This work was to be anchored in medical and biological science, but also to integrate the social sciences. To Davis's frustration, however, the committee's work was extremely conservative in the 1920s, and avoided controversial topics.

Katherine Bement Davis's 1917 appointment as general secretary of the Bureau of Social Hygiene transformed the organization. Believing that prostitution could not be understood without a more general understanding of human sexuality, Davis advocated for comprehensive research into the medical, biological, and social sciences, and formed an important partnership with the National Research Council. (Library of Congress.)

Meanwhile, with funding from the Foundation and John D. Rockefeller Jr., Davis arranged for groundbreaking research, published in 1929, on the sexuality of "normal" females. Women whose names were found in club membership directories and college alumnae lists were surveyed about "auto-erotic" practices, sexual desire, homosexuality, contraception, and intercourse. This work challenged a pervasive view derived from Victorian society that women had no innate sexual drive.

After the Bureau of Social Hygiene ceased operations in the early 1930s, the Rockefeller Foundation continued to fund the Committee for Research in Problems of Sex as part of its larger effort to promote a more scientific understanding of human behavior. The committee's 1941 decision to provide a $1,600 grant to Alfred Kinsey at Indiana University marked a major departure from its conservative past.

An entomologist by training, Kinsey developed a scheme of classifying and thus normalizing sexual behaviors that, at the time, were considered deviant. Kinsey believed that homosexuality was a variation of human sexuality, and his research refuted previously held notions of female asexuality by showing that one in four women reported achieving orgasm by age 15, 50 percent by age 20. When the results of his research were first published in 1948 under the title *Sexual Behavior in the Human Male*, Kinsey became a lightning rod for controversy. Many people were shocked, for example, by his assertion that homosexuality was more widespread than previously believed.

Leaders of the Rockefeller Foundation were deeply committed to Kinsey's work in the 1940s. Alan Gregg, the director of Medical Sciences, agreed to write the introduction for *Sexual Behavior in the Human Male*. But the controversy that surrounded the publication of the book was troubling to many Foundation leaders. When Kinsey's work was challenged on the basis of its statistical approach, the Foundation sent statisticians to Indiana to review Kinsey's methods. The Foundation continued to fund Kinsey's work for several more years prior to the publication of *Sexual Behavior in the Human Female* in 1953. Appearing at the height of a conservative, anti-communist era in American history, Kinsey's second book was even more controversial. The following year, the Foundation terminated its funding for Kinsey because of the controversy, but also because Kinsey's book had been such a commercial success that program officers felt he didn't need Foundation money to carry on with his work. Meanwhile the Foundation continued to invest in other research initiatives focused on human behavior, including the influence of heredity on personality and mental illness.

BEHAVIOR GENETICS

In the 1920s and 1930s, the Foundation had supported research into behavior genetics with the expectation that it would lead to a better society. Although some Foundation trustees were fearful that genetic research into what was then called "degeneracy" would lead to criticism that the Foundation supported the highly controversial field of eugenics, the Foundation agreed to fund research on the heritability of various mental conditions. In one study, psychiatric social workers were sent out to interview the families of 330 patients admitted to hospitals from 1928 to 1930 for conditions known today as schizophrenia and bipolar disorder. The startling results indicated that family members were two to three times more likely to have a disorder.

The Foundation also provided grants to support studies on intelligence and its heritability in dogs. John Paul Scott conducted a comprehensive analysis of data, collected over 13 years, on the performance of 300 puppies from five different breeds, rated in 30 different tests. The analysis revealed no "general-intelligence" factor. A pup's ability on one test did not correlate highly with his performance on another. None of the breeds were demonstratively better overall than any other. Motivation and physical capability, rather than breed, drove performance. Within a breed, performance was highly variable. The same held true for temperament. In short, motivation was a stronger influence than either cognitive or emotional capacity. The implication for humans was that the behavioral traits were determined not by genetics but by environment. And the best environments offered numerous possibilities and freedom of choice.

Like much Foundation research, funding was not limited to the United States. The Foundation supported research in Denmark conducted by Oluf Thomsen and Tage Kemp in the early 1930s on the genetics of psychopathology. This led to the development of a Danish twin registry composed of nearly two thousand pairs. The findings suggested that while intelligence and personality were highly correlated among twins reared apart, there was less correlation involving schizophrenia, suggesting that environment had an influence.

In Germany the Foundation supported Emil Kraepelin's biologically oriented German Research Institute of Psychiatry in Munich and Oskar Vogt's Kaiser Wilhelm Institute for Brain Research in Berlin. Kraepelin was considered by some psychiatrists to be even more important than Freud for his systematic efforts to compile enormous data sets on asylum patients and then narrow the framework for diagnosis to two basic categories: those characterized by an affective component—meaning they evidenced emotional distress—and those who were psychotic but without affective signs. The first group he described as suffering from various forms of "manic-depressive illness" and suggested that most would eventually get better. The second group had dementia praecox (later termed schizophrenia) and would not improve. Between 1932 and 1935, the Foundation also funded twin research projects at the Kaiser Wilhelm Institute for Anthropology, Human Heredity, and Eugenics. As the Nazi regime became increasingly repressive, the Foundation terminated funding to all German programs in 1938.

Research grants were also given to D.K. Henderson and T.A. Munro at Edinburgh, Scotland, to study the effects of consanguineous marriage, and Janet Vaughan at Hammersmith, England, to investigate the intersection of human heredity and psychic disturbances.

Ever interested in public health worldwide, the International Health Division of the Foundation funded international surveys of mental hygiene as early as 1938. Unfortunately, an empirical review of these and other surveys revealed methodological problems due to differences in the selection and interview processes that made it impossible to accurately compare groups. Some of the state-to-state surveys, however, did allow comparisons between urban and rural communities. For example, the rate of mental hygiene problems overall was found to be 6.5 percent in Baltimore and 6.9 percent in less-populated counties in Tennessee. Although this project did not achieve what it set out to accomplish, due to its methodological problems, it did point the way for standardization in diagnosis, which led to the International Classification of Diseases (ICD) later published by the World Health Organization.

YALE UNIVERSITY INSTITUTE OF HUMAN RELATIONS (IHR)

In 1929 the Foundation launched what Raymond Fosdick considered its "most ambitious undertaking," an integrated interdisciplinary institute at a prestigious university created to understand human behavior from as many vantage points as possible. The Foundation's support in forming such an institute transcended the disciplinary walls of academic departments, reflecting not only the science of the times regarding interdependent causation but also the Foundation's own effort to coordinate its five divisions while minimizing entrenchment among various professionals in their own programs. Beardsley Ruml, a psychologist who was the director of the Laura Spelman Rockefeller Memorial, developed the plan along with James Angell, president of Yale, and Robert Yerkes, a Harvard-trained psychologist. Foundation trustees read within the plan an expectation that the interdisciplinary nature of the research enterprise could be protected from the individual interests of the scientists.

The Foundation gave $2.5 million ($33.7 million in 2013 dollars) to create the Institute of Human Relations (IHR), designed to bridge the gap between medical and social knowledge of human behavior. The IHR appropriation was the largest made that year, amounting to one-fifth of all Foundation appropriations in 1929, more than the entire program of the International Health Division. In the next ten years, the IHR would receive an additional $4.5 million ($77.3 million in 2013 dollars).

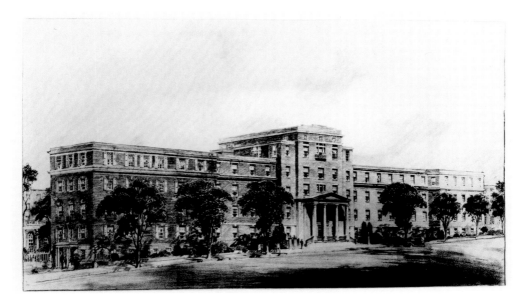

The IHR was itself an experiment. Staff attempted to maintain a centralized organization (through the directorship), regulated social arrangements (through seminars and division of research laboratories), and structured research (through a psychological metatheory of the individual and environment and a mechanized methodology). The results of this organizational pilot study revealed that integrated research units and regular seminars worked best, the latter to check the reasoning of the scientists involved. Funds were most effective when distributed to groups of scientists, not to individuals or departments. Finally, theories were valued more highly than applied work, and cooperation was rewarded more than independence.

Yale University's Institute of Human Relations was created in 1929 as a site for the interdisciplinary study of human behavior. The Rockefeller Foundation invested heavily in the institute, hoping it would develop as a new model for research in the field. (Rockefeller Archive Center.)

During the IHR's 20 years of existence, its researchers published hundreds of articles and reports that influenced subsequent research on aggression, socialization, learning, psychopathology, culture and personality, and motivation. Some of the research findings led to advances in the theory or philosophy of human behavior, while others led to more practical applications. While many of the researchers contributed to the science of human behavior, a few advanced the science by leaps and bounds.

Overall, IHR researchers were highly productive, and the institute gained a high stature within the research community. But it failed to develop a truly integrated approach for the study of human behavior. The institute closed in 1952 not because of a lack of funding, but due to the personalities involved and interdisciplinary infighting.

The Laura Spelman Rockefeller Memorial
and the Child Development Movement

With the passing of John D. Rockefeller Sr.'s wife, Laura, in 1915 at age 75, a memorial had been established in her honor. For the first several years, the Laura Spelman Rockefeller Memorial (LSRM) contributed to causes important to Laura during her life, such as churches, charities, missionary projects, and African-American education. But in 1922, with $74 million accrued in the memorial fund (more than $1 billion in 2013 dollars), Beardsley Ruml was hired—as mentioned earlier—as a permanent director to develop a plan for distribution. A psychologist with expertise in statistics who had come from the Carnegie Corporation, Ruml soon laid out a plan to support fellowships in social and behavioral sciences along with endowed social science programs at several prestigious U.S. universities—including Columbia, Virginia, Chicago, and Massachusetts—as well as at Fisk University and the Atlanta School of Social Work, which were dedicated to educating African-American students.

Perhaps the most important practical contribution made by the LSRM was to establish child development and parent education as a national movement. As research showed that the causes of juvenile delinquency were less related to biology and race than to home and school environment, the LSRM increased its funding for child development research. Ruml recognized in Lawrence K. Frank a unique individual with ideas about conducting research on toddlers that could be used to develop strategies to support normal development. Over the next decade, Frank was able to "create an entire professional scientific subculture of child development, including a half dozen research centers, several score teaching and demonstration programs in child study and parent education, a scientific society, several technical journals, a popular magazine, *Parents*, and a national post-doctoral fellowship program."

Frank also promoted child development research results through parent study groups, university extension courses, and radio programs. Frank was the first expert to advocate that parents control their own emotional reactions when disciplining children. And secondary education, Frank's investigations suggested, should focus more on "human relations" as a means of enhancing society. A more recent interpretation of Frank's approach can be seen in Daniel Goleman's *Emotional Intelligence* (1995).

With Rockefeller support, Frank also contributed to the Iowa Child Welfare Research Station, the first institute in North America established to study developmental norms. The station developed the nation's first preschool, where it found that early intervention could raise IQ scores. The findings led to the formation of Head Start and other national programs to support early child development.

In the early years of the Foundation, the trustees advocated for a distinct profession of public health, apart from medicine, which included mental hygiene in its course of study. As an organization, the Foundation rejected Cartesian dualism—the view that the mind is distinct from the body—and favored a holistic approach to treatment by a physician. It saw psychiatry as a bridge over the Cartesian gap.

Part of the problem of integrating mental hygiene and psychiatry into higher education was the "official agnosticism" of medical schools toward the science of the mind. As of 1919, the Johns Hopkins School of Hygiene and Public Health did not have a mental hygiene department because its leaders wanted to see more results from science before they would support further scientific research in the area of mental hygiene.

Efforts supported by the Foundation to disseminate and professionalize psychiatry started with Thomas Salmon, who provided the U.S. Army with a neuropsychiatric service in World War One. In 1917 the Foundation contributed to the Surgeon General's efforts to commission mental health specialists in the treatment of nervous and mental diseases of soldiers. But even with the success of these professionals in treating shell shock and aiding in personnel selection, psychiatry was not being taught in most medical schools.

In 1923, as part of an eight-lecture course on mental hygiene at Yale University, Salmon and Clifford Beers gave lectures on the mental hygiene movement as well as on mental hygiene and personal health. Also in 1923, a survey of 23 major schools of nursing revealed that none of them provided courses, training, or practical experience in treating mental diseases.

Beginning in 1933, thanks to the efforts of Foundation trustee and Dean of the Harvard Medical School David Edsall, psychiatry was increasingly integrated into medical education. Edsall was able to make his case by pointing out that more beds were taken up by the mentally ill than by other types of patients. Edsall's advocacy was supported by the Rockefeller Foundation as it invested in teaching, research, and the application of psychiatry. In 1934 the Foundation provided fellowships, along with the Commonwealth Fund, that "organized postgraduate instruction in psychiatry." The Commonwealth Fund was an independent philanthropic organization endowed by Stephen Harkness, one of John D. Rockefeller Sr.'s partners at Standard Oil.

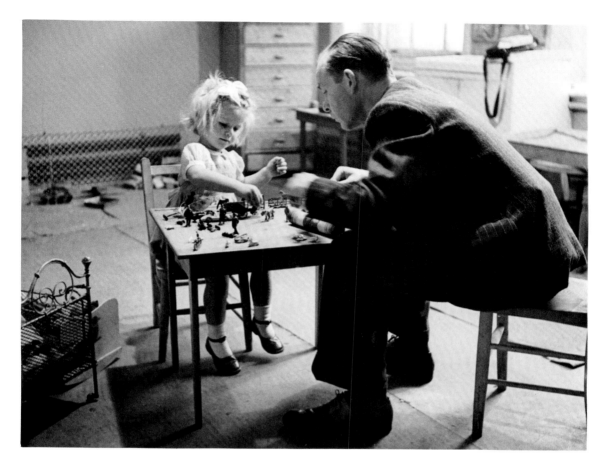

In the area of mental hygiene it followed the Foundation's lead. Together they provided grants to several universities and institutions to either teach psychiatry or foster psychiatric training programs at Colorado, Leiden, Johns Hopkins, McGill, Michigan, Pennsylvania Hospital, and Rochester.

Raymond Fosdick estimated that between the 1913 inception of the Foundation and 1933, the Foundation contributed at least four million dollars ($54 million in 2013 dollars) to psychiatry. It was responsible for starting departments of psychiatry at McGill, Tulane, Duke, and Washington (St. Louis), and broadened them at Harvard, Johns Hopkins, Yale, Colorado, Michigan, and Tennessee. Indeed, by 1943 three out of four dollars granted by the division of Medical Sciences went for psychiatry or related neurologic research or education.

Researchers at the Tavistock Clinic in London, England, studied child development and psychology. In 1946, with support from the Rockefeller Foundation, a group of these researchers formed the Tavistock Institute of Human Relations, which became a leading center for work in psychology and psychoanalysis in the United Kingdom. (Rockefeller Archive Center.)

Before 1920 the Rockefeller Foundation was one of only three philanthropic organizations that financially supported basic scientific research. In the United States, social support and reform agencies such as the National Committee for Mental Hygiene were largely dependent on the Foundation, since no support could be procured from the National Research Council, the Social Science Research Council, or the American Council of Learned Societies. Rockefeller-funded research contributed to a better understanding of social problems such as prostitution and crime, linking them to the context of the times as well as underlying medical issues like mental illness, and liberating the afflicted from the burden of moral condemnation or racial stereotyping.

Psychiatrist Esther Richards taught classes for would-be doctors and nurses at Johns Hopkins Medical School in 1939. Rockefeller Foundation support, in collaboration with the Commonwealth Fund, helped finance the adoption of psychiatry into the curricula of a number of medical schools, including Johns Hopkins. (The Alan Mason Chesney Medical Archives, Johns Hopkins University.)

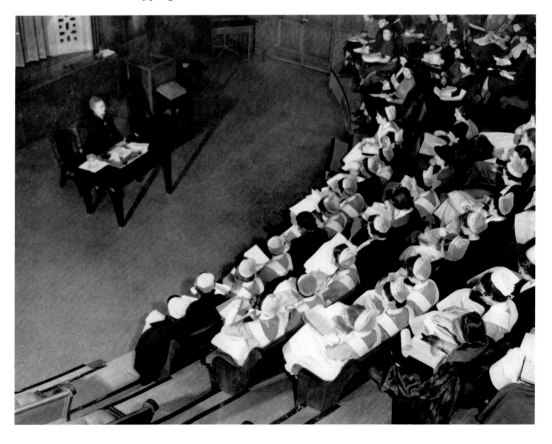

Chapter Five: The Life of the Mind

As with other Rockefeller endeavors, the Foundation's initial investments in certain areas, such as prison reform, led local, state, or federal agencies to invest as well. Thus the lesson the Foundation learned from the hookworm campaign about the power of leveraging its assets held true in the realm of mental hygiene.

Without the Foundation, the study of behavioral genetics would not be as robust as it is today. Over the years, the Foundation funded global research programs in psychobiology, mental hygiene, and psychiatry that all had as their aim the investigation of behavior from a biological standpoint.

The full effect of the Foundation's contributions would not become apparent until the unexpected importance of psychiatry was truly solidified during World War Two. During the war, one in three men was excluded from military service due to neuropsychiatric difficulties, more than one million soldiers were admitted to the hospital for similar reasons (roughly 6 percent of all admissions),

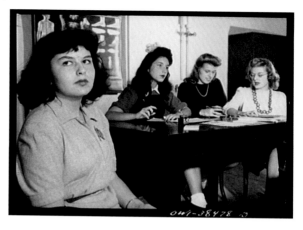

Students in a 1943 health class at Woodrow Wilson High School in Washington, D.C., participate in an assignment in which the student in the foreground has submitted her personality problems to a panel of fellow students for evaluation. Exercises like this demonstrated the increasing popularity and acceptance of psychiatry into mainstream science and culture. (Library of Congress.)

and competent mental health providers were urgently needed. On a more general level, the Foundation's investment in psychiatry played a key role in developing the field and in giving it a solid basis in science.

Thirty years after the deaths of his first wife Win and his children, Raymond Fosdick wrote: "The mentally ill merely present in exaggerated and dramatic form aspects or properties of human nature which must be taken into account by all who are responsible for the functioning of the

> "The mentally ill merely present in exaggerated and dramatic form aspects or properties of human nature."
> *Raymond Fosdick*

modern world and the design of its institutions." As the Rockefeller Foundation endeavored to adjust to the dramatic changes brought on by World War Two, these complicated and troublesome aspects of human nature would continue to shape the pattern of the Foundation's investments.

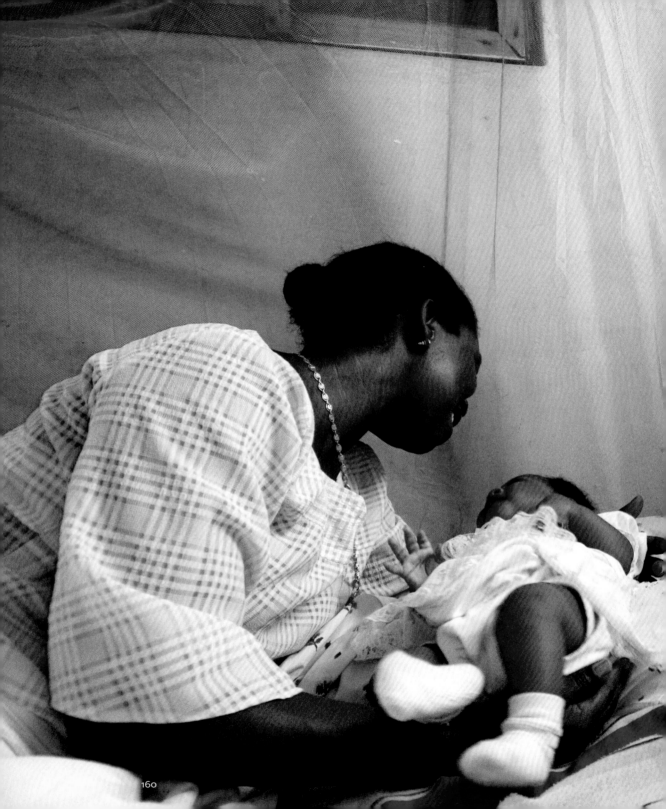

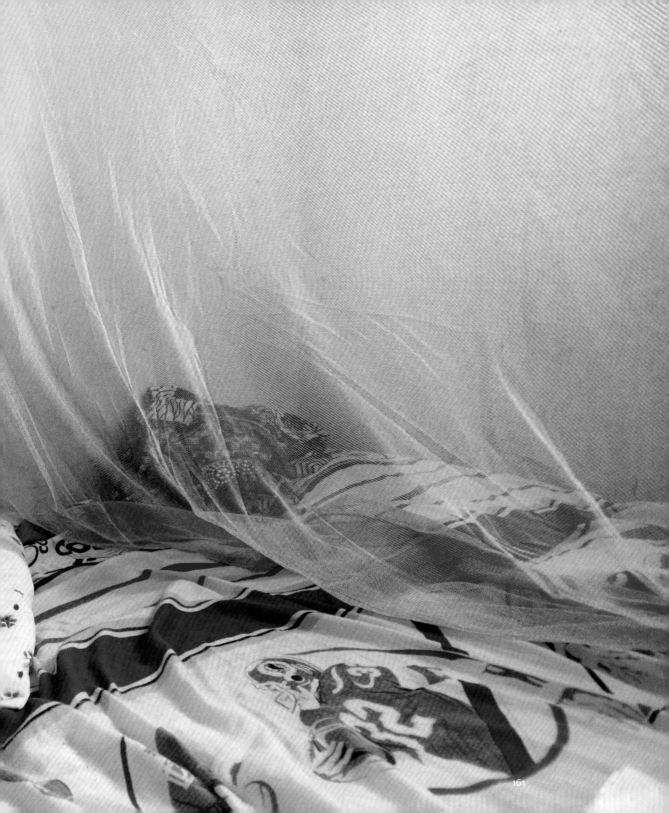

A NEW ROLE IN
THE POSTWAR WORLD

World War Two caused enormous devastation and social dislocation around the world. In Europe alone, 60 million people were displaced due to border changes, evacuation, deportation, expulsion, or forced resettlement. In many countries food shortages, inadequate shelter, and poor sanitation fueled disease outbreaks. Countries devastated by the war urgently needed to restore their health services to combat or forestall epidemics. Malnutrition, tuberculosis, and venereal disease were among the biggest threats, while typhus, malaria, and hepatitis lurked close behind. Nations had few resources with which to defend themselves. Medical professionals were exhausted, scientific and medical contacts had been broken, and the reconstruction and repair of hospitals and other public health infrastructure presented an enormous challenge.

To those involved with reconstruction, the effort to rebuild included a mandate to create a new world order that would prevent another global conflagration. "The challenge of the future," Rockefeller Foundation President Raymond Fosdick wrote in 1946, "is to make the world *one* world—a world truly free to engage in common and constructive intellectual efforts that will serve the welfare of mankind everywhere."

To support this effort, the Foundation appropriated $6 million ($77.9 million in 2013 dollars) for emergency work in Europe. "The sum was pathetically inadequate," Fosdick later wrote. "The situation was far beyond the capacity of private funds. Such funds could ameliorate some of the difficulties, but the

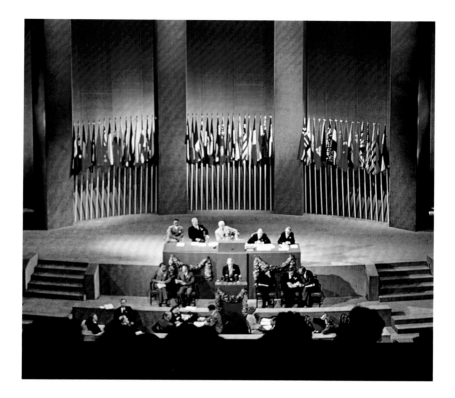

need was so universal and overwhelming that it could be met, if at all, only by governments."

The Foundation did play a part in working with governments, however, to shape a host of new international agencies that emerged to promote global cooperation and world peace. The pattern for these new organizations was established with the creation of the United Nations. When representatives from 50 nations gathered in San Francisco to draft the U.N. charter in April 1945, they also discussed the need for a global health organization. The following year, at an International Health Conference sponsored by the U.N., members approved the Constitution of the World Health Organization (WHO). It took two more years, however, for nations to ratify this constitution, which was finally adopted in 1948 in Geneva by the first World Health Assembly, the WHO's decision-making forum of representatives from its member states.

The emergence and growth of new international agencies would transform the Foundation's international role. The International Health Division (IHD) would continue to pursue its prewar objectives—research and control

In April 1945 representatives from 50 nations gathered in San Francisco to draft the United Nations Charter. Following a series of debates and meetings that took place over the next two months, the charter was unanimously passed on June 25, 1945. The next day, international delegates affixed their signature to the U.N. Charter. (McCreary. United Nations.)

of specific diseases, building efficient health services, and supporting public health education—but it would now pursue these goals in cooperation with other agencies, both private and public. And it would play a significant role in the early history of the WHO, supplying several of the WHO's early leaders.

PUBLIC HEALTH AND RECONSTRUCTION

Given the devastation wrought by World War Two, experts and specialists in medicine and science were needed as advisors. The Foundation therefore applied a portion of its resources to aid public health schools in training medical administrators, sanitary engineers, and nurses. These training programs were broadened in 1947 and 1948 to include socioeconomics and "observations on population, health, agriculture, nutrition, natural resources, and water supplies."

Reopening universities and training programs was one crucial part of early relief measures. The Foundation equipped and funded universities, libraries, and research centers, and provided support

Nursing students from Brazil, China, the Philippines, and the United States pose together at the University of Toronto, which hosted 39 percent of all Rockefeller Foundation-funded nursing fellows—more than any other institution. Fellows formed important professional networks during their international experience and returned home with the skills to help rebuild public health and nursing programs in countries that were often poor or devastated by war. (Rockefeller Archive Center.)

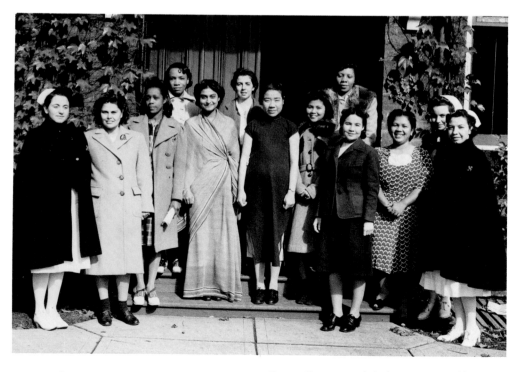

for international conferences and the purchase of scholarly journals. One grant to the Royal Society of Medicine's Central Medical Library Bureau, for example, was for $250,000 ($2.6 million in 2013 dollars). The largest fellowships and grants went to institutions and individuals in public health and in the natural, medical, and social sciences in Denmark, France, Great Britain, Holland, Norway, Poland, Sweden, Switzerland, and Yugoslavia.

The Foundation also provided funding to the National School of Nursing in Ceylon, the National School of Hygiene in Colombia, the University of Rome Engineering School, the National Institute of Health in China, and the Tacuba Training Center and Demonstration Health Unit in Mexico. The IHD continued to support schools of hygiene and nursing in London as well as the Toronto School of Nursing. In addition in 1951 it maintained one or more staff members in England, France, Italy, Egypt, India, Iran, Japan, Canada, Bolivia, Brazil, Chile, Colombia, the Dominican Republic, Mexico, and Peru. Public health projects garnered a substantial amount of Foundation funds in the postwar years, as much as 20 percent of annual appropriations. In 1946 and 1947, public health as a field received $2.45 million and $2.25 million respectively ($29.3 million and $23.5 million in 2013 dollars). Appropriations for medical programs, meanwhile, totaled nearly 10 percent of all the Foundation's grants in the postwar years.

The Foundation's efforts to meet the need for trained public health workers in China and other war-torn regions of the world went hand-in-hand with new public health campaigns to eradicate the most virulent diseases—especially malaria. And it was in the context of these campaigns that the role played by IHD staff in global health began to evolve.

Malaria Campaigns

After the Second World War, the incidence of malaria and associated mortality increased dramatically throughout the world. At one point, international health experts considered malaria the biggest threat to public health, with an estimated 300 million people infected and 3 million related deaths every year.

In the Mediterranean region, the fight against malaria had been hindered by war. A famine in Greece had contributed to the outbreak of a severe epidemic in the winter of 1941. By 1944 the Red Cross estimated that there were at least 2.4 million cases of malaria in a population of seven million people. With malaria control programs paralyzed because of the war, infection rates returned to pre-twentieth-century levels, and the crisis continued even after the war ended. Meanwhile an epidemic that broke out on Sardinia in 1944

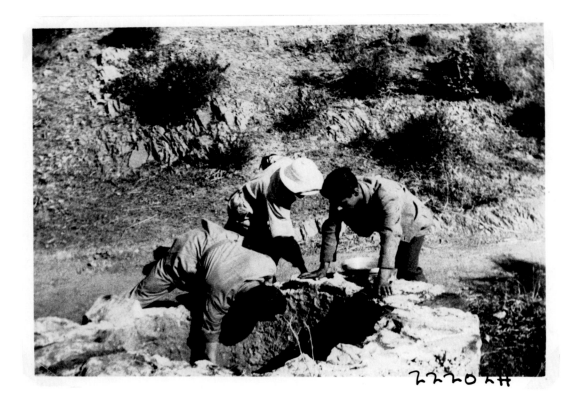

Between 1946 and 1951, an effort supported by the Rockefeller Foundation engaged more than 30,000 people and deployed 10,000 tons of DDT to rid Sardinia of malaria-carrying mosquitoes. Local men called *segnalatori* were employed to spray DDT and to search for larvae in breeding areas such as shallow wells. (Rockefeller Archive Center.)

continued over the next several years. In 1946, 74,600 cases of malaria and 169 deaths were reported, double the figures reported in 1940. Public health officials in both Italy and Greece were eager to adopt the strategies using DDT that the IHD had used with great success in Naples at the end of the war.

By that time, IHD epidemiologist Fred Soper (see Chapter IV) was widely acknowledged as the expert in malaria control. In addition to his work in Brazil, he had more than a year's experience using DDT. His techniques included detailed record keeping, efficient use of manpower, and chemical controls. Dwellings were rigorously inspected for mosquito infestation and pesticides were sprayed to leave an effective and abiding residue. At the invitation of the governments of Greece and Sardinia, Soper and the IHD began working in early 1945 on large-scale public health and sanitation measures using DDT.

To eradicate malaria in Greece, the IHD collaborated with the newly established United Nations Relief and Rehabilitation Administration (UNRRA). UNRRA had been created in 1943, before the United Nations

Chapter Six: A New Role in the Postwar World

On the Italian island of Sardinia, Rockefeller Foundation officers fiercely debated the merits of concentrating on efforts to control the spread of malaria versus attempting to eradicate *Anopheles* mosquitoes. John Austin Kerr, superintendent of the Sardinia campaign, favored a focus on controlling the disease, as he expressed in a 1946 letter to Fred Soper, director of the International Health Division. (Rockefeller Archive Center.)

THE ROCKEFELLER FOUNDATION
49 WEST 49th STREET, NEW YORK

APO 794

700
RFHC
Typhus-Malaria

Enc FLS-GKS
6/22/46

Through Dr. Strode

Rome, June 6, 1946.

AUG

GKS

Dr. Soper

Copy initialed by HHS
AJW

Letter Nº 286.

Dear Fred:

   After spending a week in Sardinia I am of the opinion that the aim of the project there should be changed from the eradication of anopheles to the __eradication__ of malaria.

   More specifically, I think the goal should be to ascertain what is the cheapest way to secure the complete control of malaria on Sardinia which can then be continued within the administrative capacities of the Italian Government in Sardinia.

   I believe that the soundest way to start is to control labranchiae by means of DDT spray-painting of all buildings on the island. Once this is done and the costs worked out, and the distribution of labranchiae and other possible vectors ascertained, then will be the time to think about spending the very large sum of money which would be involved in an attempt to eradicate anopheles in Sardinia. The very important question of reinfestation would have to be considered when assessing the advisability of attempting anopheles eradication.

   When he works with an indigenous species of anopheles an eradicationist simply must become ecologically minded. The fact that gambiae was eradicated in Brazil and in Egypt without much thought having been given to ecology does not obviate the need for very careful ecological studies regarding indigenous species of anopheles in other areas.

itself was formally established, to coordinate relief and assistance for the victims of war from its headquarters in New York. IHD Director Wilbur Sawyer left in 1944 to take charge of the new organization, which worked closely with philanthropic and charitable organizations, including the Rockefeller Foundation.

Another IHD alumnus was Daniel Wright, the head of the Sanitation Section of UNRRA's Health Division in Greece. As an IHD sanitary engineer he had worked for the Foundation in Greece throughout the 1930s. His familiarity with the IHD's methods and personnel helped ensure close coordination between the Foundation and UNRRA as the antimalarial campaign deployed nearly 300 tons of pure DDT to control the mosquito population. UNRRA provided the organizational and logistical framework, while the IHD provided technical expertise. The program led to a substantial reduction in the incidence of malaria in Greece. As Wright noted in a September 1947 letter to George Strode, who had succeeded Wilbur Sawyer as director of the IHD, "The results of 1945 and 1946 showed conclusively that even in a country like Greece which is close if not 100% malarious the disease can be brought under complete control, if not wiped out."

To eradicate malaria in Sardinia, the IHD collaborated with UNRRA, the Italian government, the local government of Sardinia, and the U.S. Economic Cooperation Administration as well as private agencies such as the Regional Organization for the Struggle against the *Anopheles* in Sardinia (Ente Regionale per la Lotta Anti-Anofelica in Sardegna, or ERLAAS). According to historian John Farley, the plan represented "the largest-scale attempt ever made to eradicate an indigenous *Anopheles* vector." At the height of the project in 1949, ERLAAS employed 33,000 people.

In Brazil, before the war, Soper had intended to kill every *Anopheles* mosquito. He changed his strategy in Sardinia, reasoning that the IHD needed to spray only 80 percent of homes in infected areas to break the cycle of malaria transmission. But some members of the team resisted this strategy. Malariologist Paul Russell, who in 1947 had returned to the IHD to oversee malaria efforts in Italy, wondered "if it is safe to leave loopholes in an eradication program where there is a much smaller margin of safety than one has in a simple malaria control project." As he wrote in August 1947, "It has always seemed to me that the success of the anti-*gambiae* project in Brazil was in large measure due to the fact that no possible loopholes were left and every feasible method of attack was pushed to the limit." What Soper and Russell shared, however, was the hope that data collected in Sardinia would lead to the development of effective anti-malaria campaigns around the world, including China, where malaria was epidemic.

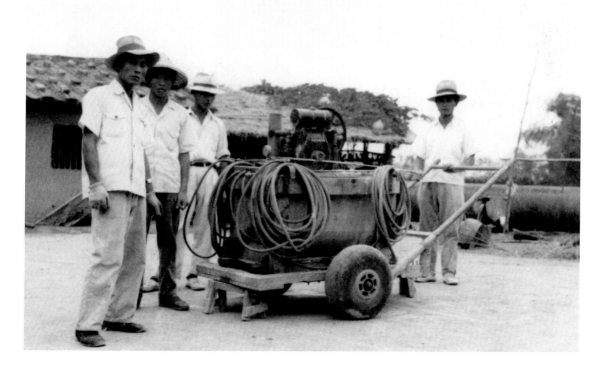

To lead the campaign in Sardinia, the IHD chose J. Austin Kerr, an IHD veteran who had started his career fighting hookworm in Tennessee, had battled yellow fever in Brazil, and fought malaria in Egypt. But the campaign was problem-ridden from the start. The extermination of *Anopheles* proved difficult, in part because each of the seven species had a different habitat. Residual spraying, which seeks to leave a residue of insecticide on surfaces like eaves and walls, also proved logistically difficult, and there was disagreement over the goal of the campaign with Strode pushing for eradication and Kerr insisting that it was only possible to control the spread of the disease. This disagreement became so profound that Kerr resigned, and William Logan succeeded him as director in September 1947.

Based on the success of the Sardinian campaign, DDT was adopted as a primary tool in eradicating malaria-carrying mosquitoes worldwide. In 1949 workers at the Taiwan Malaria Research Institute used leftover military machinery, including a U.S. Army decontamination sprayer and wheels from a Japanese bomber, to create a mobile DDT sprayer. (Rockefeller Archive Center.)

Logan understood that the IHD's reputation was at stake in Sardinia, along with the future of the IHD's strategy for fighting malaria. He increased DDT spraying dramatically in an effort to kill 95 to 99 percent of the malaria-carrying mosquito larvae. Logan was not able to achieve this goal, but the massive effort led to a virtual halt in malaria transmission in 1949. New malaria cases fell from more than 75,000 in 1946 to fewer than 10 in 1951.

These campaigns contributed important lessons for solving the problem of malaria and overcoming the challenges to eliminating the disease. They showed that substantial reductions in infection rates could be achieved. And although the IHD had not been able to completely eliminate the indigenous *labranchiae* mosquito, eradication seemed possible. Indeed, based on the overall positive results recorded in Sardinia, the Eighth World Health Assembly adopted the goal of eradication in 1955. The assembly also voted to adopt DDT as the primary tool in the fight against malaria.

Amid the celebration of DDT's success, however, there were signals that raised concern. One involved acquired resistance to insecticides, which emerged during early malaria control programs. The first documented resistance to DDT occurred in 1945. By mid-1955, resistance to DDT among malaria-carrying *Anopheles* was reported in Greece, Indonesia, and parts of Africa and South America. It was believed that the mosquito population needed about six years, on average, to become resistant to DDT.

Another area of concern was the dangers of DDT and its long-term environmental effects, which were brought to light in subsequent investigations of the Rockefeller malaria control strategy. Sardinia, where 10,000 tons of DDT had been used during the five-year campaign, became a favorite site for studying DDT's toxicity. Researchers discovered that the spraying program affected the island's ecosystem. Bee colonies and fish populations had been destroyed, and farmers complained that their sheep had been poisoned. These concerns would become increasingly important in later years, but DDT's ability to prevent millions of malaria-related deaths seemed nothing short of miraculous in the mid-1950s.

Leadership Transitions

With the creation of UNRRA and the development of multi-agency anti-malaria campaigns in the Mediterranean during and immediately after the end of World War Two, the Rockefeller Foundation's historic place in global health began to give way to a more collaborative model, and many of the IHD's leaders played an important role in the new multilateral agencies that took center stage.

The IHD's Paul Russell, for example, would make invaluable contributions to shaping the WHO's malaria program. While overseeing control efforts in Italy, he had been a member of the Expert Committee on Malaria created by the WHO's Interim Commission in 1947, attending its first session in Geneva in April of that year. The committee's aim was to assist the WHO and the United Nations in carrying out international public health functions related to researching and eradicating malaria, viewed as the most preventable disease of the tropics and subtropics at the time. The committee endorsed DDT as an effective, economically viable tool to control malaria, placing its hopes in the technique of residual spraying.

In 1948 Russell was also the U.S. delegate to the first World Health Assembly, mentioned earlier, which placed the highest priorities on programs for malaria, tuberculosis, maternal and child health, venereal diseases, nutrition, and environmental sanitation. In its first two decades, the WHO would also initiate mass campaigns against single diseases—not only malaria and tuberculosis, but also yaws, syphilis, smallpox, leprosy, typhoid, schistosomiasis, onchocerciasis, and trachoma.

Fred Soper left the IHD in 1947 to become the director of the Pan American Health Sanitary Bureau, which became the executive agency of the WHO's Regional Office for the Americas after 1949 and was renamed the Pan American Health Organization ten years later. During his 12-year tenure he was the main proponent of the WHO's Global Malaria Eradication Program, and it was under his leadership that malaria control evolved to incorporate a global eradication plan.

The loss of Wilbur Sawyer, Paul Russell, and Fred Soper to the emerging international agencies was part of a major transition taking place in the field of global health. The loss of other IHD personnel—including in-country field scientists and engineers like Daniel Wright, for example—illustrated the extent of this transition. For the Rockefeller Foundation's leaders, these losses seemed to signal the end of an era.

The End of an Era

The heady days of the Foundation's search for a yellow fever vaccine in the laboratories of New York and the tropical forests of West Africa had given way to a wartime sense of urgent practicality during World War Two. Even while the Foundation faced those demands, however, President Raymond Fosdick hoped that the Foundation would return to its traditional ways after the war.

Fosdick believed that heavy investment in basic research could, if the commitment held long enough, result in practical applications for humanity. He wrote passionately about the Foundation's role in supporting the research that had taught scientists how to use penicillin to treat infection and had unlocked the secrets of blood plasma. The research had been "abstract and theoretical" for 15 years, he wrote, without any clear practical value. But eventually researchers had broken plasma into its component parts, including albumin

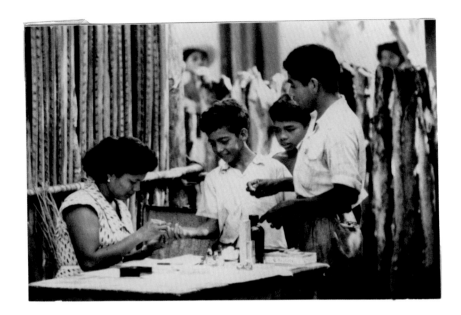

and clotting agents. The process had been "painstaking" and "abstruse," but the Foundation had persevered in its commitment and the practical results had revolutionized the way surgeons do their work.

Staff from the Foundation's International Health Division interviewed children in Mexico in 1950 as part of an effort to assess the prevalence of malaria. (Rockefeller Archive Center.)

In the immediate aftermath of the war, Fosdick and the trustees continued to support this basic research in medical science. Grants by the Medical Science and Public Health programs of the Rockefeller Foundation, which included the IHD, accounted for 58 percent of annual appropriations, including commitments in the fields of psychiatry and molecular biology, and Fosdick looked forward to a postwar golden age of medical research. "When the war is done," he had written earlier, "men will again have access to all knowledge, wherever it may be found, and armed guards will no longer protect the secrets of research that might bring health and a better life to the race. Laboratories surrounded by barbed wire are ugly monuments to the intellectual and moral distortion of our time."

For Fosdick and many members of the board and staff, the medical sciences and basic research were transcendent. They fit Fosdick's view of what the Foundation should be doing in the highly politicized world of the emerging Cold War. "Public health work carries no threat to anybody, anywhere," Fosdick wrote. "Cancer and scarlet fever have no political ideology. There is no Marxian method of eliminating *gambiae* mosquitoes as distinguished from a western democratic method."

In their last effort to return to the world they had known before the war, the trustees appropriated $10 million in 1947 to rebuild Peking Union Medical College into the most prestigious medical training facility in Asia. Fosdick described the commitment as a "leap of faith" that medicine can be one of the "bridges across the gulf that separates this frightened present from a saner and better balanced future." Two years later, revolution swept communists to power, and the Rockefeller Foundation retreated from China for almost a half-century.

After Fosdick retired in 1948, a new generation of Foundation leaders was increasingly recognizing just how deeply the world had changed. With the Cold War leading to open conflict in China, Korea, Indochina, and Europe, they moved quickly to restructure the Foundation's medical and health programs to respond to the emerging needs of developing nations.

The End of the International Health Division

As the new leaders of the Rockefeller Foundation struggled to redefine the Foundation's work and role in the postwar world, they undertook a major review of the International Health Division, which had represented the primary face of the Foundation in developing countries for decades. With the creation of the United Nations and new groups like the World Health Organization, the Rockefeller Foundation no longer played the only major role in international health. In fact, its resources for global disease eradication efforts paled in comparison to those of the new agencies. Moreover, new priorities in agriculture and the social sciences seemed to demand a reallocation of resources. Given all of these considerations, the board of trustees reached an historic decision to close the International Health Division in 1951 as an independent agency.

Some of the IHD's staff—like Paul Russell and Fred Soper—had already departed to lead the emerging organizations. Others were transferred to the newly reconfigured Division of Medicine and Public Health. The Foundation's new president, Chester Barnard, optimistically noted that "the new division is designed to meet today's larger concept of medicine, in which the formerly distinct boundaries between curative and preventive medicine are rapidly disappearing." In reality, this age-old tension between the priorities of William Welch and Wickliffe Rose continued to challenge the Foundation and the world, even as the Foundation continued to strengthen the field of public health.

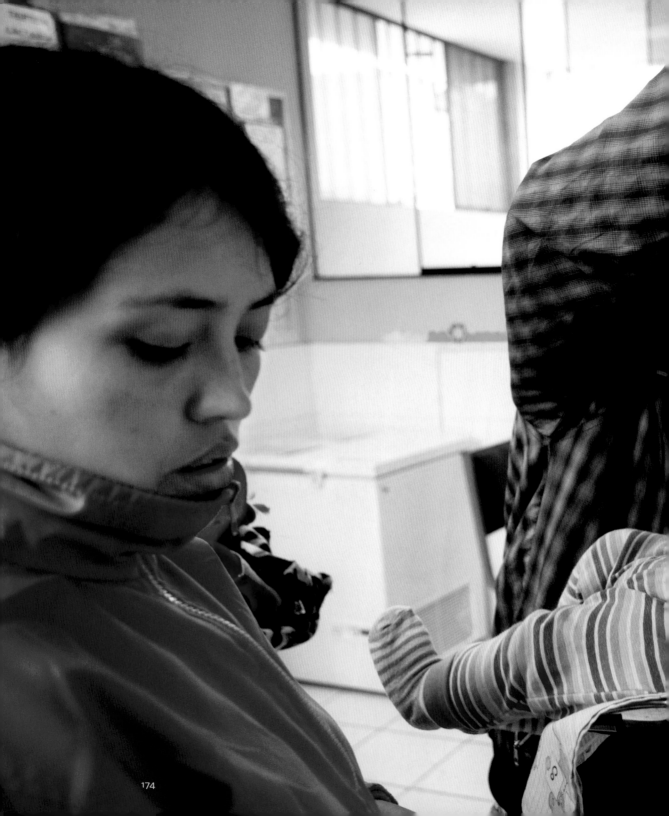

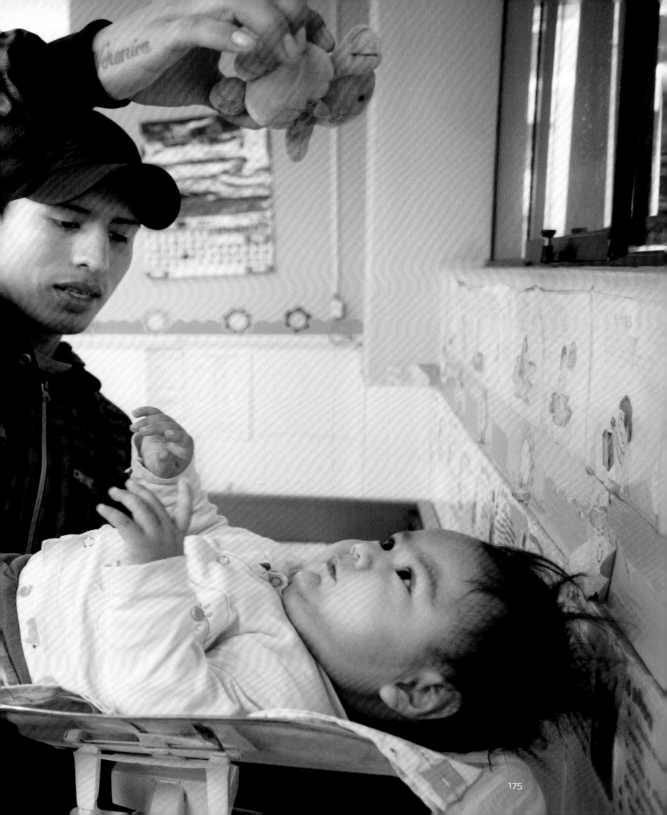

RETURNING TO HEALTH
IN COMMUNITY

The closing of the International Health Division (IHD) coincided with the rise of a major new initiative for the Rockefeller Foundation—the application of science to prevent widespread famine in the world's developing countries. This effort, which began in Mexico in 1943, became known by the Foundation as the Conquest of Hunger program and by the world as the "Green Revolution." Although the Foundation's grants and field staff focused primarily on increasing agricultural yields, the program also prompted new ways of thinking about health and population.

The growth of human populations had been an academic problem in the 1930s. By the 1950s the global population was exploding, and the highest rates of growth were in the postcolonial new countries of Asia and Africa. In the developed world, improvements in public health had resulted in dramatic declines in death and disability from infectious disease. But in these burgeoning countries in the developing world, food scarcity and the threat of famine lowered resistance and heightened the potential for epidemics. In these countries especially, health care issues were inextricably bound to poverty, a lack of educational opportunities, and unsanitary systems for water and sewage.

Among the new generation of leaders at the Rockefeller Foundation, a handful were keenly aware of these issues. John D. Rockefeller 3rd, the grandson of the founder and son of the Foundation's long-time chairman,

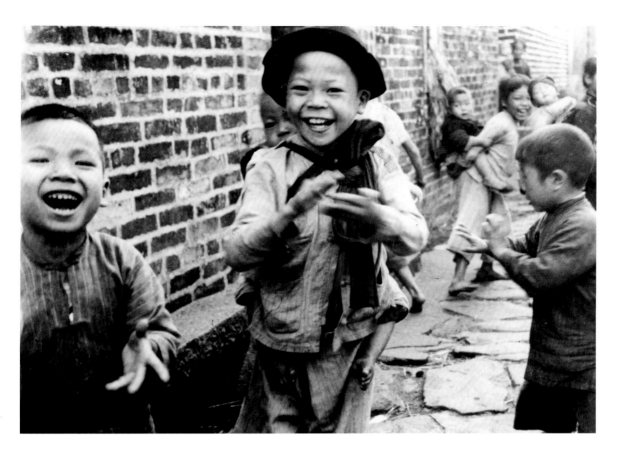

had served on the board of trustees since 1931. He had been deeply concerned about global health and population issues for nearly two decades. He became chairman of the board in 1952, the same year that the Foundation welcomed a new president—Dean Rusk. A Rhodes Scholar and former U.S. Assistant Secretary of State, Rusk believed that the emerging nations of the developing world posed critical challenges to the future of the world order. As he wrote in his first presidential review in 1952, "Both research *and statesmanship* are required if the great benefits of medical science are to be brought effectively to the service of the people."

In the 1950s a dramatic rise in population growth among postcolonial and often poverty-stricken countries of Africa and Asia compelled the Rockefeller Foundation to invest in programs designed to improve agricultural output in an effort to stave off potential famines. Agriculture and health were intrinsically linked, given that hunger and malnutrition increase one's susceptibility to disease. (Rockefeller Archive Center.)

To some it seemed that statesmanship superseded the emphasis on science and public health over the next two decades, as the Foundation spent a smaller share of its resources on medical education and medical science. To be sure, grants for biomedical research continued. The Foundation also invested heavily in university programs in the developing world to build capacity in agriculture, education, and health. These efforts complemented the investments the Foundation had made in medical education and public health training in the 1920s and 1930s. But for those who remembered heroic campaigns to eradicate hookworm, yellow fever, or malaria, or expected research in the Foundation's laboratories to produce Nobel Prize-winning breakthroughs in vaccine development, the turn away from the traditions of the past was disappointing. What they did not expect is that these two decades would lay the groundwork for a dramatically different approach to health in the last quarter of the twentieth century that would at last emphasize Wickliffe Rose's vision of a multifaceted, integrated public health system over the biomedical approach of William Welch and others at the beginning of the century.

Confronting a Growing Population Crisis

As Dean Rusk pushed for a focus on emerging nations, the problem of expanding human population came to the Foundation's attention. In the villages of Asia and Africa, populations were doubling every 30 to 40 years. The explosion was a function of improved standards of living, stable supplies of food, and improvements in basic hygiene. But the consequences threatened to undo a half century of medical and public health work. Infant and maternal mortality rates were high, and a specter of famine appeared. There seemed no way for emerging nations to climb out of poverty unless they managed population growth.

Population had long been a concern for John D. Rockefeller 3rd. In the years immediately following World War Two and before he became chairman, he had tried to interest the Foundation's trustees in the issue. Ironically, the Foundation had been accused of helping to promote this population boom by fighting yellow fever and malaria. While he was still president, Raymond Fosdick showed some interest in the problem. "Population problems are worldwide, ever present, and of first importance," he wrote in 1948. "They underlie many critical national, class, and racial conflicts."

It was a paradigm straight out of the emerging science of human ecology and population biology. Populations of all species grow when they have plentiful food and are able to avoid disease. But when a population outgrows the carrying capacity of its environment, famine and disease threaten collapse. Leaders of the Foundation believed that civilization had a moral obligation to break the inevitable cycle that would lead to famine and epidemic, but no one had a clear idea of how to proceed.

The trustees authorized some exploratory grants. In 1948, in addition to funding for the Office of Population Research at Princeton University and the International Union for the Scientific Study of Population, the Foundation commissioned a study of population issues in the Far East. This research laid the groundwork for population control efforts in the 1970s. The staff also began to explore the idea of creating a program in "Human Ecology" that would fuse the traditional work of the IHD and the Medical Education Division. At that time, however, these explorations failed to spur the trustees to embrace what seemed to be an intractable and politically explosive problem.

Frustrated by his inability to enlist his fellow trustees or win support from key members of the Foundation's staff, Rockefeller used his own money to establish the Population Council in November 1952 as an international organization to stimulate interest and research in human fertility and population questions. The council quickly

In 1952 John D. Rockefeller 3rd created the Population Council in an effort to confront issues of fertility and population growth that he believed were directly linked to achieving global health and security. Since its inception the council has sponsored successful family planning and health programs in numerous countries. (Rockefeller Archive Center.)

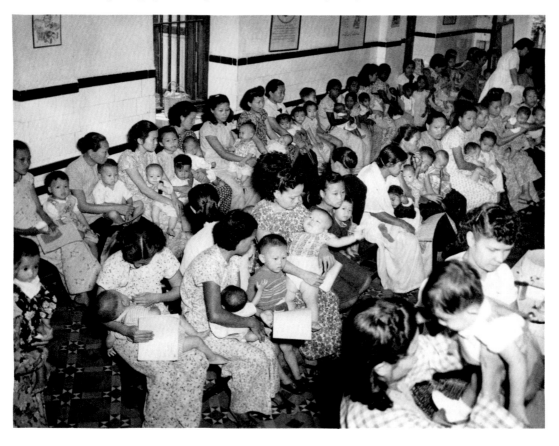

garnered additional financial support from the Ford Foundation to help fund research fellowships. The Rockefeller Brothers Fund provided $540,000 to help the Population Council create a biomedical research laboratory at Rockefeller University. With these resources, over the next eight years, the council funded work in the lab and in the field to understand the biological and sociological dimensions of population growth.

While the Rockefeller Foundation did not participate in most of this work in the 1950s, it did make limited grants to fund other population-related studies. In 1953, for example, the Foundation gave a grant to the Harvard School of Public Health for a population study in India. And by the early 1960s, with the demonstrated success of the Population Council and a growing interest in tackling the problem head on, the Foundation began to play an active role in encouraging the U.S. government to support family planning programs in the developing world. John D. Rockefeller 3rd, as chairman of both the Population Council and the Rockefeller Foundation, even met with President Lyndon B. Johnson in 1968 to appeal for support.

As this interest grew, the Foundation appropriated and disbursed $333 million between 1963 and 1972 (more than $1.86 billion in 2013 dollars) for population research, policy initiatives, and stabilization measures. With these funds, the Foundation supported basic research into the physiology of reproduction and the development of birth control technology as well as demographic studies and fellowships.

Foundation leaders recognized that the complex problem of population was not, strictly speaking, a problem of science. It was a social and economic problem, a problem of culture and even religion. According to the Foundation's annual report in 1963, "In the last analysis the decision on population stabilization must be made by society. It cannot be imposed by force of law but must come from understanding, individual conviction, and public action. Action must involve educational and research institutions, religious organizations, and governmental and civic groups—in short, all levels of social endeavor. Only then will the problem be capable of solution; only then will it be possible to make available to each individual the information and materials necessary to permit rational family planning within his own cultural and social environment."

The problem with a social perspective was that most developing countries did not have time for the slow transitions of society and culture to take place. Famine threatened, and malnutrition was at the heart of disease and poor health. "Many conditions that emerge in the clinic as specific diseases are, in fact, merely symptoms of a single underlying condition—a disordered food supply," the Foundation reported. Health was inextricably tied to food. Tens of millions of humans in the world's poorest communities were starving, and half the human population was malnourished or chronically hungry. By the mid-1960s, the problem looked as if it could only get worse. For the leaders of the Rockefeller Foundation, a rapid expansion of the production of nutritious food was the key to health, and that is where the Foundation was increasingly investing its resources.

THE GREEN REVOLUTION

The initiative that came to be known as the Green Revolution started in Mexico in 1943 with a simple focus: to dramatically increase agricultural production by developing higher-yielding varieties of basic food grains like wheat and corn, by improving irrigation, and by enhancing fertilizing techniques. Working closely with the national government, the Foundation supported the training of a generation of Mexican agronomists and scientists to lead and sustain a permanent increase in food production.

The basic elements of the program were rooted in years of practice that were closely allied with the Foundation's work in health. Even before the Foundation was created in 1913, the Rockefeller-funded General Education Board had combined support for agricultural research with community education programs to teach farmers in the United States ways to increase their yields. In China in the 1930s, the Foundation funded a rural reconstruction program that also included education and research programs to improve rural health and increase agricultural productivity.

During the 1930s, the Foundation's leaders were increasingly interested in the close relationship between malnutrition and disease. The Foundation had begun making grants in 1935 to study this relationship, as well as nutrition's influence on human behavior and well-being. Laboratory projects focusing on Atabrine, protein, calcium, and riboflavin led to the first nutrition-related public health grant, to the Provincial Bureau of Health in Quebec, Canada. This work sparked a growing interest in the systemic effects of nutrition on poverty, education, and health, and set the stage for an innovative approach to development.

The Foundation's trustees saw the agriculture project in Mexico "as a natural outgrowth of the [Foundation's] interest in public health and the biological sciences." Although it was operated in conjunction with the Mexican Ministry of Agriculture, Foundation staff were deeply involved with research and the transfer of new knowledge to farmers in the field. J. George Harrar, an agricultural scientist hired to run the Mexican Agricultural Program, assembled a talented team of scientists, technicians, and geneticists who developed

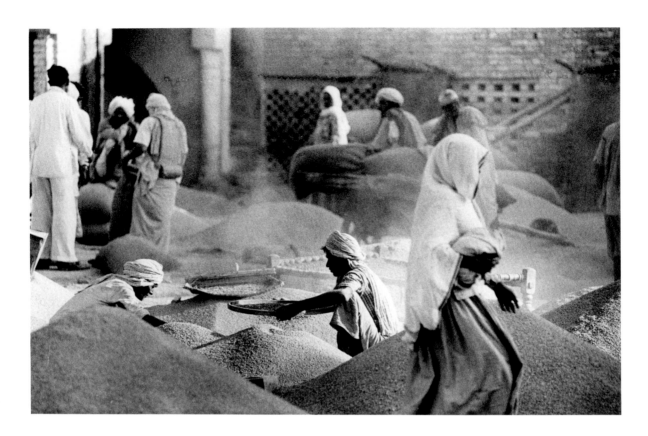

distinctive, high-yielding wheat and corn crops that grew well in differing climates. The team included Norman Borlaug, who would win a Nobel Peace Prize in 1970 for his research on behalf of the Rockefeller Foundation.

The Mexican Agricultural Program was enormously successful (see *Food & Prosperity* in the Rockefeller Foundation Centennial Series). In little over a decade, Mexico became self-sufficient in the production of wheat and maize. The model was soon exported to other countries in Latin America and Asia. Using hybrid seeds bred for high yield and high nutritional values—combined with irrigation, pesticides, and synthetic fertilizers—the program that became known as "Conquest of Hunger" played a key role in the Green Revolution. It helped transform modern agriculture and, at least in the short term, stabilize the global food supply. Indeed, by preventing widespread famine, the increase in food production alone is estimated to have saved over one billion lives.

One of the Rockefeller Foundation's primary goals in the 1960s was to alleviate hunger and malnutrition in an effort to improve global health. To this end, the Foundation supported a number of global studies and field projects to increase agricultural yields for wheat and other staple crops. The Foundation also provided grants to benefit vulnerable populations, like expectant mothers and children, who were given access to a balanced diet. (Raghubir Singh. Rockefeller Archive Center.)

J. George Harrar succeeded Dean Rusk as president of the Rockefeller Foundation in 1961, and oversaw a fundamental realignment of the Foundation's program two years later. This realignment recognized five major goals for the Foundation, including three that were focused on the developing world: overcome malnutrition, stimulate the development of strong universities, and stabilize the growth of populations. Significantly, for the first time, in the wake of this realignment the Foundation did not have a major program or goal aimed specifically at health. Instead, the Foundation's efforts to promote medical education and public health were subsumed by a major effort to develop human capital in a number of important fields in nations recently freed from the bonds of colonialism.

University Development

In 1963 the Rockefeller Foundation launched an ambitious program to advance higher education in a selected group of developing countries. As with other Foundation programs at the time, the University Development Program (UDP), later known as the Education for Development Program, was international in scope and well-funded. The 16-year, $125 million initiative sought to create higher-education institutions in the developing world that would provide expert local human capital to help tackle the numerous long-term problems plaguing countries trying to develop economically and socially. Many of the countries selected for the program lacked the homegrown engineering, agricultural, medical, economic, and management talent needed to solve development problems. Through the UDP, the Rockefeller Foundation sought to create self-sustaining institutions to train future generations of specialists and scholars who could engage over the long term in helping to address problems that faced the developing world.

In health, the UDP focused on two fronts: training health care professionals and developing clinics to provide hands-on training opportunities, develop new strategies for delivering health care, and meet the needs of poor, often rural, communities. In the early 1960s, the Foundation recognized that the critical problem in the developing world was one of providing access to vaccines, treatments, and basic health services to people who lived in poor communities that were either underserved by or without health care professionals. Drawing on the operational model developed in Mexico for agriculture, the UDP sent Rockefeller Foundation scientists to work as administrators and faculty in medical schools in developing countries. It also encouraged the creation of adjunct community health centers where young doctors could be exposed to the real-world

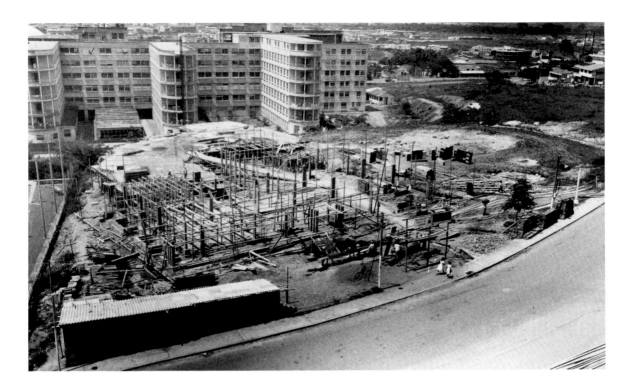

problems of their nations. In several universities—
including Mahidol University in Thailand, Makerere
University in Uganda, and Universidad del Valle in
Colombia—the Foundation's UDP initiatives built
upon previous efforts to promote an integrated,
interdisciplinary approach to community medicine.

At the Universidad del Valle, for example, the
Foundation had supported the medical faculty and its
innovative community medicine program since 1953.
When Universidad del Valle was chosen to become a
UDP site in 1961, the regional influence and strength
of its medical school weighed heavily in the university's favor, overcoming
the perceived weakness of its social science departments and lack of an
agricultural school. According to James Coleman, a key UDP strategist,
the Foundation appreciated the Universidad del Valle because the medical
school was led by Colombians; emphasized an "interdisciplinary orientation"
where students functioned "as members of a health team rather than as
isolated practitioners"; trained non-physician health care providers, such
as nurses and paramedics; and taught preventive medicine and community

The Rockefeller Foundation had
supported Colombia's Universidad del
Valle since 1953, and the university's
inclusion in the 1961 University
Development Program (UDP) helped to
make its medical school among the best
in Latin America. UDP funds supported
physician training and medical support
staff as well as the construction of new
facilities, including a nursing school in
1963. (Rockefeller Archive Center.)

Chapter Seven: Returning to Health in Community

development along with basic science and curative clinical medicine. The Foundation also valued the national government's strong support for the university and the medical school, and recognized the important presence of a "critical mass" of well-trained, experienced Colombian medical leaders—many of them trained in the United States—who believed in the principles of community medicine. These local commitments, in combination with Rockefeller Foundation support, helped make the medical school at the Universidad del Valle one of the best in Latin America by 1971, in part because of its required rotation at a rural health center to focus on family planning, well-baby care, nutrition, and hygiene.

While the Universidad del Valle was an obvious UDP choice for its health programs, the Foundation's commitment to Mahidol University was initially more problematic. The Foundation had deep roots in Thailand, a geopolitically important nation and close ally of the United States, but no single university fit the criteria for UDP support. Kasetsart University was the national center of agricultural education, Thammasat University in Bangkok was the national center for social science, and Mahidol was the national center for health sciences and medicine. The initial survey team

Nurses in Colombia used a chart devised by Rockefeller Foundation staff member and physician Joe D. Wray to diagnose malnutrition in children. The chart worked by plotting a child's weight against his or her age. In the 1960s, malnutrition among preschool-age children was identified as one of Colombia's most pressing problems. (Joe D. Wray. Rockefeller Archive Center.)

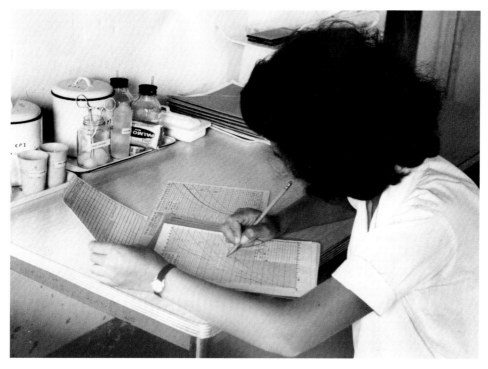

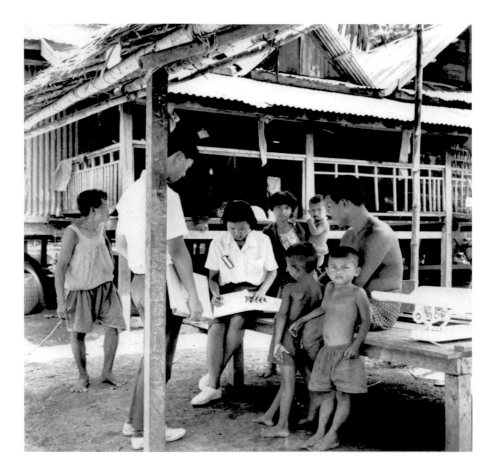

from the Foundation doubted that a UDP center could succeed, given the challenges involved in trying to foster interdisciplinary work. Even Thai officials were skeptical, and it took several years to come to an agreement on the idea that the three separate schools would attempt to coordinate their work.

In the end, however, Foundation officers liked Mahidol precisely because it did not have "ingrained traditions." As James Coleman wrote, "In the Thai situation, the greater plasticity [that] a *tabula rasa* promised was reinforced by the absence of any penetrative and weighty colonial hangover or imprint." Progress would be all the more measurable as a result.

The Foundation helped develop six life science departments in the Faculty of Science at Mahidol. It sponsored 30 fellowships for the most promising Thai medical students to study in the United States. Twenty-two Rockefeller

Thai medical students visit villagers to discuss health issues and to measure and weigh local children. In 1966 the Faculty of Medicine at Thailand's Ramathibodi Hospital became the leader in offering medical students a curriculum focused on a community-based approach to healthcare. (Joe D. Wray. Rockefeller Archive Center.)

Foundation field staff served as faculty. Altogether, the Foundation spent $11 million in Thailand, the largest UDP investment in any single country. The program was a striking success because it was able to build local capacity. By 1975 the academic staff at Mahidol was entirely Thai.

There were disappointments in Thailand as well. The medical program at Mahidol did not quickly develop as a regional center for medical education in Southeast Asia, something Foundation officials had hoped for. Between 1964 and 1974, 20 Ph.D. candidates enrolled at Mahidol came from other Southeast Asian countries. By 1974 the number had dropped to zero, reflecting less regional participation. A second disappointment, according to Coleman, was that the Mahidol experiment had focused heavily on scientific research at the expense of community health. For many years, he wrote, "the preclinical sciences being taught to future medical students were designed to serve a western system of medical education inappropriate for a developing country like Thailand." The problem was solved in 1966 when the Faculty of Medicine at Ramathibodi Hospital turned its attention to community-based clinical medicine. Mahidol focused on the training of scientists, while Ramathibodi prepared physicians, and the Rockefeller Foundation supported both. "Thus," Coleman concluded, "the Foundation became simultaneously involved in supporting both orientations—building the best science faculty in Southeast Asia in the Western tradition and seeking to introduce into the medical curriculum the concepts and practice of community medicine in rural areas."

The tension between curative medicine and community health, however, was not unique to Thailand. For the Foundation, of course, these issues stretched all the way back to Wickliffe Rose and William Welch. And the same issues surfaced at almost every institution that participated in the UDP's health initiatives.

At the University of East Africa, which was spread across three campuses in three different countries, UDP planners faced a different challenge. Unlike Colombia and Thailand, Kenya, Uganda, and Tanzania had recently been British colonies. Despite pressures to assert their sovereignty, none of the countries had the individual capacity to establish a medical school without expatriate faculty from Europe or the United States. With Rockefeller Foundation support, each school retained a core liberal arts and science faculty, but Royal College in Nairobi became the seat of veterinary medicine; Tanzania's University College, Dar es Salaam, became home to the law school; and Makerere College in Kampala, Uganda—the oldest university in British East Africa—became home to the medical and agricultural faculties. While the distances between the three countries were greater, and the schools more politically isolated from each other, the organizing principle was similar to that in Thailand. With UDP support, the University of East Africa worked to combine the scattered resources of several institutions into a coordinated, holistic, interdisciplinary strategy. The experiment in East Africa lasted only seven years before the stresses of patriotism compelled each nation to go its own way, but the investment in the medical school at Makerere would prove important over the long run.

Working with the Foundation, the medical faculty at Makerere established one of Africa's preeminent community health centers at Kasangati. Unfortunately, political instability in Uganda under- mined the program's success for a time. When many members of the expatriate and Ugandan faculty fled following the rise of Idi Amin, the medical school was starved for resources. In the 1990s, however, long after the Foundation had concluded the UDP and Amin had fallen from power, the Foundation was able to reinvest in Makerere's program and faculty, building on the legacies of the UDP era. Over time both the medical school and the Kasangati health center became living testament to the efforts of a small handful of dedicated physicians, nurses, and scientists to keep medical education alive in Uganda.

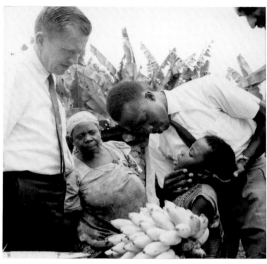

Dr. George Saxton and Mr. Letihaku, a health educator, examine a patient at the Kasangati rural health center in Uganda. With funds from the University Development Program, the medical faculty from Makerere University built Kasangati into one of Africa's best health centers. While the center suffered during Idi Amin's presidency, the Rockefeller Foundation reinvested in it during the 1990s. (Rockefeller Archive Center.)

Initially, Foundation professional staff in all UDP centers conceived of and directed or administered their programs, supplemented by non-Foundation "visiting professors." Many of the staff and non-staff were expatriates who could easily secure local input and, eventually, support. As the UDP training sites matured, they were expected to secure funding from sources other than the Foundation. As the former students became teachers and administrators, postgraduate teaching and research were stressed, along with multidisciplinary programs cooperating with non-academic agencies, all working on problems of population stabilization, public health, food production, diet, and finances.

The Foundation attempted to influence population issues through the UDP by "encouraging universities both in the United States and abroad to consolidate population studies into an independent academic discipline,

Chapter Seven: Returning to Health in Community

embracing demography and the social sciences as well as the basic natural sciences and medical disciplines relevant to human production." The hope was to "give work on population problems more scientific leverage and wider scope as well as more professional prestige."

By the late 1970s, under the aegis of the UDP and other initiatives, the Foundation was supporting research in reproductive biology, contraceptive technology, public policy, and population program evaluation in developing countries. This financial support continued through the 1980s, as the Foundation sought to "advance cooperation among developing countries in the population sciences and reproductive health." A major goal was to create an international consortium for this purpose, and the Foundation appropriated $1 million to "sustain collaborative research, training courses, workshops, publications, and other activities which encourage exchange and cooperation among Third-World scientists and family-planning experts."

In 1973 Mechai Viravaidya (center) founded the Population and Community Development Association (PDA) to promote family planning and condom use among Thailand's rural poor. His community-based approach has often included attention-grabbing tactics like condom-blowing contests. PDA has received the support of a number of philanthropic organizations, including the Rockefeller Foundation. (Rockefeller Archive Center.)

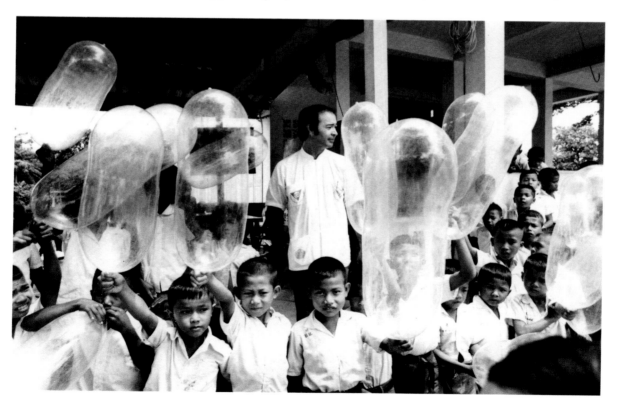

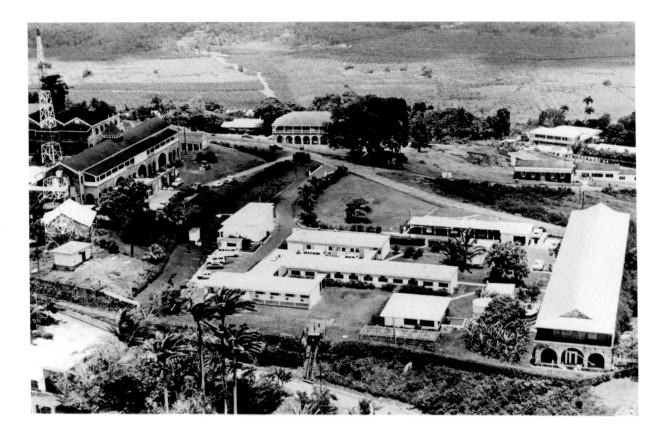

Nearly all UDP sites were encouraged to focus on population and demographic issues. At the Universidad del Valle, for example, medical students collaborated with instructors, OB/GYN department staff, and public health officials to advise families on birth decisions. At Mahidol University the Rockefeller Foundation supported the creation of the Center for Population and Social Research within the Faculty of Public Health.

In the 1970s a number of factors combined to bring an end to the program that had been known first as University Development and later as Education for Development. Many development specialists had grown disenchanted with the idea of investing in higher education as a way to meet the needs of the poor in the developing world. They increasingly turned their attention to primary and secondary schools instead, and searched for agricultural development and health strategies linked more directly to communities. At the same time, the Rockefeller Foundation came under financial pressure as a downturn in the equities markets coupled with

The Rockefeller Foundation initiated the schistosomiasis control project in St. Lucia in 1965. Through the cooperation of both foreign and local experts, and by combining programs in health, science, and agriculture, the project took an integrative approach to combating the parasitic disease. (Rockefeller Archive Center.)

rapid inflation diminished the Foundation's ability to finance expensive field operations. By 1975 most UDP site funding was curtailed or ended, and in 1977 the board voted to terminate all support by 1983.

Many years would pass before the real impact of the UDP could be seen in the growth and development of strong universities in emerging nations around the world. But within the Rockefeller Foundation itself, the program left a profound mark on the ways in which the organization approached problems related to community health. This new approach developed in particular as agricultural scientists and health care experts learned from one another.

COOPERATION BETWEEN HEALTH AND AGRICULTURAL PROGRAMS

Initially, in 1963, the Foundation's medical science program had focused on population stabilization through research on "physiology of reproduction, endocrinology, human genetics, the biochemical effects of diet, . . . demography and cultural attitudes" as well as "pilot operations and studies in areas where population density poses especially difficult problems and where there is a desire for help." By 1965 the Foundation had begun to integrate its efforts in development, combining medical science, medical education, public health, and agriculture programs. This new integrative approach was epitomized in the Foundation's efforts to fight schistosomiasis on the Caribbean island of St. Lucia.

On August 16, 1965, President J. George Harrar announced that the Foundation would "undertake field studies aimed at the control of schistosomiasis," a parasitic disease commonly known as snail fever that can result in liver fibrosis or kidney failure. The disease was and is prevalent in tropical and subtropical areas, especially in poor communities without access to safe drinking water and adequate sanitation. Indeed, Harrar characterized schistosomiasis as "one of the great unconquered parasitic diseases afflicting man and animals" and noted that it posed "a major obstacle to increased food production in many parts of the world," since the disease spread through snail larvae in waterways that were often developed for irrigation. Given research suggesting that the prevalence of schistosomiasis increased with the proliferation of large-scale irrigation projects throughout Africa and the Middle East as part of the Green Revolution, the Foundation had an especially strong interest in this problem.

As with hookworm in British Guiana in 1915, the Foundation envisioned an intensive program aimed at eradication. This time, according to the Foundation, the campaign would combine professionals working in public health,

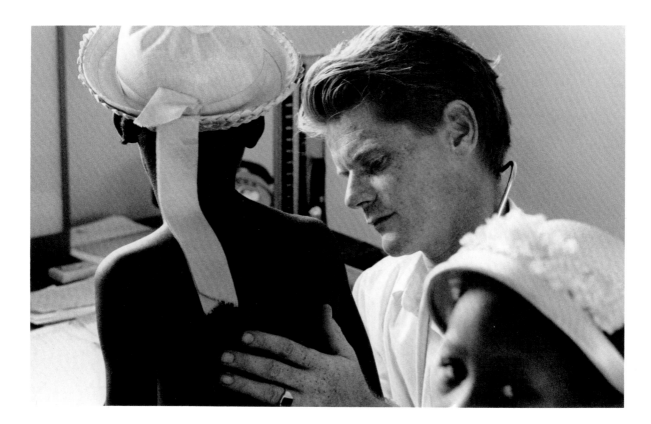

nutrition, and the environment to attack a "disease [that] has crippled the agricultural populations of large areas of Japan, the Philippines, Brazil, Venezuela, and some of the Caribbean islands for more than a century, and in Egypt for many hundreds of years." The program would be conducted in close cooperation with the government and local public health officials, with the Rockefeller Foundation providing funds for facilities and laboratories and the government supporting most of the project's staff.

The schistosomiasis control project in St. Lucia was one of the great medical success stories for the Rockefeller Foundation. The project dramatically reduced rates of infection and transmission on the island, and provided a model for future public health campaigns. (Rockefeller Archive Center.)

St. Lucia proved ideal for testing different methods of controlling the disease, in part because schistosomiasis was endemic. Snails were present in banana field drainage ditches, but isolated valleys allowed researchers to test and compare different control methods. Three principal methods were used: biological control of the snails (*Biomphalaria glabrata*), screening and chemotherapy for the infected, and reducing exposure by providing a domestic water supply separate from that for irrigation, sanitation facilities, and health education.

The project also compared the cost effectiveness of each strategy. Chemotherapy, at 88 cents per person per year, proved to be the most affordable, and effective intervention. Improving water supplies, on the other hand, was more expensive. While it did lead to a reduction in the transmission of schistosomiasis, the cost of providing household water as well as for laundry and shower facilities was $4.80 per person per year. This information helped public health officials in other parts of the world devise strategies for lowering schistosomiasis transmission rates.

In part, the project's success derived from the Foundation's ability to enlist other financial partners. In 1974, for example, the Edna McConnell Clark Foundation committed $32.4 million over 20 years to achieve effective control of schistosomiasis and reduce its importance as a major disease. Over the next several years, the two organizations collaborated to prioritize grants for "research, whether biological or sociological and cultural"; to create leaders; and to support "direct field operations" and individual fellowships.

The schistosomiasis program on St. Lucia provided a model for a more integrative approach to disease mitigation and public health that embraced the fields of medicine, community development, and agriculture.

Overall, the St. Lucia program was extremely successful, but it took many years. In 1962 an estimated 25,000 islanders were infected with the parasite, and the rate of schistosomiasis prevalence varied from 17.9 percent to 74.1 percent. At the end of the program in 1981, schistosomiasis prevalence varied between 4 and 14 percent. Foundation leaders deemed it "one of the largest and best controlled experiments involving human subjects," and today the rates of transmission are very low.

Of equal importance to the Foundation, the schistosomiasis program on St. Lucia provided a model for a more integrative approach to disease mitigation and public health that embraced the fields of medicine, community development, and agriculture. These insights provided support for a renewed commitment to strengthening the field of public health, which began with the arrival of a new president in the 1970s.

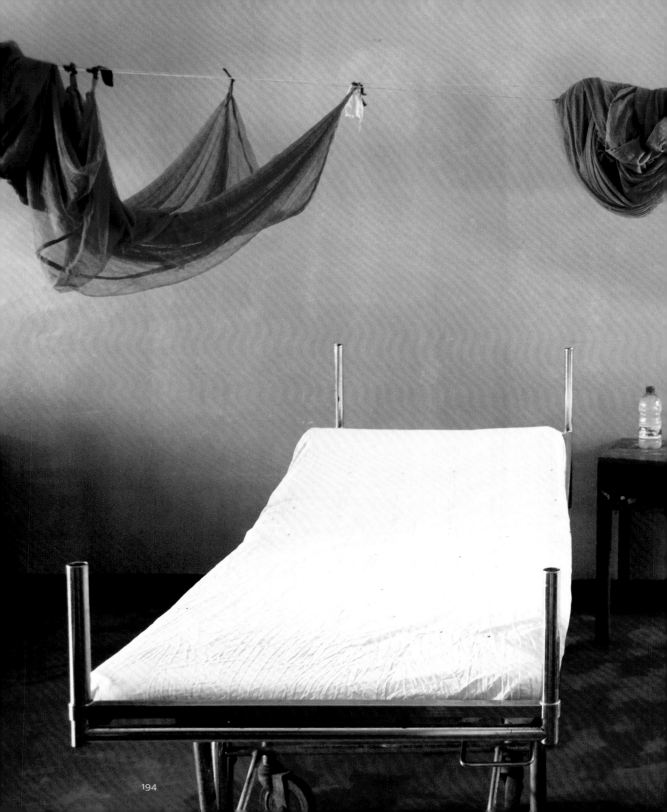

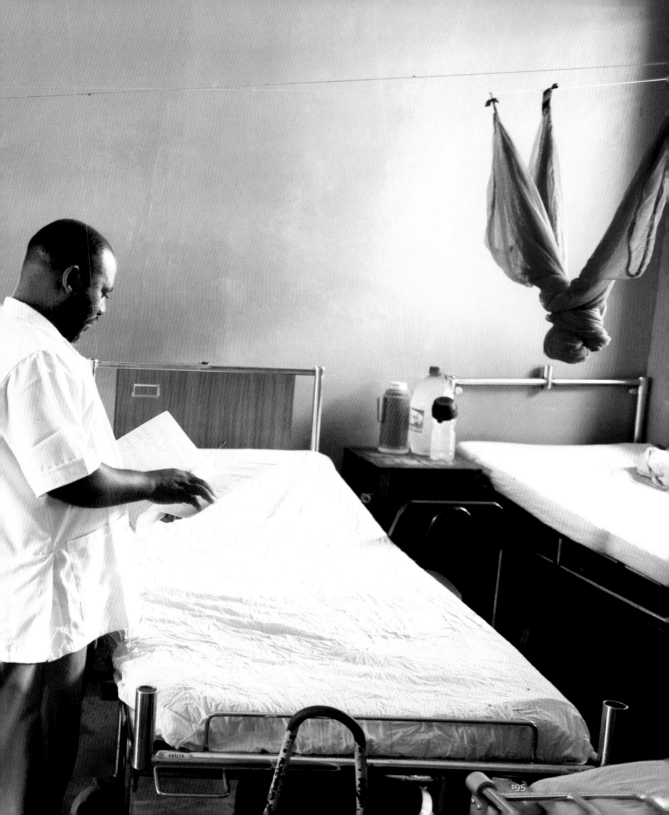

AN EMERGING PARADIGM

When John D. Rockefeller 3rd retired from the Rockefeller Foundation's board in 1971, he chided his fellow trustees for not leading the Foundation to realize its potential to change the world. "Our board has not consistently made the contribution of which it is capable," he asserted. The Foundation would be more efficient if the trustees were available "to a much greater extent as a sounding board" for officers to discuss "more true issues" about policy. He also believed that trustees should play a greater role in the critical grant review process and allow subordinates "the privilege of dissent." Rockefeller hoped that a new president would help change the organization's culture.

The board appointed John Knowles, a professor of medicine at Harvard Medical School and the youngest-ever director of Massachusetts General Hospital, to succeed J. George Harrar as president of the Rockefeller Foundation. Knowles was a powerful advocate for health insurance for all Americans, a politically controversial cause that had cost him a high-level position in the U.S. Department of Health, Education, and Welfare under President Richard Nixon. A champion for preventive medicine, he urged hospitals to work more closely with their communities. He believed policymakers interested in health needed to do more to address the many social and economic problems that hampered overall well-being. He was also deeply concerned about the effects of climate change on health, but he was not especially well versed in international health. Except for one trip to

South Vietnam to evaluate the health of the civilian population, Knowles had done no professional work abroad.

Although he could be headstrong and outspoken, the trustees had decided that Knowles was just the kind of change agent the Foundation needed. Waldemar Nielsen, the most well-known commentator on private foundations in the United States, suggested that "the choice promised important, possibly radical changes in direction for the staid old battlewagon of the Rockefeller philanthropic fleet."

Knowles immediately ordered an extensive review of the programs in each of the Foundation's five divisions. His main goal was to examine the efficiency of the Foundation's internal organization, funding allocation, and public relations. The trustee committee tasked with this effort included John D. Rockefeller 3rd, who continued to serve on the board as a non-voting trustee. Knowles, as chair of the committee, asked its members to consider whether the Foundation should continue its operational focus on pure research, become a think tank or a consulting firm, or limit its activity to making grants. "The question is," said Knowles, "what is the best balance of functions?"

One major impetus for Knowles's call for a comprehensive programmatic review—aside from his own insights and Rockefeller's critical comments—was the Tax Reform Act of 1969, which had mandated that private foundations disperse at least 5 percent of the fair market value of their investments annually. Under the new law, the government also taxed a foundation's investment income at 4 percent (later reduced to 2 percent). These two rules, along with rising global inflation, cut into the Foundation's income and alarmed its Finance Committee.

Another factor was a significant reduction in available funding. Between 1964 and 1974, the Rockefeller Foundation's portfolio experienced the greatest decline in its history, from roughly $860 million to $610 million

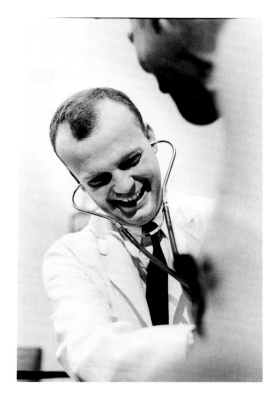

A staunch supporter of preventive medicine and universal medical coverage, John Knowles was a controversial choice for the Rockefeller Foundation presidency in 1972. The first medical doctor to head the Foundation, Knowles was also concerned with social and economic issues and saw them as intrinsically linked to the Foundation's work in health, agriculture, and population growth. (Daniel Bernstein. Rockefeller Archive Center.)

($6.5 billion to $2.9 billion in 2013 dollars). Adjusted for inflation, this decline represented a 55-percent drop in purchasing power, meaning that the value of the Foundation's portfolio was roughly equivalent to what it had been during the Great Depression. Moreover, the inflation that was cutting into the Foundation's income was also causing a precipitous increase in costs associated with social and biological experimentation.

Not only was the Foundation under intense financial pressure, but it also found itself overshadowed by the rise of international development agencies. In 1974 the World Bank pledged $4.4 billion ($20.8 billion in 2013 dollars) for agricultural development and $1 billion ($4.7 billion in 2013 dollars) for education, many times the total value of the Foundation's entire portfolio. Even greater amounts were allocated to services and research concerned with human welfare by various United Nations agencies—FAO, UNDP, UNESCO, and the WHO, for example—as well as U.S. governmental agencies like the National Academy of Sciences, the Environmental Protection Agency, the National Endowment for the Humanities, the National Endowment for the Arts, and the Departments of Labor, Agriculture, the Interior, and Health, Education, and Welfare.

Against the backdrop of these changes in the institutional landscape and the economy, the Rockefeller Foundation struggled to determine how it could best contribute to the well-being of humanity. Knowles even wondered if the Foundation had outlived its purpose.

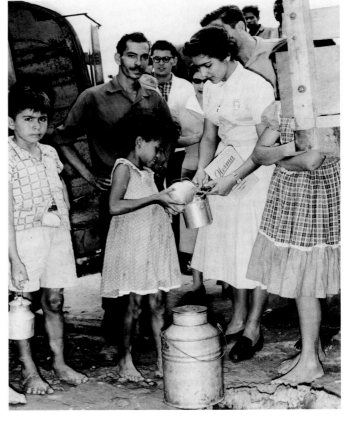

To promote community health, a nurse and social worker in training at the Medical School at the Universidad del Valle in 1957 observed and documented local systems for selling and dispensing milk in Colombia. Insights gained from this kind of training program led to the development of population-based health programs in the region in the 1960s. (Rockefeller Archive Center.)

Chapter Eight: An Emerging Paradigm

Published in 1974 as *The Course Ahead*, the trustees' 38-page review articulated a new role for the Foundation in light of the changes taking place. Where the International Health Division and the Conquest of Hunger programs had deployed staff around the world to treat patients and work with farmers, the new strategy emphasized the Foundation's "ability to influence policy and the allocation of resources" and to cultivate leaders in a variety of disciplines. Knowles was quick to say that this did not mean the Foundation was abandoning all "direct operations"—field experience fed the entrepreneurial nature of the Foundation's work—but the Foundation needed to find the right balance for a new era in its history, when influence would play a larger role than direct intervention.

Specifically, the new vision focused on seven substantive program interests: Arts, Humanities, and Contemporary Values; Conflict in International Relations; Conquest of Hunger; Education for Development; Equal Opportunity for All; Population and Health; and Quality of the Environment. Structurally, five divisions collaboratively addressed these pursuits: Biomedical Sciences, Natural and Environmental Sciences, Agricultural Sciences, Arts and Humanities, and Social Sciences.

In the field of health, Knowles acknowledged that, with the growth of large international agencies like the World Health Organization (WHO), the Foundation had been relieved of its "unique, historic role of targeting attacks on the control of specific diseases." But he also believed that "our activities in developing countries vis-à-vis health should be strengthened and increased." Indeed, he suggested that the Foundation's health-related initiatives "should be more attuned to the interaction of social determinants." Knowles wanted to move the Foundation into community medicine and focus on problems related to maternal and child health, sanitation, infectious diseases, population dynamics, family planning, and health care delivery systems, "each in the context of a defined population and with due consideration of related socio-economic and cultural factors," according to the Foundation's annual report.

The new vision was revolutionary, although rooted in many past experiments with community medicine. In fact, according to historian Paul Cruickshank, "the boardroom of the Rockefeller Foundation became the central forum for exchanging ideas for all of the most senior leaders in international health in the 1970s and 1980s."

As described in *The Course Ahead*, the Foundation resolved to renew its emphasis on health in close coordination with its other major programs. To illustrate the need for this new approach, Knowles talked of the World

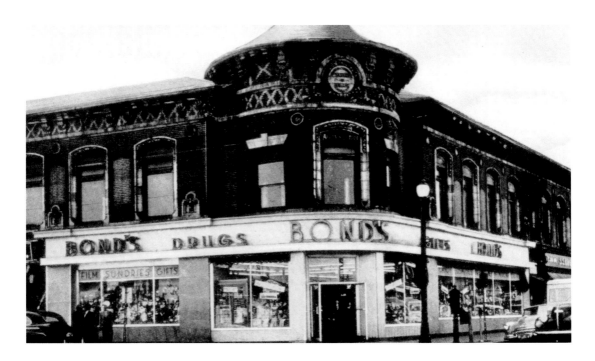

Bank's onchocerciasis or "river blindness" control program in Upper Volta (now Burkina Faso) in West Africa. Disease-spreading blackflies had been quickly controlled and the disease eradicated. Yet new health problems soon appeared in the region with the construction of a hydroelectric power station and new drainage and irrigation systems, which spread waterborne diseases such as schistosomiasis and malaria. Having read the World Bank's 1969 report on international advancement, "Partners in Development," Knowles observed that planning for economic growth had failed to include health outcomes. He believed that economists and engineers had erroneously assumed that economic growth would "trickle down" and improve health. "Whether on moral or humanitarian grounds, or purely utilitarian and practical grounds," Knowles wrote, "this defect can no longer be defended." For Knowles and many others in the early 1970s, the mere absence of disease no longer satisfied the criteria for health. Instead, health policymakers needed to focus on whether individuals lived in healthy communities, a concept that included their physical, social, economic, and political environments. These ideas were reinforced by new research that challenged the traditional paradigm for health care.

Since 1948 residents of Framingham, Massachusetts, have been the subject of a major ongoing study to determine the impact of genetics, lifestyle, and environment on cardiovascular disease. The study's first phase, completed in 1971, revealed poor diet and a lack of exercise as significant risk factors. Today the town continues to be a site of research among a third generation of subjects. (National Library of Medicine.)

Chapter Eight: An Emerging Paradigm

A New Way to Understand Health

By the mid-1970s, new attitudes toward the causes of disease and its prevention had emerged. Research showed that lifestyle factors such as smoking, sedentary habits, poor nutrition, and stress contributed to cancer, cardiovascular problems, and cerebrovascular lesions. These new findings suggested that the "cure" often lay in nonmedical remedies, including changes in personal behavior and social policy—factors later known as the social determinants of health. New approaches to medicine integrated clinical and community-based interventions to address individual lifestyle choices.

Several large-scale studies on lifestyle and health unequivocally identified the causes of leading chronic diseases. One of the first American studies of cardiovascular disease was the Framingham Heart Study, conducted in Framingham, Massachusetts. Beginning in 1948, researchers examined more than 5,000 residents of the town between the ages of 30 and 62 every two years until the end of the study's first phase in 1971. The goal was to determine the influence of genetics, lifestyle choices, and environmental risk factors on cardiovascular disease. By 1970 more than 80 articles had been published based on the collected data. Major risk factors identified by the study included poor diet, lack of exercise, and high

A woman at the World Health Organization unpacks autopsy specimens of coronary arteries to be used for research. Since the second half of the twentieth century medical researchers have undertaken a number of important studies that examine the relationship between lifestyle choices, physical and social environment, biology, and chronic disease. (Tibor Farkas. National Library of Medicine.)

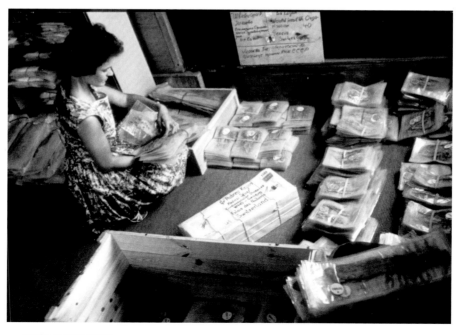

blood pressure. The study was subsequently broadened to include participants' adult children, their spouses, and grandchildren, as well as a more
racially diverse group of participants, with similar results.

Like the Framingham study, the British Doctors Study tracked the influence
of behavior on health over a long period of time. The study's coordinators
recruited 40,000 physicians—more than two-thirds of all those registered in
the United Kingdom—to participate in the first prospective cohort study of
the effect of smoking on disease. A connection between smoking and illness
had previously been suspected, but earlier studies had been inconclusive due
to small sample sizes. The British Doctors Study's first follow-up indicated that
roughly 50 percent of all smokers died of lung cancer, myocardial infarction
(heart attack), or a related disease, and that these smokers died as much as ten
years earlier than nonsmokers.

The 1958 Seven Countries Study widened the examination of the influence of lifestyle factors on cardiovascular disease by including cross-cultural
differences in occupation and diet among more than
12,000 participants in the United States, Finland, the
Netherlands, Italy, the former Yugoslavia, Greece, and
Japan. Like other surveys, the Seven Countries Study
showed that smoking was directly connected to cardiovascular disease, as were total serum cholesterol, blood
pressure, weight, and activity level.

A poster from the City of Toronto's
Department of Public Health warns
its readers, "Don't Start." In the 1950s
smoking was proven to dramatically
increase one's risk of lung cancer
and other diseases. In response,
public health practitioners turned to
marketing campaigns in an effort to
influence personal behavior.
(National Library of Medicine.)

In 1974 the Lalonde Report, officially titled *A New
Perspective on the Health of Canadians*, examined the
impact of smoking, diet, and exercise on disease, as well
as the contribution of various environmental factors like
exposure to toxins in air or water. It was based on available morbidity and
mortality data from university hospitals and medical insurance programs
across Canada. The report concluded that overall health is determined not
only by the health care system, but by four interrelated factors: human
biology, environment, lifestyle, and health care organization.

"Human biology," according to the report, "includes all those aspects of
health, both physical and mental, which are developed within the human
body as a consequence of the basic biology of man and the organic make-up of
the individual," including genetics, the aging process, and the internal organ
systems. The second factor, environment, covers "all those matters related to
health which are external to the human body and over which the individual
has no control," for example the physical and social elements of environment such as food, drugs, cosmetics, air, water, and noise pollution, as well
as safety features and working and housing conditions. Individual decisions

Chapter Eight: An Emerging Paradigm

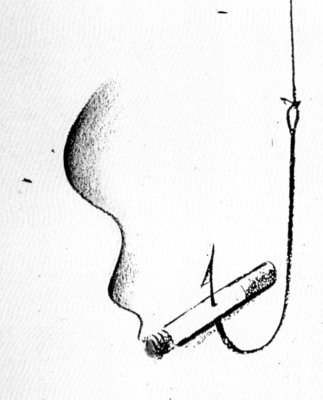

Don't Start

CITY OF TORONTO DEPARTMENT OF PUBLIC HEALTH

made by citizens "which affect their health and over which they more or less have control" were categorized as lifestyle, the third factor. Examples include consumption of toxins (alcohol, smoking, psychotropic drugs), poor diet, lack of exercise, and stress. Finally, health care organization included medical practice, hospitals, nursing homes, medical drugs, ambulances, and other health care services.

The Lalonde Report was controversial. It indicated that the health care delivery system was only one component in a much larger health-policy framework that included human biology, environment, and lifestyle. It also suggested that allocating federal and provincial dollars to the larger framework might reduce morbidity and mortality more effectively than current health care spending patterns. The report ignited a debate in Canada and elsewhere over the role that government should play in shaping the context of community health.

Lifestyle Behavior, Environment, and Health

The findings of the Lalonde Report were in line with Knowles's own views on lifestyle, behavior, and health. He would soon be the editor of the widely distributed report *Doing Better and Feeling Worse: Health in the United States*. A compilation of articles originally presented to the Commission on Critical Choices for Americans, headed by Nelson Rockefeller, the report highlighted the shortcomings of the health care system in the United States. The book's central theme was the relationship between health and illness. "It can be shown numerically," Knowles said in a speech in 1977, echoing the theme of the book, "that the massive sums which Americans have expended on medicine in recent decades have not been attended by a proportional increase in the health of individual Americans." Knowles suggested that the lack of any commensurate decrease in morbidity and mortality reflected the fact that large sums were being spent on technological innovations that benefited a relatively small population. Had that same money been spent on environmental changes and efforts to encourage individuals to adopt healthier behaviors, the outcome per invested dollar might have been much greater.

In 1975 the United States spent 8.3 percent of its gross national product on health care. "These millions of dollars," Knowles argued, "have not been used to explore the causes of most disease: environmental conditions and lack of individual responsibility." Before 1900 improved nutrition and decreased exposure to air- and water-borne infectious materials led to dramatically improved health and decreased morbidity. After 1900, however, preventive medical advances such as vaccines led to only a 10-percent reduction in mortality, and

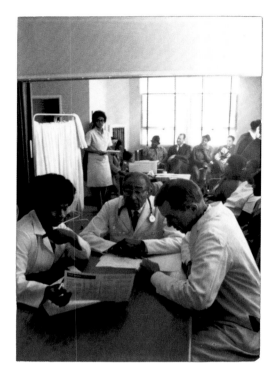

Doctors from the University of Mississippi Medical School work with a patient at a family planning clinic in Durant, Mississippi. John Knowles believed that investing in initiatives that encouraged patients to develop healthy behaviors had an overall greater impact on public health than investing in medical technologies that benefited very few patients. (Matt Herron/Take Stock/The Image Works. Rockefeller Archive Center.)

the introduction of antibiotics and innovative surgical procedures contributed less than 10 percent. On the other hand, behavior changes such as improved hygiene (hand washing) and safe sex practices (condom use), along with environmental changes (food inspection, milk pasteurization, water purification, and sewage disposal) had contributed greatly to post-1900 reductions in morbidity and mortality.

Knowles questioned why America had not invested more heavily in efforts to influence personal health-related behaviors and the environment. In 1977 only 2 percent of the $140 billion spent on health in the United States was aimed at prevention; 0.5 percent was spent on health education; and 0.25 percent was spent on environmental improvements. Knowles answered his own question by acknowledging a Western cultural bias in favor of curing rather than preventing disease; the influence of various lobbies, such as the American Medical Association; and a push for technological rather than social solutions.

Like Wickliffe Rose two generations before him, Knowles believed that more primary-care practitioners were needed to address the growing health care crisis in the United States. Before he became president, the Rockefeller Foundation had backed the development of the first physician's assistant training program at Duke University. Other types of health assistants, such as those of Project Hope in Laredo, Texas, were trained in four months. These kinds of programs addressed the critical shortage of health care professionals practicing community medicine.

Knowles and others believed that strategies for improving health should include preventive environmental measures as well as individual and community education campaigns, because healthier habits could save lives and money. "The individual," Knowles wrote, "has the power—indeed the moral responsibility—to maintain his own health by the observance of simple prudent rules of behavior relating to sleep, exercise, diet and weight, alcohol and smoking." In addition he supported structural changes to improve the health of the poor. "Here we must rely on social policies *first* in order to improve education, employment, civil rights, and economic levels, along with efforts to develop accessible health services."

Implementing the New Paradigm

The new paradigm for health care in the developing world had been articulated by a Rockefeller Foundation fellow several years before Knowles became president. John "Jack" Harland Bryant was on the medical faculty at the University of Vermont in the early 1960s when he accepted an invitation from the Foundation to conduct a study across 27 countries. Bryant then analyzed and documented his findings while serving as a Foundation-appointed professor of medicine in Thailand. His report, *Health and the Developing World*, published in 1969, called attention to the fact that many people in the world—perhaps more than half of the population—had no access to health care, and that "the most serious health needs cannot be met by teams with spray guns and vaccinating syringes." Bryant's book inspired a new generation of students and professionals in global health.

Under the influence of these emerging ideas, the Rockefeller Foundation increased its support in the 1970s for community medicine in the developing world. Specifically, the Foundation began to target infectious diseases, maternal and child health, family planning, care delivery systems, nutrition, sanitation, and demographics. The Foundation also emerged as a leading voice in a debate between proponents of two different strategies for reducing disease morbidity and mortality globally: primary health care versus selective primary health care.

Primary health care is defined as "essential health care based on practical, scientifically sound and socially acceptable methods and technology made universally accessible to individuals and families in the community through their full participation and at a cost that the community and country can afford to maintain at every stage of their development in the spirit of self-reliance and self-determination." Inspired in part by the barefoot doctors of China, whose work had been launched by the Rockefeller Foundation-supported rural reconstruction movement in the 1930s, the model of primary health care includes attention to all areas that play a role in health, such as the physical and social environment and access to high-quality health services.

Selective primary health care, in contrast, is a strategy to obtain low-cost solutions to very specific and common diseases in developing countries. It has concise, measurable, and easily observable targets and effects, focusing on interventions to address high-priority, easily remedied diseases that have dramatic impacts on infant and child mortality.

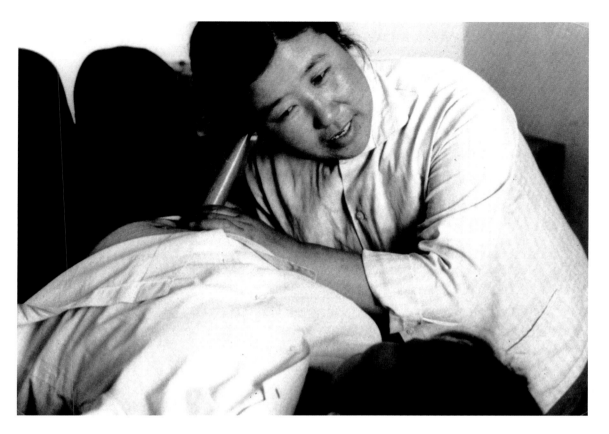

The tension between the primary health care and selective primary health care approaches was particularly evident with regard to immunization, one of the targeted interventions emphasized in the selective primary health care approach. Prior to 1974, great advances had been made in vaccine development, such as oral polio in 1963 and combined tetanus and diphtheria toxoids in 1970 for children older than seven. Also released in 1970 was a combined vaccine for diphtheria, tetanus, and pertussis, followed in 1971 by a combined vaccine for measles, mumps, and rubella. The development of malaria and tuberculosis vaccines had also given rise to programs that targeted eradication of one disease for one group, employing a massive intervention such as inoculating all children under age five.

A "barefoot" doctor listens to a fetal heartbeat through a fetoscope. "Barefoot" doctors were introduced during China's rural reconstruction movement of the 1930s to deliver medical care to rural villages. "Barefoot" doctors, named for the farmer-doctors who worked barefoot in rice paddies, treated common illnesses and educated villagers on sanitation, family planning, and disease prevention. (D. Henrioud. National Library of Medicine.)

The limitations of this approach, however, were quickly apparent. Vaccines have a limited impact on overall health if the individual being vaccinated lives in an area plagued with poverty and malnutrition, making him or her susceptible to opportunistic diseases. Calling instead for a system of health care that was integrated with other components, including economic development, community education, and improved housing—the primary health care model—the WHO and UNICEF, under the leadership of the WHO's director-general Halfdan Mahler, issued the Alma-Ata Declaration of 1978, which set an idealistic goal of "health for all" by 2000.

Knowles was among those who believed that "health for all" by 2000 was not feasible. Given his experience at Massachusetts General Hospital and the Harvard Community Health Plan (now Harvard Pilgrim Health Care), and with the U.S. Agency for International Development's (USAID) State Department Medical Investigation of South Vietnam, Knowles was well informed about cost-effective health care strategies. No cost-effective strategies to implement such broad primary health care goals had yet been identified, and he was skeptical of proposals to provide minimal training to new cadres of community health volunteers.

Knowles and others at the Rockefeller Foundation were also aware that diarrhea as well as diseases that are readily preventable by immunization were most common among infants in developing countries. Approximately 4.6 million children died of diarrheal dehydration every year. And while immunization rates in the Americas and Europe averaged about 50 percent, global rates were only 18 percent, while rates in Africa, Southeast Asia, and the Western Pacific were as low as 5 percent.

To identify more tangible goals and more effective strategies for attacking these primary causes of disease and mortality, Knowles invited a group of key leaders for a weekend meeting at the Foundation's office in mid-March 1979. The group included David Bell, executive vice president at the Ford Foundation; John Evans (a future Rockefeller Foundation chairman) from the World Bank; Rockefeller Foundation staff; and representatives from several other foundations and universities. Tragically, on March 6, 1979—less than two weeks before the gathering—Knowles succumbed to pancreatic cancer at the age of 52. Sterling Wortman, who stepped in as interim president of the Foundation, chaired the meeting. The discussion was extremely fruitful and helped to frame a larger convening organized by the Rockefeller Foundation the following month.

This conference, "Health and Population Development," was held April 18-21 at the Bellagio Center in Italy. It was formulated around a white paper titled "Selective primary health care: An interim strategy for disease control in developing countries," written by Julia Walsh of Harvard University and the Foundation's new health sciences director, Kenneth S. Warren (who will be discussed in greater detail in Chapter IX). A number of attendees from the

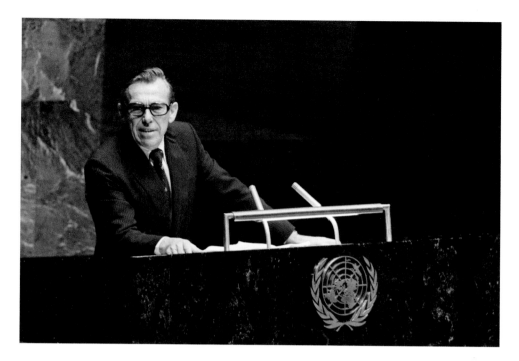

March meeting were joined at Bellagio by several heads of international agencies, including Robert S. McNamara, president of the World Bank since 1968 and former Secretary of Defense under the Kennedy and Johnson administrations; Maurice Strong, chairman of the Canadian International Development Research Centre; and USAID administrator John J. Gilligan. The WHO's director-general Halfdan Mahler attended as well, although he was skeptical of the organizers' implicit challenge to the approach outlined in the "health for all" by 2000 initiative he had announced in 1978.

The Bellagio conference led to the initial development of the concept of selective primary health care, guided by the paper by Walsh and Warren. The focus would be on four critical, low-cost interventions in poor communities and the developing world, collectively referred to as GOBI: growth monitoring, oral rehydration treatment, breastfeeding, and immunization. Organizations working with this concept would eventually add three more areas of intervention—food supplementation, female literacy, and family planning—referred to altogether as GOBI-FFF. These new low-cost, high-impact focus areas represented the beginning of a major transformation in the global approach to public health.

In debating health for the developing world, two well-meaning, but opposing viewpoints predominated. Primary health care advocates urged economic and social development as part of an overall effort to improve health. Halfdan Mahler of WHO advocated this approach. Proponents of selective primary health care, including the Rockefeller Foundation, sought more realistic and cost-effective goals for the developing world, including a program of targeted vaccinations. (Yutaka Nagata. United Nations.)

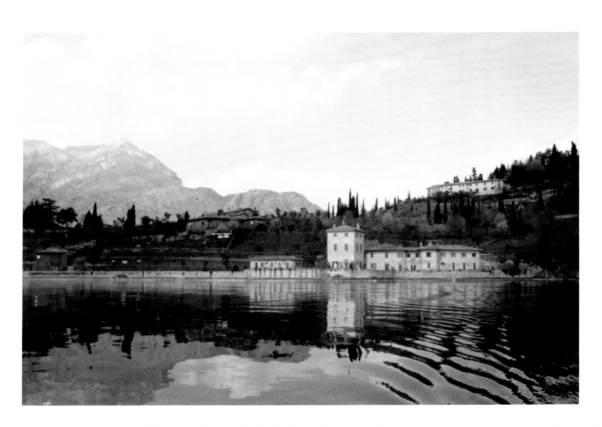

One of the attendees at the Bellagio conference, who would soon become the head of UNICEF, was particularly impressed by the idea of selective primary health care. Born in Beijing in 1922, James "Jim" Pineo Grant was the son of John Black Grant, the Rockefeller Foundation doctor who had pioneered community health programs in rural China (see Chapter III). After leaving China, the younger Grant had served as U.S. deputy assistant secretary of state for Near Eastern and South Asian Affairs; director of U.S. Economic Aid Missions; and assistant administrator of USAID. Leaving USAID in 1969, he founded the Overseas Development Council (ODC), which he saw as a neutral extension of USAID that would be free to investigate modes of development avoided by government agencies or more conservative philanthropies. The Rockefeller and Ford foundations decided to underwrite the ODC, providing more than half of its initial funding. Some ODC members, like Theodore M. Hesburgh and Clifton Wharton, also sat on the Foundation's board, and Grant himself had become a Rockefeller trustee and executive committee member on February 6, 1978.

The Bellagio Center has been the site of many important international meetings, including the 1979 conference on "Health and Population Development." The conference advanced a program of selective primary health care for the developing world that included low-cost, high-impact initiatives that would specifically affect the lives of women and children. (Rockefeller Archive Center.)

Using the concepts developed at Bellagio, Grant launched what became known as a "child survival and development revolution" in 1983. He helped mobilize international, national, and local initiatives to bring life-saving, cost-effective techniques—including all four GOBI interventions—to the care of children in developing countries. This "revolution" saved the lives of an estimated 20 million children by the end of the 1980s. Meanwhile the idea of selective primary health care would drive a host of new initiatives at the Rockefeller Foundation over the next several decades.

Community Medicine and Family Planning

In one sense, the community health movement had been inaugurated by Rockefeller philanthropies in 1910, when local governments, public-health advocates, physicians, and scientists came together to fight hookworm, a disease that was a direct result of poverty. This coalition reduced the incidence of hookworm in the United States and also sparked the transformation of the nation's infrastructure and health systems, which resulted in improved health among the poor. In many ways, the effort revolutionized the field of public health in the United States.

In the 1930s, the International Health Division had supported community development programs in China that addressed local public-health problems while also addressing larger social and economic issues in rural communities. In the 1960s, the Foundation supported schistosomiasis control programs in the British West Indies that considered larger community issues such as agriculture, sanitation, and environmental stewardship. All of these initiatives were very much in keeping with the vision that Wickliffe Rose and other trustees of the General Education Board and the Rockefeller Foundation had articulated in the early 1910s.

Building on this approach in the 1970s, the Rockefeller Foundation financed surveys to help establish health-status baselines. In the rural Ban Chang district not far from Bangkok, for example, initial surveys performed in conjunction with the University Development Program revealed that as many as half of all infants were malnourished. Once a need like this was revealed, Foundation staff would begin work in the community, either among local officials and university or medical college staff or at the national level, to develop training and implementation programs for auxiliary health care personnel. These rural community health initiatives were also launched in Zaire (now Democratic Republic of the Congo), Brazil, and Indonesia. In Bahia, Brazil, for example, the Foundation supported the federal university's transformation into a center focusing on local political, social, and medical development

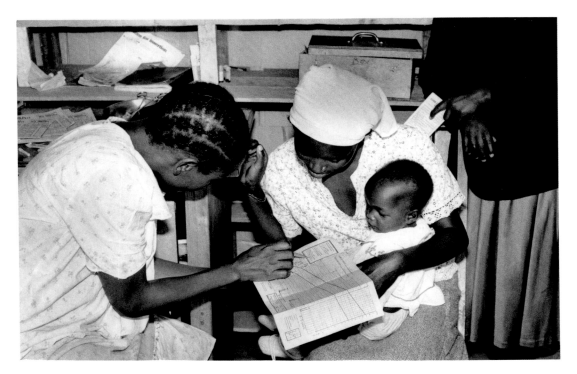

Beginning in the 1970s the Rockefeller Foundation included family planning counseling in its maternal health programs and began to contribute significant funding to research the development of safe, affordable, and effective contraceptives. (Wendy Stone. Rockefeller Archive Center.)

needs. The medical goal was to develop an "inexpensive health system for poor people in rural areas," which could only be secured through an educational system that provides "the greatest amount of education and training in the shortest possible time."

In bolstering health care delivery systems, the Foundation attempted to decentralize the provision of care. In the Laguna province of the Philippines, a program provided training in rural health care to students in medicine, nursing, dentistry, sanitation, and related fields while extending care to 75,000 citizens. The Foundation also included rotations in sanitation in Philippine health care training programs for medical students. In other locations, the need was for better organization rather than more health care providers. At Harvard's Center for Community Health and Medical Care, the Foundation supported an exhaustive record-keeping and evaluation system to monitor a wide array of cooperating programs in the greater metropolitan area of Boston, providing the programs with information they needed for better administration, which ultimately led to greater access to existing services.

The success of all of these interventions, however, continued to be threatened by the explosive population growth around the world. By the 1970s, the

Chapter Eight: An Emerging Paradigm

Foundation included family planning counseling in its conception of caring for mothers, because higher birth rates were associated with poorer maternal health. The Foundation also wanted to link contraceptive services with maternal and infant health. Knowing that women would need access to the best forms of contraception, the Foundation funded research on spermicides, hormones, and the ideal size and shape of intrauterine devices, in an attempt to identify the most effective protection with the fewest side effects. The Foundation supported efforts by the Population Council's International Committee for Contraception Research to test 14 devices and 39 compounds, including progestin, which is now common in oral contraceptives.

These efforts to address the scientific and technological aspects of human reproduction, however, were increasingly balanced by efforts to address the social and economic forces that contribute to rapid population growth. The Foundation provided technical assistance to governments focusing on the reciprocal impact of population and economic and social policies as well as research, through the Population Council's Demographic Division, on the social, economic, cultural, and behavioral determinants of population growth. This new approach was reflected in a statement by John D. Rockefeller 3rd that "the only viable course is to place population policy solidly within the context of general economic and social development in such a manner that it will be accepted at the highest levels of government and adequately supported."

ENVIRONMENT

Population growth had a major undeniable impact on the larger dimensions of community health. But by the mid-1970s, a growing number of policymakers recognized that the environment also played a key role in public health and medicine. To many Americans in the 1970s, the environment no longer felt safe. Concerns both real and fictitious surrounded potential exposure to natural and manmade toxins such as lead, pesticides, and radioactivity in the water and the air.

In its Quality of the Environment Program, the Foundation applied industrial-organizational principles to pollution. It proposed to support any organization capable of contributing to the creation of a "balance sheet" for "residuals"—the leftovers from production processes—as well as research on larger ecosystems. The Foundation also financed numerous efforts to reduce pollution. These included finding alternatives to chemical pesticides, developing pesticides with greater specificity or controllable degradation properties, using insect pheromones to distract insects away from crops, and using hormones to keep insects in their juvenile stage.

The Foundation funded research on ways to change the environment to reduce pollution levels. For example, researchers tried to design a workable system of sewage disposal and community water management using a series of lakes and ponds with different plants, aquatic insects, and microorganisms to help filter out pollutants. The Foundation also funded innovative approaches to reducing air pollution from industrial plants, such as systems of underground tunnels containing pollution exhaust filters or systems to filter contaminated air through different soil types.

The Rockefeller Foundation-funded Candelaria Rural Health Center in Colombia was an early pioneer in population-based community health in the mid-1960s. In rural communities, auxiliary nurses were trained to collect demographic and epidemiological information to improve community health services. (Rockefeller Archive Center.)

Throughout its history, the Rockefeller Foundation had implemented numerous training programs to foster the development of technical skills in medicine, research, and public policy. These technical training programs were typically endowed over several years to ensure that they could produce a large enough cadre to sustain a given field well into the future. Similarly, in order to create a legacy of environmental protection, the Foundation supported universities in establishing multidisciplinary environmental research programs to ensure that a sufficient number of technicians would be available for the monitoring and control duties necessary in both public and private agencies.

All of these environmental initiatives contributed to the growing holistic approach to community health that incorporated a view of an entire population within a specific environment responding to social and economic forces, as well as the care and treatment provided by health care professionals. Within this emerging paradigm, the measure of success was no longer just the health of the individual but rather the health of both the individual and the community.

With the addition of this facet to the research and clinical approach to chronic diseases, old core beliefs and traditional interventions began to collapse. A single discipline was unlikely to make significant improvements in community health. As the evidence accumulated about the multiple social determinants of health, the Rockefeller Foundation increasingly searched for new interdisciplinary research programs to address the health of individuals and their communities.

Ultimately, the 1970s saw the Foundation reshape its traditionally vertical programmatic approach—which included campaigns against a single disease or disease vector—into a multidisciplinary effort that spanned all divisions and was geared toward what were deemed the most important aspects of developing nations: community health, population growth, and environmental issues. Although there was a great deal of trial and error and learning by doing, these programs would lead to major new initiatives anchored in the ideas of community medicine and epidemiology.

Chapter Eight: An Emerging Paradigm

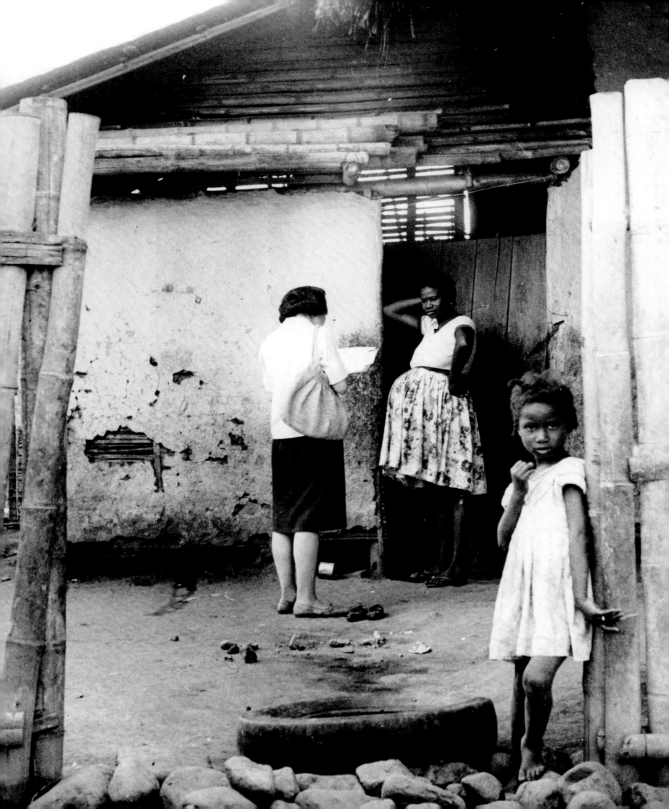

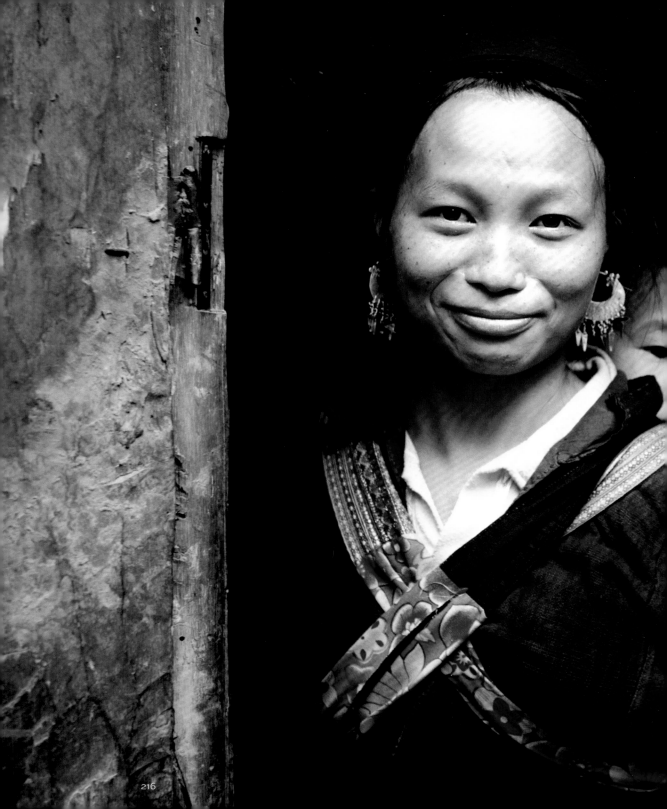

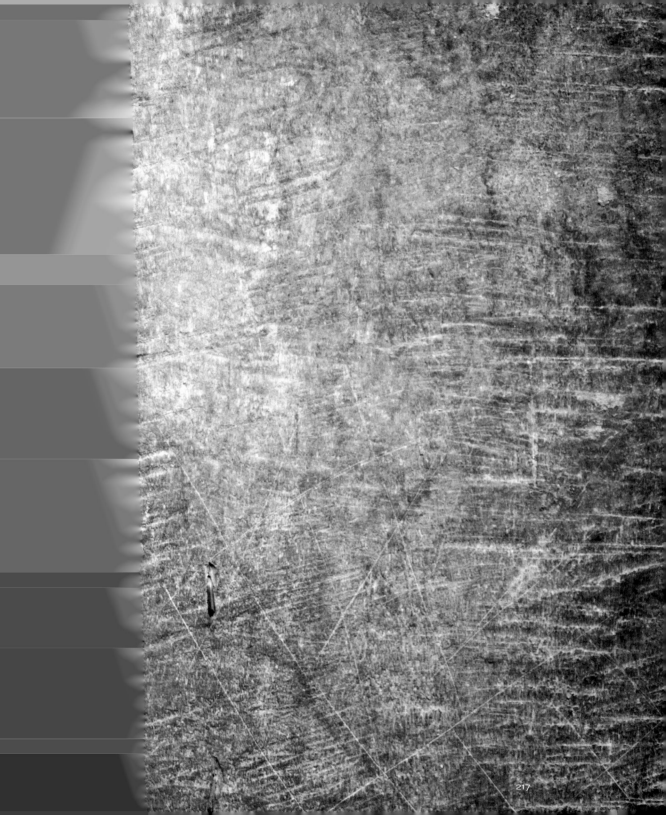

THE PENDULUM
SWINGS BACK

In 1918, when the Rockefeller Foundation provided funding to the first American school of hygiene and public health at Johns Hopkins University, Wickliffe Rose believed that medical training alone was insufficient to meet the demands facing public health administrators. He and other Foundation trustees hoped to develop a new cadre of experts who understood the interactions among bacteriology, biostatistics, epidemiology, sanitary engineering, and public health administration. But by the 1970s, according to Foundation President John Knowles, the training of physicians had been weakened by medical schools' lack of attention to fields related to public health. As Knowles advocated for a community approach to health, he asked two long-time senior vice presidents to assess the state of medical education and public health training and propose new strategies for the Foundation's programs in health and population.

In their report, Sterling Wortman and Laurence Stifel noted that the Foundation's work in population and health was at a turning point. Several key long-time staffers were retiring, and the schistosomiasis program in St. Lucia, after winning international acclaim, seemed to be coming to a natural end. As the Foundation assessed its ability to shape public health internationally, it continued to face a problem of scale. It no longer had the resources to launch and staff projects in the developing world, as it had with hookworm and yellow fever. But the Foundation's reputation in the field of international or global health was significant, and, according to Wortman

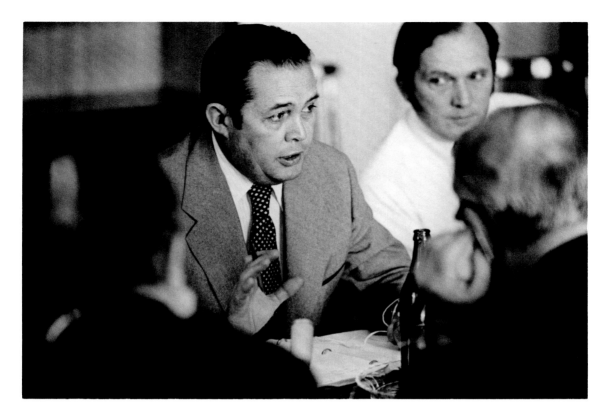

and Stifel, it represented a critical asset that could be leveraged in the context of efforts to convene others for collaborative action.

Wortman and Stifel recommended that the Foundation help to organize a global campaign to increase basic research on "great" or important diseases that had been "neglected" because they generally affected poor people in developing countries. Wortman and Stifel also called for "the development of medicine oriented to populations of people rather than individual patients." They suggested exploring new ways of managing and exploiting the burgeoning volume of information in the health sciences. Knowles and the board of trustees embraced these recommendations. To pursue the new agenda, Knowles recruited Kenneth Warren to serve as director of a new Health Sciences Division.

A Brooklyn native, Warren had earned a bachelor's degree in history and literature at Harvard, writing his thesis on the poet T.S. Eliot, before attending Harvard Medical School. Throughout his life he was interested in

Sterling Wortman joined the Rockefeller Foundation as an officer in the Mexican Agricultural Program. He went on to help found and direct the International Rice Research Institute and the Consultative Group on International Agricultural Research. Later, as vice president, Wortman made recommendations regarding medical training that helped to shape modern Foundation initiatives in health. (Rockefeller Archive Center.)

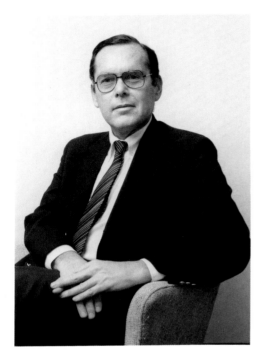

Kenneth Warren helped to revitalize and transform the Rockefeller Foundation's approach to controlling disease in the developing world. His approach, known as population-based medicine, concentrated on communities rather than individuals. Warren emphasized the inclusion of epidemiology—the study of patterns of diseases in populations—and today epidemiology remains a central tenet of public health. (Rockefeller Archive Center.)

the creative processes that inspired scientists and artists. In medical school, Warren had become fascinated with tropical diseases. He did postgraduate work at the London School of Hygiene and Tropical Medicine and became an expert on schistosomiasis. He later worked in Africa, Asia, and the Caribbean, and taught at Case Western Reserve University before joining the Rockefeller Foundation as director of Health Sciences in 1977 at the age of 48. Knowles hoped that Warren would be able to help direct the Foundation's efforts in tropical medicine and international public health.

Soon after arriving at the Foundation, Warren read a paper by the health economist R.N. Grosse, who concluded that the major factors affecting life expectancy were not medical per se, but economic and social. Warren embarked on a research project with Rockefeller Foundation research fellow Julia Walsh to determine the key factors affecting morbidity and mortality in the developing world. As noted in Chapter VIII, Walsh and Warren presented their paper at the 1979 Rockefeller meeting on "Health and Population Development" at the Bellagio Center and later published it in the *New England Journal of Medicine.*

The authors defined new cost-effective and efficient approaches for primary health care in the developing world. They believed that focusing on populations and communities, rather than individuals, could stretch health care dollars and reduce global disparities in health outcomes. Their approach became known as *population-based medicine*, which Warren defined "as an integration of epidemiology, biometry, demography and mass [preventive] or therapeutic intervention programs."

Epidemiology was at the time considered a backwater in medicine. An area that deals with the patterns, causes, and possible control of diseases, epidemiology had fallen out of favor early in the twentieth century with the rise of biomedical research, as scientists focused on the cellular and molecular causes and manifestations of disease rather than the environmental or social context. Although Foundation statistician Persis Putnam had pushed

Chapter Nine: The Pendulum Swings Back

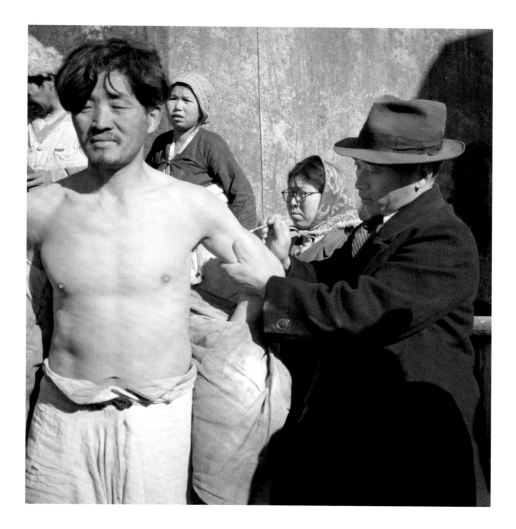

the staff of the International Health Division to be rigorous in their statistical methodology, she was not able to invigorate the division's interest in epidemiology. After World War Two, however, statisticians used increasingly rigorous methods to correlate risk factors with the incidence of chronic disease. As historian Paul Cruickshank explained, "The framework of analysis and action that underpinned postwar epidemiology prioritized highly quantitative and systems-based styles of thinking."

Along these lines, Warren and others believed that paying close attention to the patterns of outbreaks would make possible strategic interventions to stop the spread of disease. Lewis Thomas, president of the Memorial

Refugees fleeing the war in Korea arrived at Koje Island in January 1951. All of the island's permanent residents, as well as newly arriving refugees (between 3,000 and 5,000 per day), were systematically vaccinated against smallpox and typhus in order to avoid potential outbreaks. (Gordenker. United Nations.)

Sloan-Kettering Cancer Center and author of *The Lives of a Cell*, agreed. As he wrote in *Science* in 1977, the same year that Warren began his work at the Foundation, "medicine must be building, as an essential part of its scientific base, a solid under-pinning of biostatistical and epidemiological knowledge."

Warren hoped to institute a revolutionary reform in clinical medical training. He proposed a campaign to introduce epidemiology to medical school curriculums at the point when students receive training in bedside care. He wanted to ensure that epidemiology would not be taught as an independent discipline. It was to be imparted routinely, he hoped, as a methodology of bedside medicine in all clinical disciplines, training students "not what to think but how to think."

At the September 1977 meeting of the Rockefeller Foundation Board of Trustees, just months after he started work, Warren had laid out a tripartite program. He wanted to improve research on major diseases in less developed nations, establish clinical epidemiology within medical schools, and improve health-related information systems. The trustees approved this three-part initiative, but, instead of taking on the medical education establishment in industrialized nations, the Foundation chose to focus on low-income countries.

In 1978 Kerr L. White joined Warren's team as head of the Health of Populations program. White was a pioneer in the field of health services research. He had earned degrees in economics, political science, and medicine at McGill, Yale, and Dartmouth Universities. As assistant professor of internal medicine at the University of North Carolina at Chapel Hill for ten years, he collaborated with statisticians and epidemiologists, developing his ideas about how to get "physicians to think more broadly about disease and medical care." Among the hundreds of articles White published, one of the most influential was his 1961 referral study, "The Ecology of Medical Care," published in the *New England Journal of Medicine*, which coined the term "primary medical care." White had been considered for the post of Surgeon General of the United States during the Johnson administration and was instrumental in persuading Senator Edward M. Kennedy to include language in the 1973 Public Health Authorization Bill that ensured Congress received an annual update on the health of the nation.

White was also a champion of population-based medicine. After joining the Rockefeller Foundation, he began his effort to build a population health education program by first investigating the University of Pennsylvania's pilot program, which had been training Rockefeller fellows for several years.

While working with the International Health Division, Persis Putnam encouraged staff to keep well-documented statistics in an effort to correlate risk factors with disease and to control potential outbreaks. Putnam was a pioneer in the field of statistics and epidemiology. In these graphs, spanning a ten-year period, rates of pulmonary tuberculosis are recorded among Tennessee's rural and urban populations. (Rockefeller Archive Center.)

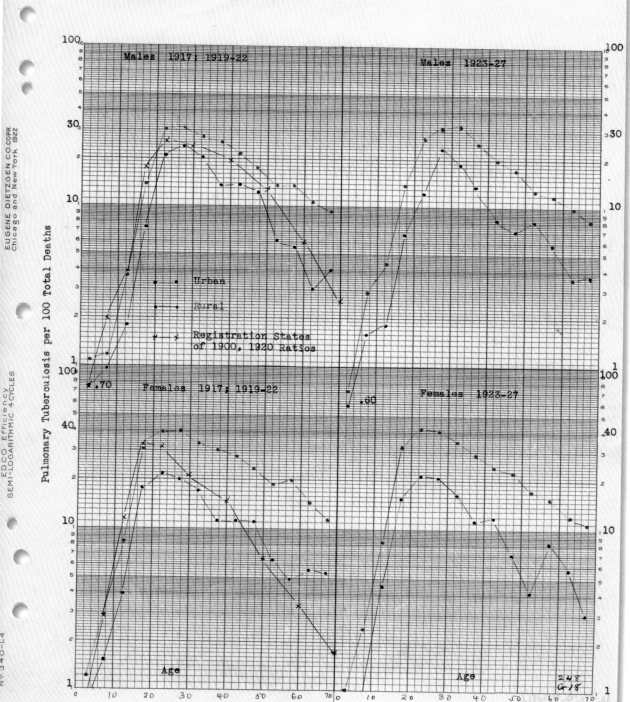

Figure 1

Tennessee: Comparison of Urban and Rural White Pulmonary Tuberculosis
Death Ratios by Age for Two Five-Year Periods

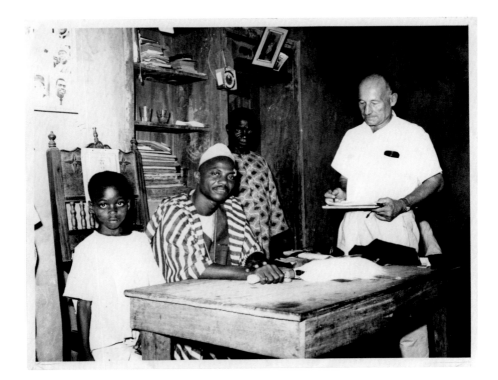

White, Warren, and others at the Foundation envisioned a capacity-building project that would include the establishment of preeminent epidemiologic research and training centers at a few select medical colleges in developed host nations. Subordinate clinical epidemiology units, composed of several research physicians, would be identified in developing countries. After physicians from those units were trained in epidemiology at one of the research and training centers, they would return to their home countries as part of a cadre of researchers who would disseminate the epidemiological perspective and campaign for additional training courses and funding.

With this massive undertaking, the Rockefeller Foundation intended to once again shift the paradigm of public health, medical education, research, and policy, this time from one in which epidemiology had little relevance to the practice of medicine, to one in which it was intrinsic to all aspects of clinical care. In the meantime, however, Warren and the Foundation took a page from the Foundation's history to promote new efforts to address health problems affecting the poor around the world.

A researcher from University College of Ibadan in Nigeria conducts a health survey with a local village leader in 1959. In 1977 the Rockefeller Foundation drew upon its past experiences when initiating a program to improve health research and health systems through the introduction of courses in epidemiology. (Rockefeller Archive Center.)

Chapter Nine: The Pendulum Swings Back

In the mid-1970s, the Foundation's leaders had realized that many of the most prevalent and pernicious diseases in the world were not receiving attention from pharmaceutical companies because these diseases primarily affected the poor and thus offered little opportunity for the drug companies to make a profit. Because of this lack of attention, these pathogens were poorly understood. "We couldn't even begin to think of a vaccine because we didn't know what was going on," Warren would tell a Congressional committee in 1985.

Other institutions were also struggling with this issue. The WHO's Special Program for Research and Training in Tropical Diseases and a similar initiative at the Fogarty International Center for Advanced Study in the Health Sciences were looking for ways to address diseases that affected primarily the poor in developing countries. But these efforts were still straining to receive support.

To help move these efforts forward, the Foundation's trustees allocated $10 million in December 1977 for a new initiative focused on these "Great Neglected Diseases of Mankind" (GND), including schistosomiasis,

Scientists at the National Institutes of Health work in a snail culture room, conducting research on tropical diseases. With the launch of the Great Neglected Diseases of Mankind program, the Rockefeller Foundation provided support to persons and institutions undertaking research on the most prevalent and deadliest tropical diseases affecting some of the world's poorest regions. (National Library of Medicine.)

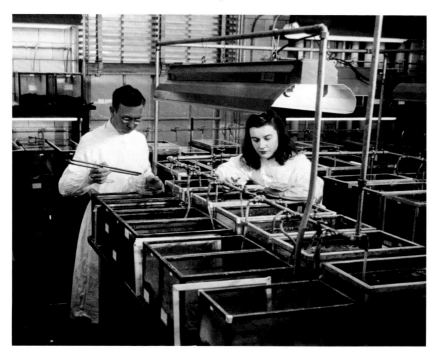

hookworm, malaria, and amoebic dysentery. In launching the program, the Foundation once again became a major player in international health and tropical medicine.

Warren initiated the GND program amid great advances in bacterial and viral disease research. In 1972, for example, the causative agent for leprosy, *Mycobacterium leprae*, had been discovered in armadillos, offering hope for an animal model and ultimately for mass production of *M. leprae* to facilitate research and development. In 1976 the malaria parasite *Plasmodium falciparum* had successfully been cultured *ex vivo* (outside of a living organism), opening the door for another vaccine development. In addition, the ten-year global vaccination campaign against smallpox had finally succeeded, the last case having been discovered on October 31, 1977, in the port town of Merca, Somalia.

The GND program used innovations in molecular biology—a field incubated and developed in the 1930s and 1940s by the Rockefeller Foundation—to unearth mysteries of tropical parasitic diseases such as malaria, schistosomiasis, African sleeping sickness, and hookworm, as well as diarrheas and respiratory ailments—the greatest killers of children at the time.

One of the core requirements of Warren's GND program was to link "the bench with the bush" through applied research and collaborations among investigators in developed and developing countries. That idea was controversial at the time. The concern was how to bring disparate groups into a unified program and how to interest Western scientists in the research. Warren wanted to recruit researchers from various disciplines such as biochemistry, molecular biology, and immunology. He called for establishing research units at universities, medical schools, and scientific institutes. With new resources, he also hoped to encourage young scientists to enter previously neglected fields of research.

The program quickly succeeded, generating great interest and support for basic and applied research in "tropical" illnesses. "Scientists now consider such research exciting rather than mundane," wrote Leslie Webster, head of the pharmaco-parasitology group at Case Western Reserve University. Within the GND program, ten research units were formed during the first year, each of which established as promptly as possible a "critical mass of investigators" in parasitic diseases to provide career opportunities for young investigators with new perspectives. By the end of the second year of the program, the Foundation was supporting dozens of investigative units in the United States, Europe, and Australia, and provided training for 47 outstanding scientists. Each team received a limited sum—up to $15 million total—to spend over a period of eight years.

Minor challenges arose along the way. For example, many developing countries lacked modern laboratory facilities. Warren was concerned that once these nations received funding, some portion of the funding dedicated to the epidemiological investigative units would be siphoned off to other areas of research. Warren overcame this obstacle by mandating that resource allocations remain under the Foundation's control.

One key factor in the success of the GND program was an annual conference held in New York City. The first meetings were uneasy, in part because "nobody quite knew what anybody else was doing," recalled David Weatherall, head of the GND unit at the University of Oxford. Within a few years, however, the GND communication network was functioning efficiently. Members discussed latest work in their labs and constructively criticized the ideas of others. "They would also help, assist and work together within the network," commented Gerald Keusch, who was at Tufts University School of Medicine, "to enlarge the scope of inquiry for all." Investigators established close friendships. "Every annual meeting," said Carlos Gitler of the Weizmann Institute of Science, was like "a reunion, or perhaps a family meeting."

The group's familial feeling had the effect of increasing friendly competition and accelerating the pace of innovation. "Every group wanted to show that they had been working hard over the past year and had established new and important scientific findings," recalled Anthony Cerami of Rockefeller University. "Everyone wanted to look their best." New avenues of thinking, research, and collaboration opened up when participants met socially in evening activities that "mixed scientists as people."

The GND program was a prime example of the "wedge," or leveraging tactic, that Wickliffe Rose had first described in 1910 with regard to the Rockefeller Sanitary Commission's campaign to eradicate hookworm in the United States. As a result of the Foundation's efforts, nearly $17 million in new investment ($41 million in 2013 dollars) flowed to GND research.

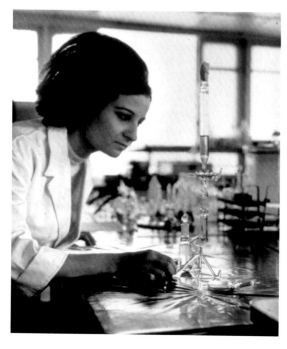

A researcher isolates the schistosoma parasite at the Institute for Schistosomiasis Research at Cairo University. Considered one of the world's great neglected diseases, schistosomiasis is a chronic disease that continues to be a major health threat in tropical and subtropical countries, where its impact is second only to that of malaria. (D. Henrioud. National Library of Medicine.)

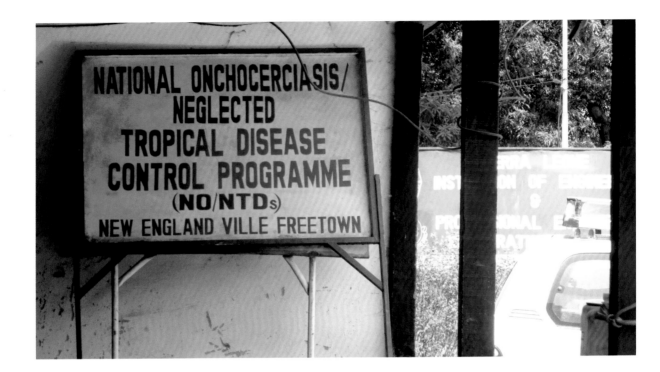

Eventually 157 grants were given to 67 different institutions in 23 countries, and a number of five-year career development grants of $50,000 per year ($120,000 in 2013 dollars) were awarded to scientists. By the end of the program in 1987, other organizations had donated a total of five times the amount invested by the Foundation.

Overall, the GND program significantly improved basic knowledge about tropical diseases, many of which had been poorly understood at the time. It also played a critical role in increasing the number of talented young scientists interested in studying the problems of the developing world. After eight years, the staff at the research units included 161 senior scientists and clinicians as well as 360 trainees, including 150 from the developing world. Many of the scientists eventually secured positions of major responsibility and leadership in the field.

Nonetheless, the GND program fell short of meeting the Foundation's goal of creating research capacity in tropical countries, because it primarily (though not exclusively) used American researchers at American labs to study the diseases. In addition—as Tim Evans, who served as the director of the

A Neglected Tropical Disease Control Programme office in Freetown, Sierra Leone, provided treatment for onchocerciasis or "river blindness." Transmitted by parasitic blackflies, onchocerciasis causes itching and lesions on the eye that can result in a loss of sight. Onchocerciasis is second only to trachoma, another neglected tropical disease, as the leading cause of preventable blindness. (Romina Rodríguez Pose. Overseas Development Institute.)

Foundation's Health Equity program in the late 1990s, has pointed out—no set strategy was identified for converting the knowledge gained from research into vaccines. Moreover, even if the advances in basic research had led to opportunities for new drugs, most developing countries lacked the delivery infrastructure needed to benefit from this high-end science. Thus, vaccines did not get to the people who needed them most.

The primary lesson learned from the GND program, however, was that the goal of controlling neglected diseases was broadly valued by stakeholders. Sixteen years after it ended—according to Gilbert Omenn, a professor of internal medicine, human genetics, and public health at the University of Michigan—the GND provided the foundation for the 2003 Gates Foundation Grand Challenges in Global Health. That initiative sought to promote scientific breakthroughs for preventing, treating, and curing diseases that annually kill millions of people, especially children, in developing countries.

INCLEN Is Born

The clinical epidemiology project that Knowles, Warren, and White had dreamed of in 1978 developed alongside the GND program. In July 1979, months after Knowles's death, the Foundation's Executive Committee approved a $300,000 grant ($965,000 in 2013 dollars) to the University of Pennsylvania for three years of funding to design and establish a clinical epidemiology research and training center, with the expectation that those trained at the center would form an international clinical epidemiology network (INCLEN, as the program later became known). The Foundation wanted to explore how best to disseminate "a quantitative population-based approach to medicine including biometry, epidemiology, and demography as an integral part of clinical medical education."

Following a long tradition, the Rockefeller Foundation had begun the effort that would lead to INCLEN with a survey. Kerr White collected data from medical schools in Southeast Asia, China, Latin America, and Africa to identify where to base research and training centers to train physicians in sophisticated approaches for assessing the health needs, priorities, resources, and outcomes of a given population. He also sought potential sites for subordinate clinical epidemiology units from which to draw mid-career physicians dedicated to a population-based perspective; they would be educated at the research and training centers and then return to conduct research and influence policy. Following Knowles's untimely death, however, White's efforts, except for the grant to the University of Pennsylvania, were put on hold until a new president could be picked.

Richard Lyman became president in 1980. A historian with a Ph.D. from Harvard, Lyman had taught at Washington University in St. Louis before moving to Stanford in 1958. He later became provost and then president of the university in 1970, during the height of the Vietnam War protests. On campus, Lyman was known for being tough with protestors, but he also worked hard to increase minority enrollments and launched a $300 million fundraising campaign, the largest in the history of higher education.

As a member of the Foundation's board of trustees for several years before becoming president, Lyman understood the tensions within the board and the staff. But he also took over during a tough time of transition as the Foundation continued to struggle with the financial consequences of inflation and the decline of its endowment in the 1970s. As he began to develop his vision for the organization, he moved the Foundation away from basic research to focus on the use and dissemination of existing scientific knowledge instead. Given INCLEN's goal to train future generations of researchers, some staff members were concerned that Lyman might not support the project, but he saw the practical benefits and chose to move forward.

INCLEN faced a number of challenges, however, as it was being developed. The program was designed, according to Kerr White, to address the fact that "departments of community, preventive, or social medicine, and schools of public health have, for the most part, failed in their efforts to provide all physicians with the population perspective." Furthermore, it sought "to change the thinking about health policies and practices by medical educators, politicians and the public." The INCLEN project proposed to establish a handful of key clinical and epidemiological research and training centers and a broader network of clinical and epidemiological units, but no one could agree on what expertise was needed to make these centers and units successful.

In the fall of 1980, White gathered 25 senior researchers from medical schools in developing countries to discuss selection of INCLEN research and training centers, epidemiology units, sponsors, and potential trainees. The group included researchers from the Rockefeller Foundation-funded project at the University of Pennsylvania, which would serve as the first of INCLEN's centers. Criteria were developed based on feedback from this group, and, later that year, another research and training center was established at McMaster University in Hamilton, Ontario, along with a third center at the University of Newcastle, Australia.

One of INCLEN's first goals was to provide all trainees with the necessary tools to investigate the health of their countries' populations. Basic information about death and disease was often lacking. Medical funds were allocated more readily to urban centers, where they often benefited only a few. In rural

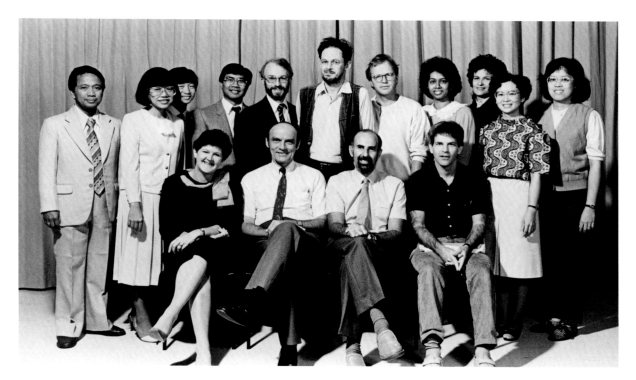

areas, where public health needs were greater, medical funds were often inadequate or lacking altogether. National health data could provide crucial information to help direct health funds where they were needed most. One of the first things INCLEN ensured was that all trainees had access to computers and that all research data and teaching methods and materials were computerized and accessible to the trainees for sharing and analysis.

The staff and students of the Asian and Pacific Centre for Clinical Epidemiology at the University of Newcastle, Australia, in 1986, including Scott Halstead from the Rockefeller Foundation (seated front row, second from left). With support from the Foundation, the center focused on teaching epidemiology to doctors from developing nations in Southeast Asia. (University of Newcastle.)

As the network grew, international trainees worked alongside their domestic partners at the clinical and epidemiological research and training centers, thus broadening the exposure of both groups to their mutual needs and resources. The commitment among participants deepened, and INCLEN attracted attention from other leaders in the field of global health. The development boards or agencies of Australia, Canada, and the United States contacted INCLEN representatives, as did the Special Program for Research and Training in Tropical Diseases (sponsored by the WHO, the U.N. Development Program, and the World Bank), which had previously joined forces with Rockefeller's GND program. Most important, INCLEN garnered the support of an outspoken and entrepreneurial physician and leader from Canada.

John Robert Evans was a remarkable pediatrician. Born in Toronto in 1929, the youngest of six children, he had been raised by his siblings after both of his parents died before he reached the age of ten. The experience made him very independent. After graduating high school, he went straight to medical school at the University of Toronto and then continued his training in Canada, the United States, and the United Kingdom as a Rhodes Scholar. At the age of 35, he became the founding dean of the faculty of medicine at McMaster University. Evans introduced an innovative curriculum at McMaster, emphasizing "problem-based learning," a hands-on approach in sympathy with the Rockefeller Foundation's focus on the application of knowledge in the world. He also provided for instruction in population-based medicine and clinical epidemiology. From McMaster, Evans returned to the University of Toronto, where he was president from 1972 to 1978. In 1979 he became head of the Population, Health and Nutrition Department at the World Bank, where he was increasingly concerned about the dominant paradigm for managing public health in the developing world.

John Evans and David Sackett were pioneers in the development of problem-based learning when they helped to establish the School of Medicine at McMaster University in Hamilton, Ontario, in the late 1960s. Both played an important part in the creation of INCLEN. Evans also served as a trustee and chairman of the Rockefeller Foundation. (Mike Lalich. McMaster University.)

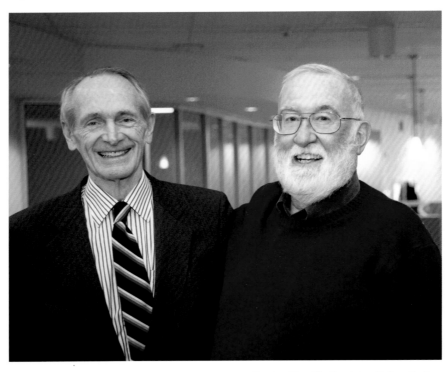

Chapter Nine: The Pendulum Swings Back

Evans was recruited to serve as an advisor to the Rockefeller Foundation by John Knowles shortly before Knowles died. In 1981, with a grant from the Foundation, Evans prepared a report entitled "Measurement and Management in Medicine and Health Services" that provided a basic framework for INCLEN's continued development.

Evans's report positioned the need for INCLEN against a backdrop of disappointment in the field of public health. He criticized the lack of innovation in public health curriculum in the 1970s, suggesting that the discipline the Rockefeller Foundation had done so much to create had grown stale. According to Evans, the field had narrowed its focus to "technical and regulatory issues at the expense of the major health problems."

Evans exhorted physicians to work with health administrators and public health officials in developing countries to address population health needs. He suggested that schools of medicine should put more emphasis on "measurement and management," alongside diagnosis and cure. "The challenge," he wrote, "is to move from the use of epidemiology by a small cadre of specialists as a research method or disease identification technique, to its use by policymakers, managers, and practicing physicians as a disciplined way of thinking in quantitative terms and with a population perspective about health problems, the selection of interventions, and allocation of resources."

The nascent INCLEN program, from Evans's point of view, was providing scientists in developing countries with critical skills, technology, and intellectual support to design, accomplish, disseminate, and champion high-level research on health issues endemic to their home communities.

Recognizing a powerful ally, Richard Lyman recruited Evans to join the Rockefeller Foundation's board of trustees in 1982. With Evans's insight into INCLEN's potential risks and benefits, Lyman became an increasingly forceful advocate for the program. In 1983 he described the project as the "kind of high-risk, high-payoff undertaking in which a private foundation with international health interests should be substantially involved."

The risks were considerable. The Foundation's investment might be for naught if the medical community refused to embrace this new approach. Personal interests, customs, and traditions tended to dominate the culture of medical schools and hospitals, making them resistant to change. But if the gamble paid off and INCLEN succeeded, the proliferation of training and research with a population-based approach could revolutionize health policy, resource allocation, and clinical practice.

Aware of the risks, in 1983 the Foundation board decided to move forward and build upon the success of the initial University of Pennsylvania program. It awarded grants totaling $1.4 million ($3.3 million in 2013 dollars) to the clinical and epidemiological research and training centers (CERTCs) in Canada and Australia, as well as the University of Pennsylvania. As Kenneth Warren and Kerr White had imagined, these training centers functioned as hubs in the emerging INCLEN network. Physicians recruited as fellows from developing countries spent a year at one of the centers, then returned to their home countries to train other health care professionals in epidemiological methods and conduct research that would guide national health policy. If these fellows could develop institutional capacity at home, then the Foundation would provide funding to establish a clinical and epidemiological unit within a local medical school that would promote effective and efficient care directed to the health of populations.

The challenge was how to guarantee that any INCLEN unit would support and participate in the network. The solution emerged at the first annual INCLEN meeting, held in 1983, when subordinate epidemiology unit selection criteria were established. Attendees concluded that each unit had to have as a representative a "senior faculty sponsor with strong ties to policy makers and government leaders." This representative would pledge to promote the influence of the network vertically, throughout all levels of the health system. At the time, 18 of INCLEN's 28 subordinate research units (64 percent) had as sponsors deans of medical schools. Associate deans, department chairpersons, hospital directors, or research directors represented the remaining units. The backing by local, regional, and national policymakers demonstrated that there was high-level support for the Foundation's endeavor and would prove critical to INCLEN's continued growth and development.

Transitions

After Kerr White retired from the Foundation in 1983, Scott Halstead, a former professor and chairman of the Department of Tropical Medicine and Medical Microbiology in the University of Hawaii's medical school, directed INCLEN as the Rockefeller Foundation's associate director of Health Sciences. Born in India to missionary parents, Halstead had spent years thinking about the health care needs of poor countries, and understood the vital role that health information could play in addressing those needs. He helped lead INCLEN to sustainability in the mid-1980s.

To make the transition, however, Halstead would have to rely on the patience of the Foundation's president and board. In 1984 the Foundation's Executive Committee called for an assessment of INCLEN's progress and plans. After Halstead presented his review, the board decided to continue funding for both INCLEN and its annual conference despite the fact that Lyman and the trustees were cutting field staff and operations to balance the budget. Indeed, swayed by Halstead's advocacy, the board recognized that INCLEN's success or failure could not be accurately measured in the short term. Fellows and clinical units would have to be in place for at least ten years before their impact could be assessed.

The board's patience and support seemed to be rewarded the following year when ministers of health, some of whom attended INCLEN's annual conference, praised the organization's work and spurred training conferences and workshops within their own countries. Funding from new partners followed. Based on the number of INCLEN-trained physicians in Thailand and China, USAID awarded $2.1 million ($4.5 million in 2013 dollars) to India to establish an INCLEN research and training center.

INCLEN built upon this success by raising standards. The leadership committee added a requirement that a subordinate epidemiology unit must consist of six clinicians and one biostatistician trained in epidemiology, as well as a health economist. To assure continued commitment from INCLEN members, new fellows were required to collect population health data in their home countries before their training commenced.

With this support and rising standards, INCLEN moved from start-up to expansion and independence. It gained additional funding and political legitimacy when the World Bank endorsed the network and funded a clinical and epidemiological research and training center, as well as several clinical and epidemiological units, in China. In 1985 the three schools that housed the CERTCs began to award degrees in clinical epidemiology, further enhancing INCLEN's legitimacy. Several Latin America governments also promised to support any clinical and epidemiological research and training centers or clinical and epidemiological units established in their countries. Meanwhile the network expanded its training agenda, adding courses in health economics and the social sciences to existing courses in epidemiology in an effort to help fellows play a key role in shaping health policy in their home countries.

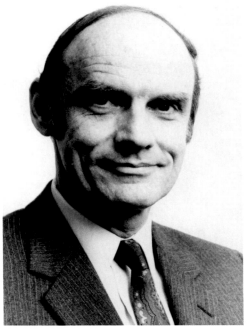

As associate director of Health Sciences, Scott Halstead advocated for the long-term support of INCLEN. In 1987 he, Julia Walsh, and Kenneth Warren edited the Foundation's publication *Good Health at Low Cost*, based on the proceedings at the Bellagio conferences in 1984 and 1985. The book played an important part in building support for selective primary health care. Halstead also helped launch the Children's Vaccine Initiative. (Rockefeller Archive Center.)

By 1986, 27 INCLEN clinical and epidemiological units had been established along with an additional CERTC at the University of Toronto. In many cases, the data and information developed by these teams provided fresh insight into the issues affecting the health of their communities. The CERTCs also began to schedule site visits six months after INCLEN fellows graduated and returned to their home stations, during which a preceptor—a kind of mentor—provided additional assistance. Preceptors would guide the fellows in their ongoing research and help assure they had the material and intellectual support of their home institutions by advocating on their behalf to the institutional sponsor, typically the dean of the medical school.

The Foundation's board of directors, along with the leaders of the research and training centers and units, further refined INCLEN in 1987 by funding social scientists to help develop cost-effective means of preventing and treating the most serious health problems with consideration of the social, political, cultural, and behavioral determinants of health. These added refinements raised aspirations for INCLEN even more. It was hoped

Cooperation between national governments, international organizations, and philanthropies has helped to improve health in the developing world. For example, a joint initiative between the United Nations Development Program and the governments of seven countries in the Upper Volta region of Africa has helped to dramatically lower rates of onchocerciasis, or "river blindness," in the region. (Kay Muldoon. United Nations.)

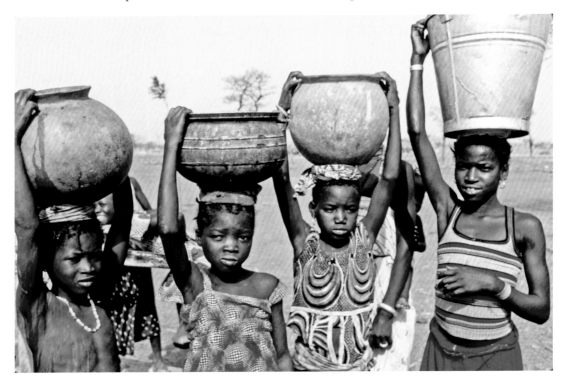

Chapter Nine: The Pendulum Swings Back

that nonprofit organizations would emerge to support and use the network in advising the governments of developing nations on their health care issues. As INCLEN continued to gain recognition at community and international levels, governmental and commercial agencies sent their executives for training clinical epidemiology.

By 1987, then, INCLEN was expanding in size and influence. A survey of clinical and epidemiological units demonstrated their growing legitimacy, since all were located within medical departments, affiliated with multiple specialties, or set up as national training and research centers. Several INCLEN research groups received invitations to make presentations—not only on their research but also on INCLEN as a whole—from international associations of health care, epidemiology, and public health.

But perhaps the watershed moment marking INCLEN's arrival in the world of policy was the 1987 election of a clinical and epidemiological unit sponsor, Prawase Wasi, as president of the new National Epidemiology Board of Thailand. Wasi soon established various committees that included INCLEN fellows or sponsors to develop policy on communicable diseases, environmental health, and community health. These efforts culminated in the publication of *Review of the Health Situation in Thailand: Priority Ranking of Diseases*, which became the model exported to other nations.

INCLEN's Growing Independence

The ultimate aim of the Foundation in promoting programs such as INCLEN was for the enterprise to achieve financial independence. At the beginning of the second quarter of 1987, the Foundation board awarded $1.45 million ($3 million in 2013 dollars) to continue INCLEN's work and help it transition to independence. And in 1988 INCLEN established collaborative relationships with funding bodies such as the WHO, the United Nations, the U.S. Centers for Disease Control and Prevention, and the World Bank.

But as INCLEN developed, some segments were growing faster than others. In Thailand, for example, where the number of units had grown quickly, officials were able to launch a national clinical epidemiology network, capable of conducting research and guiding regional and national agencies on making health policy. These agencies also provided grants to sustain the work. In other parts of the world, networks developed much more slowly.

To help foster a sustainable system, the Rockefeller trustees relied on the partners in the CERTCs to guide INCLEN's strategy. Moreover, as clinical and epidemiological units gathered sufficient resources, they could become

CERTCs and begin acting as the center of their own clinical and epidemiological network within their own country. In some ways, this system followed the path paved by the Foundation's Conquest of Hunger program in agriculture in the 1960s and 1970s, which had promoted the development of agricultural research institutes in regions around the world.

With additional INCLEN units established in Africa, Latin America, and Asia, and with ten national and international agencies funding the organization's activities in 1988, INCLEN incorporated. After identifying a director and nominating a board of directors, it set out to increase the number of participating medical schools as a way to continue to expand the network and ensure its long-term viability.

The success of the project was evident at the annual conference of 1989. Compared to the 22 members who had come to the first meeting, mostly from the West, INCLEN VI attracted more than 500 international attendees, nearly two-thirds

Kenneth Prewitt and Peter Goldmark (right) of the Rockefeller Foundation. As president of the Rockefeller Foundation from 1987 to 1997, Goldmark sought to make its finances sustainable. He believed that the Foundation could no longer support large-scale ventures on its own, as it had in the past, and that collaboration was vital to its future. (Rockefeller Archive Center.)

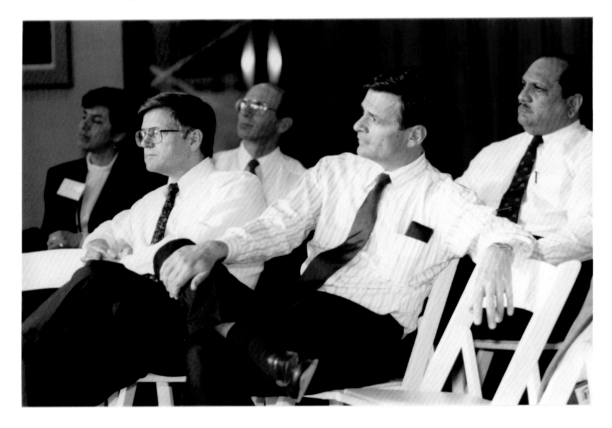

Chapter Nine: The Pendulum Swings Back

of whom were not directly affiliated with INCLEN. The attendees were interested in the quality and the content of the scientific presentations.

Meanwhile China inaugurated its INCLEN units as an independent national network, ChinaCLEN, as did Indonesia and India. Several subordinate epidemiology units also began conducting their own training in 1990, rather than rely on the supervising CERTCs, and helped other medical schools within their respective countries establish epidemiology units.

INCLEN's success was apparent from other perspectives as well. A review of the fellowship program, for example, revealed that 98 percent of INCLEN fellows had landed in influential positions in their home countries. And network units were already affecting policy. In Thailand, for example, the Health Department adjusted its hepatitis B program based on INCLEN research. By the late 1980s, however, INCLEN's costs imposed a heavy burden on the Rockefeller Foundation.

In 1987 Peter Goldmark succeeded Richard Lyman as president of the Foundation. Unlike his predecessors in the president's office, who came from academia or public service, Goldmark had worked in the corporate sector, where he was a senior vice president for the Los Angeles-based Times Mirror newspaper company, supervising the company's eastern operations and magazine publishing business. Even before he had stepped into his new role, he acknowledged the challenge of confronting a new era in the Foundation's history. "There isn't much room for solo acrobats any more," he told the staff, acknowledging what many already recognized—that the era when the Rockefeller Foundation could go it alone in the world was over. Partnerships and joint ventures, like INCLEN, were the key to the future. But for a foundation with limited resources, these partnerships had to come with the ability to exit a project once its success or failure had been proven.

With Kenneth Warren's retirement just months before Goldmark arrived, INCLEN had lost an influential champion. The new president initially supported continued funding for INCLEN—the Foundation appropriated $4.5 million as late as 1991 ($7.7 million in 2013 dollars)—but Goldmark was increasingly concerned that the Foundation could not and should not sustain this level of commitment, and that year he recruited Robert Lawrence to direct Health Sciences.

Lawrence was a Harvard-trained physician who, from 1984 to 1989, had chaired the first U.S. Preventive Services Task Force, an independent body of primary care physicians that came to play a major role in regulating quality control in the U.S. health system. As a founder of Physicians for Human Rights, Lawrence had also demonstrated a deep concern for the rights of patients in other parts of the world. But he was also a pragmatist.

Goldmark asked Lawrence to accelerate INCLEN's transition to independence and to wind down the Foundation's support for the Great Neglected Diseases program as well. With these goals in mind, Lawrence encouraged the transfer of power that had begun with INCLEN's incorporation in 1988. The devolution of authority also continued. Meanwhile a review conducted by the Council on Health Research for Development bolstered prospects for outside funding by recommending that programs such as INCLEN be supported and linked with other programs to build the capacity of developing nations for conducting research.

The Rockefeller Foundation ended its core programmatic support for INCLEN in 1998, with a final injection of $14 million ($20 million in 2013 dollars) to support its long-term viability. A year later, as much as $10 million ($14 million in 2013 dollars) came from other agencies to support INCLEN's continuing operations. In 2000 the INCLEN Inc. board established the INCLEN Trust—governed by representatives from the various INCLEN training centers and epidemiology units as well as host-nation governments and NGOs—to ensure continuing support for the network and to enable it to meet the needs of the most disadvantaged populations.

LOOKING FORWARD

The success of the networks created by Warren, White, and other Foundation staff in the Great Neglected Diseases (GND) program and INCLEN contributed to an emerging Foundation strategy. For a majority of the twentieth century the Foundation had independently financed international health initiatives, one of the few private philanthropies to do so. But as GND and INCLEN proved, joint international ventures could work. Their success set the stage for larger, more powerful relationships to come, allowing the Foundation to leverage its assets with organizations that had much greater resources, including the WHO, the World Bank, and UNICEF. These kinds of collaborations would become critical as public health officials geared up in the face of pandemics such as HIV/AIDS and SARS. These collaborations also proved essential as the global health community embraced the idea that solving basic community-related problems and providing access to good information were crucial to public health, and sought to create systems that would distribute information in ways that would allow practitioners to be strategic about their work.

The relative success of the GND program and INCLEN ultimately rested on balancing tensions: "hard science and social science, local vs. central, global vs. in-country." Whereas the GND program used hard science

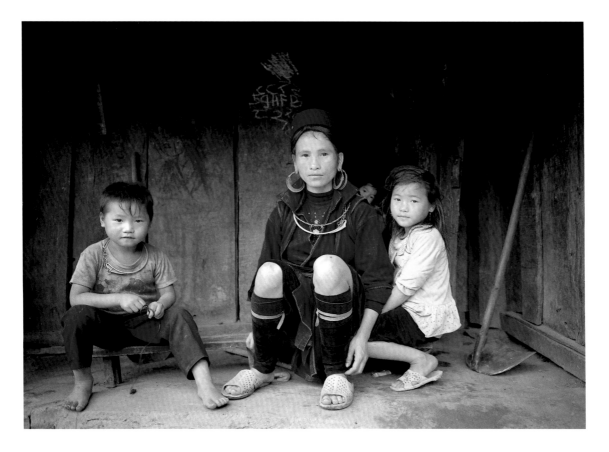

centrally and globally, INCLEN drew scientists from the developing nations and, once they had been trained at a premier center, returned them to their home countries. A key to INCLEN's success was the "network" that was required, encouraged, and rewarded by the Foundation; indeed, by 1999 the Rockefeller Foundation had invested more than $75 million in the initiative. In this sense, INCLEN built on the Rockefeller Foundation's long history of developing new fields to improve the well-being of humanity.

A mother from an indigenous Hmong group in Vietnam poses with her children. Development programs, including those that focus on health, economic growth, and improving the status of women, have led to an overall decrease in fertility rates worldwide. (Kibae Park. United Nations.)

Even as INCLEN continued to grow, however, the Foundation had moved on to a new global health crisis. In this instance, its ability to bring others to the table to develop new knowledge and breakthrough innovation would be tested in a way that was reminiscent of the fight against yellow fever. But unqualified success would be elusive.

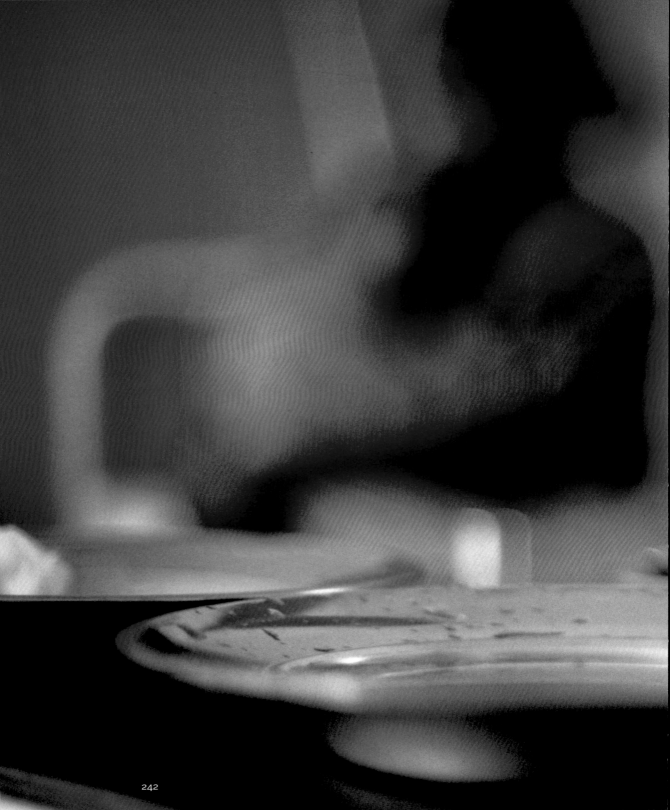

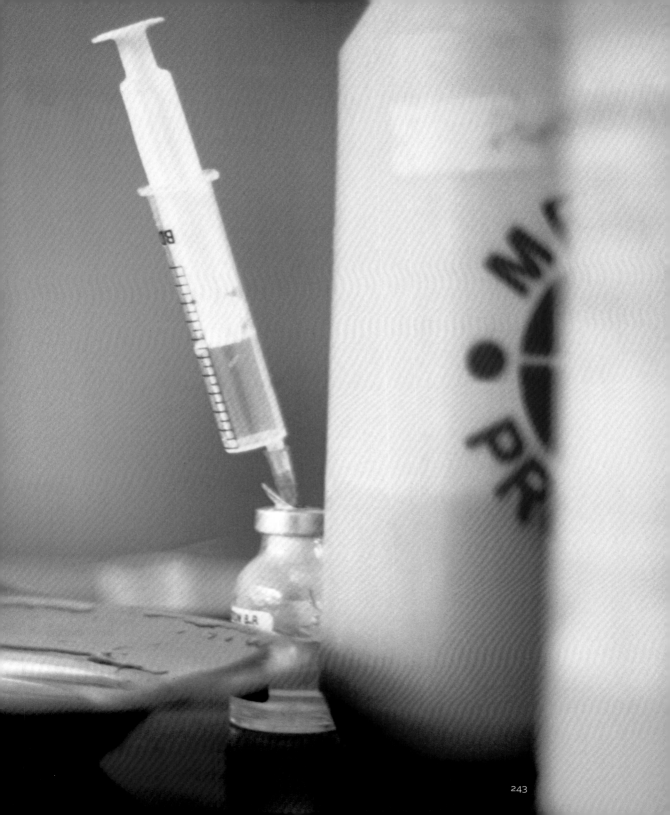

AIMING HIGHER THROUGH COLLABORATION

B y the mid-1980s, after decades of advancement in the creation and delivery of vaccines to the developing world, infectious diseases were still proliferating. Although life expectancy in many countries had begun to climb significantly and child mortality figures had dropped, in 1986 alone, 3.5 million children died from vaccine-preventable diseases because they had not been immunized.

More often diseases disproportionally affected poorer regions in the world because no organization was working on improving existing vaccines or developing new ones. The diseases that were spreading in developing nations had already been controlled in more developed countries. But in Latin America, Africa, and much of Southeast Asia, many millions were dying because available vaccines could not reach them. And for those diseases, like malaria, that had been controlled by means other than vaccines in the developed nations, no vaccines were expected to be created for less developed countries. There was no profit for the pharmaceutical industry in working on such vaccines, because the governments of poorer nations could not afford to pay what developed nations could.

At the same time, new opportunities emerged with new vaccine technology. The Foundation had operated alone as a philanthropic colossus for most of the first half of the twentieth century, driving development internationally and domestically through its financial and intellectual investments in education, training, agriculture, and health care. But with the rise of

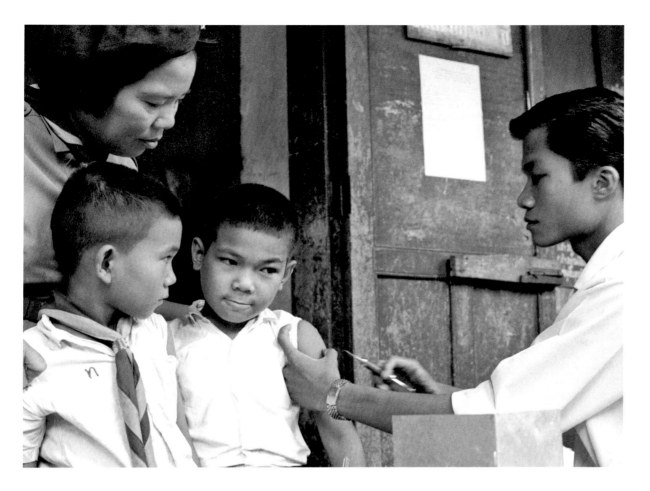

international organizations such as the World Health Organization (WHO), the United Nations, and the World Bank, Foundation leaders realized a new opportunity was at hand to join forces with these institutions to better leverage resources and address neglected "wedge" issues (to use Wickliffe Rose's term) such as childhood immunization and vaccine initiatives in the develop-

Children in Thailand in 1964 were vaccinated for tuberculosis under a program launched by the World Health Organization. By 1986, however, millions of children were still dying from vaccine-preventable diseases like TB. (United Nations.)

ing world. From the mid-1980s through the 1990s, the Foundation would spearhead several vaccine initiatives, the most important of which were Universal Childhood Immunization and the Children's Vaccine Initiative. These new initiatives revived and carried forward the Foundation's historic efforts to develop vaccines for diseases that threatened people in developing nations in the tropical regions of the world.

D espite closing the International Health Division in 1951, the
Rockefeller Foundation had not completely abandoned its own
laboratory research. Many of the scientists who had dedicated
their lives to the yellow fever campaign moved into a new effort to explore
unknown viruses, particularly the group called "arboviruses" that are borne
by arthropods—most often mosquitoes, ticks, sand flies, and midges in this
case—that transmit yellow fever, dengue fever, and St. Louis and Japanese
encephalitis. The Rockefeller Foundation Virus Program was established
in 1951 with the creation of the Virus Laboratory located at the Rockefeller
Institute laboratories in New York. The Foundation also sponsored research
centers in Africa, Asia, and Latin America. If new viruses
triggered new epidemics, they would most likely erupt in
emerging nations.

In contrast to earlier virus or vaccine research
programs, the new arbovirus program was not geared
specifically towards a single infectious agent or disease.
Researchers took a "shotgun approach" towards collecting, typing, and cataloguing numerous viruses from

Hermetia illucens, the "Black soldier" fly,
is a member of the phylum Arthropoda,
and a carrier of myiasis, an intestinal
disease. At the Rockefeller Foundation's
Virus Laboratories, researchers
catalogued more than 200 arthropod-
borne viruses and pathogens. (Centers
for Disease Control and Prevention.)

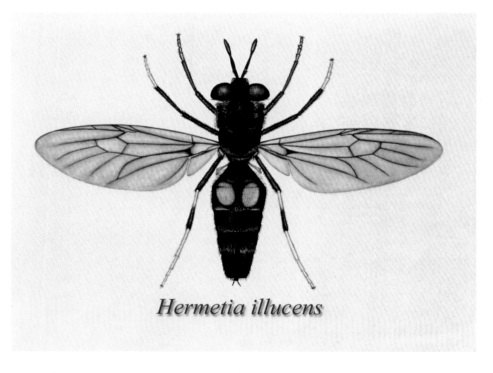

Hermetia illucens

Chapter Ten: Aiming Higher Through Collaboration

around the globe. Research at the Virus Laboratory built on new discoveries in biomedical science, one of which was the discovery by Enders, Weller, and Robbins in 1949 that poliovirus could be propagated successfully in non-neural cell cultures (for which they received the Nobel Prize in Physiology or Medicine in 1954). Their experiment had practical implications for poliovirus research and paved the way for the development of polio vaccines by Jonas Salk in 1955 and Albert Sabin (a former Rockefeller Institute scientist) in 1957. With these breakthroughs, it became much easier to study and culture viruses and to develop vaccines against communicable diseases.

The Rockefeller Foundation's Nobel Laureate Max Theiler directed the Virus Laboratory from 1952 to 1964, and established field laboratories in Brazil, Colombia, Egypt, India, Nigeria, South Africa, and Trinidad. The Virus Laboratory explored the relationship between arthropods and their viruses in each of these different geographic locales.

The Foundation also initiated in 1959, and supported until 1962, the publication of the *Catalogue of Arthropod-borne Viruses of the World*, by the American Committee on Arthropod-borne Viruses (ACAV). The catalogue contained a vast amount of information on 204 viruses, their geographic location, and their vertebrate hosts. This baseline information helped public health officials develop strategies to control the various insects or vectors that carried these potentially lethal diseases.

Through the 1960s and early 1970s, as multinational health agencies like the WHO and the Pan American Health Organization established themselves as successors to the Foundation in the field of global health, the Virus Laboratory and its field units gradually transitioned from Rockefeller Foundation support and sponsorship to become affiliated with these new multinational agencies. In 1964 the Foundation moved its Virus Laboratory from New York to the Yale Medical School in New Haven, Connecticut, where it became known as the Yale Arbovirus Research Unit. The unit was designated as the World Health Organization International Reference Centre for Arboviruses in 1966.

The Rockefeller Foundation continued to provide significant funding through this transition period. In fact, with continuing support from the Rockefeller Foundation in 1969, the center was able to identify the Lassa fever virus, which infected an estimated 300,000 West Africans, resulting in approximately 5,000 deaths per year even in 2013. By 1971 the Yale Arbovirus Research Unit had the "largest collection of viral agents and immune sera in the world" and functioned "as an international reference center and clearing-house for the investigation of viral agents and their carriers and as a training ground for virologists."

At the same time, as the main Virus Laboratory migrated to Yale and then became a World Health Organization reference center, the field laboratories also took on new roles. With the University Development Program in full swing in 1966, the Foundation facilitated the integration of the Virus Laboratory's field labs with medical colleges in Colombia, Brazil, India, Nigeria, and Trinidad, as well as California. Foundation specialists were assigned to these colleges to help train a future cadre of researchers. Meanwhile, the Trinidad Regional Virus Laboratory in Port of Spain, Trinidad, first established in 1952 with the aid of the Foundation, became the Caribbean Epidemiology Centre (CAREC) in 1970. It too became associated with a multinational health agency when it was reorganized as an important regional health institute administered by the Pan American Health Organization (PAHO) for the West Indian region.

Altogether, between 1950 and 1970, the Rockefeller Foundation contributed approximately $30 million to the arbovirus program. Although the Foundation continued to provide funding for the program's research initiatives through 1974, these changes reflected the Foundation's complete transition from a manager of laboratory research to a funder. As a funder, however, the Rockefeller Foundation continued to be interested in virus research and vaccines, particularly as a revolution in biotechnology—made possible by the Foundation's development of the field of "experimental" or molecular biology in the 1930s—promised to usher in a new era in vaccine development.

New Opportunities

In the late 1970s, biotechnology transformed the nature of vaccine research and development. New knowledge and laboratory techniques, such as recombinant DNA for genetic engineering, made it possible to identify, analyze, produce, deconstruct, and replicate infectious agents for the purpose of vaccine development. But even though scientists were extremely excited about taking advantage of these innovations, there was little political and financial support for vaccine research and development. Vaccines generally require a high initial investment and produce a relatively low profit margin. There were also potential liability issues if the vaccine went awry. In the 1960s and 1970s, for example, vaccine manufacturers had been inundated with disability claims attributed to immunizations. Threats of litigation made most investors nervous. In contrast, basic research in genetic engineering—such as for agriculture—seemed to offer huge commercial rewards and was protected from liability by government policies.

Given the reluctance of politicians and vaccine manufacturers, less than 5 percent of children around the world had received available vaccines by 1974. To improve the situation, the WHO launched its Expanded Program on Immunization (EPI) that year to immunize all children against tuberculosis, diphtheria, neonatal tetanus, whooping cough, poliomyelitis, and measles by 1990. This program was inspired by the success of the effort to eradicate smallpox, which was the first of only two diseases to be eliminated in human history (the other disease was rinderpest, which primarily affected livestock). In 1974 indications were that the six targeted diseases were killing millions of children each year. EPI called on pharmaceutical companies to improve the quality of vaccines for developing countries but also promoted self-reliance among developing nations to ensure the delivery and administration of those vaccines.

Although there was political support following the WHO's announcement of the creation of EPI, some scientists believed that a solitary focus on vaccine delivery was

As policymakers debated strategies for childhood immunization campaigns in the 1980s, physicians and researchers pressed the need for continued research to develop more effective and easily administered vaccines. (John Isaac. United Nations.)

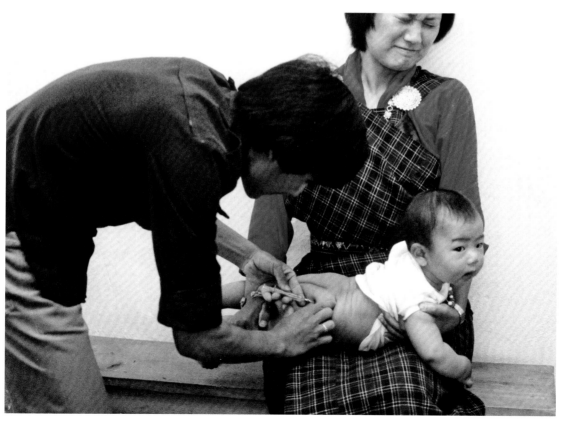

insufficient. By 1984 groups were stressing the need to direct EPI resources to basic research in vaccine development in order to take advantage of ongoing breakthroughs in biotechnology. In the middle of this growing awareness of how crucial the biotechnology revolution would be, the Rockefeller Foundation sponsored a forum to energize and transform existing international vaccine research and development.

At that time, the Foundation's Health Sciences Division was already supporting the Great Neglected Diseases program, which had established a biomedical research and training network that focused on the major diseases of the tropical world with the goal of aiding developing nations in building better tools and techniques for prevention and treatment. INCLEN provided a complementary network for the exchange of epidemiological information and intelligence.

The Health Sciences Division had also supported programs that brought cost-effective health care ideas and techniques to local communities in developing countries, saving millions of lives. As described in Chapter VIII, one of these was the selective primary health care approach popularized by John Knowles and operationalized by UNICEF using the acronym GOBI. Under its director Kenneth Warren and associate director Scott Halstead, the division now set out to accelerate global immunization strategies that would help make the Expanded Program on Immunization a success.

To do so, Warren needed to ignite interest within the international community for a renewed effort to address childhood diseases, and he coordinated a conference at the Foundation's Bellagio Center in Italy. Convened in March 1984 and known as "Bellagio I," the conference included senior leaders and public health experts from the WHO, UNICEF, the World Bank, and the United Nations Development Program, as well as key individuals from major bilateral donor agencies. Sir Gustav Nossal, director of the Walter and Eliza Hall Institute of Medical Research in Melbourne, Australia—who had been knighted for his groundbreaking work in immunology—delivered the call to action.

Nossal was concerned that the Expanded Program on Immunization concentrated on delivering health services and current vaccines without putting money into basic research. He reminded the scientists and policymakers in the room that biotechnology was beginning to open new strategies for vaccine development. "Dreams of great daring are being dreamt," Nossal enthused, "extending the concept of vaccination from viruses and bacteria to single-celled or multi-cellular parasites and even to non-infectious diseases like cancer and multiple sclerosis. The sky seems to be the limit."

One major result of Bellagio I was the formation of the Task Force for Child Survival, which included the Foundation's Scott Halstead as a member. The task force articulated a new goal of 1990 as a deadline for the Universal Childhood Immunization initiative, which had been designed to have an immediate impact and to do the greatest good for the greatest number of people. Where the Expanded Program on Immunization had called for the vaccination of all children, Universal Childhood Immunization (UCI) sought a more realistic goal given the resources available. UCI aimed to immunize 80 percent of all children under the age of one by 1990 with the six vaccines—tuberculosis, diphtheria, neonatal tetanus, whooping cough, poliomyelitis, and measles—at a cost of five dollars per child. Furthermore, the initiative put in place strategies to increase vaccine coverage and reduce the dropout rates between the first and last immunization. These strategies included national campaigns—conducted with intensive publicity and media support—to promote immunization and involve religious leaders, teachers, and other community leaders in these efforts.

The Task Force for Child Survival also helped to eliminate bureaucratic issues and reduce institutional rivalries among the U.N.'s subordinate health agencies, where tensions had been running high over the future direction of the Expanded Program on Immunizations. With the creation of the task force, international health leaders found an alternative vehicle for accelerating EPI's immunization activities in the form of Universal Childhood Immunization. The Rockefeller Foundation committed $879,200 ($2 million in 2013 dollars) over ten years to this initiative.

The Foundation's involvement in accelerating EPI was hardly surprising. Universal Childhood Immunization reflected the strategies inherent in selective primary health care, the approach developed by Kenneth Warren and Julia Walsh, supported by former Foundation president John Knowles, and championed by Jim Grant, UNICEF's executive director and a Foundation board member. One of Universal Childhood Immunization's core strategies was mobilizing politicians and government officials, usually coordinated by Grant, who often visited heads of state and held participating countries up to global standards to benefit children.

Even as the Foundation and its new partners worked with multinational agencies to expand the delivery of vaccines to the world's poor, it looked for ways to leverage the skills and financial resources of the private sector to expand basic research related to new vaccines. To stimulate investment, for example, the Task Force for Child Survival offered commercial manufacturers and public institutions financial assistance to help offset the high research costs of vaccine development. In exchange, the task force asked commercial producers to guarantee lower vaccine prices and to promote production of affordable vaccines for the developing world—so-called orphan vaccines. The task force developed these relationships by soliciting proposals from potential manufacturers and public institutions.

In the 1960s, Donald "D.A." Henderson led the international effort to eradicate smallpox. Attending Bellagio II in Cartagena in October 1985, he asserted that of the six vaccines in use by the Expanded Program on Immunization, none were fully satisfactory and continued research was needed as part of a global vaccination campaign. (Centers for Disease Control and Prevention.)

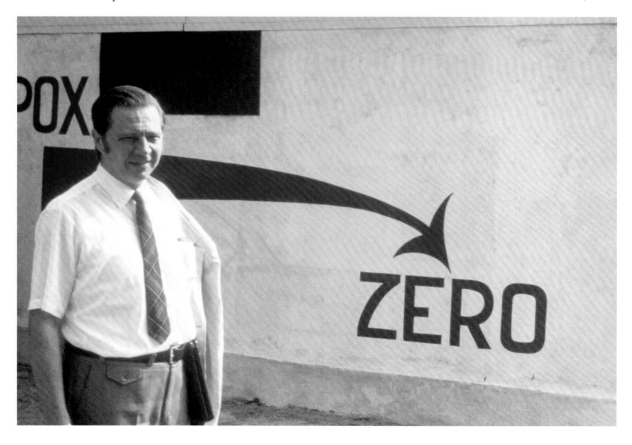

The enthusiasm ignited at Bellagio I in March 1984 continued in October 1985 with "Bellagio II," which was actually held in Cartagena, Colombia. At this second Rockefeller Foundation conference, scientists offered arguments for the importance of furthering biotechnology and vaccine development. At the time, the Expanded Program on Immunization was still delivering vaccines for polio, tuberculosis, diphtheria, pertussis, tetanus, and measles. At Bellagio II, Donald Ainslie "D.A." Henderson, dean of the Johns Hopkins School of Public Health, echoed the concerns raised earlier by Gustav Nossal and others. An epidemiologist who had played a key role in the worldwide eradication of smallpox, Henderson suggested that vaccine delivery could not be separated from basic research, and he reminded the group that smallpox could not have been eradicated without such work. He asserted that "Not one of the [six] vaccines we are using in the [EPI] program is fully satisfactory."

Henderson's comments and the broader discussion at Bellagio II helped policymakers and potential donors focus on the real costs of providing universal vaccine coverage, which were estimated at $1.5 billion a year ($3.26 billion in 2013 dollars). They concluded that $200 million to $300 million per year ($434 million to $651 million in 2013 dollars) would have to come from external (non-target-nation) donors.

These numbers and the renewed focus on the issue catalyzed by the conference helped bring potential donors to the table. A conference summary publication distributed worldwide, "Protecting the World's Children: Vaccines and Immunization within Primary Health Care," helped generate nearly $230 million ($499 million in 2013 dollars) pledged by Rotary International, the Government of Italy, and various foundations.

Kenneth Warren supported Henderson's call for more vaccine research. Warren hoped biotechnology would solve the difficulties with existing vaccines. Because the oral polio vaccine was perishable, for example, it required cold-chain delivery methods to survive in the tropics. The cost of refrigerated transportation was exorbitant in that part of the world. Similarly, the rabies vaccine was expensive and difficult to administer because it demanded serial administration of multiple doses to reach clinically effective immunity levels. Other vaccines had toxic side effects, which, when word spread among those already vaccinated to those requiring vaccination, reduced participation rates. The Foundation was also highly sensitive to issues concerning vaccine safety, given its history with chenopodium and hookworm patients (see Chapter II). The underlying question posed by basic research advocates was whether ongoing investigations might lead to solutions to these problems or, ideally, to new vaccines that were both singularly potent and weather-resistant, with fewer side effects.

Warren also pushed public-sector institutions to involve themselves in vaccine development. In 1984 he had helped create the Program for Vaccine Development—as a special group within the WHO—which had its origins in a discussion between Warren and Fakhry Assaad, the director of the WHO's Division of Communicable Diseases. Soon after that discussion, Warren was contacted by the Pew Charitable Trusts, which collaborated with the Rockefeller Foundation to provide $4 million as seed money to launch the project. A precursor to the Children's Vaccine Initiative, the Program for Vaccine Development encouraged vaccine research and product development, but this was a small step compared to the great strides that were needed.

As was often the case, the Foundation's involvement was not only financial. Scott Halstead brought his expertise in tropical infectious diseases to the project as a member of the WHO Advisory Committee on Dengue, which was working on the development of a dengue vaccine. Halstead later took over from Warren the Strategic Advisory Group of Experts (SAGE) on Immunization that advised the Program for Vaccine Development, which received $3.7 million in funding from the Foundation from 1984 through 1989. By 1990 this program oversaw 87 projects in 19 countries dealing with general problems of vaccine effectiveness.

Warren had hoped that the Program for Vaccine Development would promote both product development and basic research, but the project—and the WHO in general—emphasized basic research at the expense of product development. "We could not get those guys to be practical," Warren said. "They were acting like basic scientists.... They were doing bits and pieces without putting it together." In addition, the program struggled to raise the funds it needed to expand its impact on vaccine research and development. Despite these disappointments, the effort did help spark a new wave of research in vaccines, and from this research new vaccines were developed that would prove effective, both clinically and in the field.

THE SEARCH FOR IMPROVED VACCINES

At Bellagio II, a tall, bearded epidemiologist painted a picture of the ideal vaccine. William Foege was the chairman of the Task Force for Child Survival. A renowned physician, he had helped manage the global strategy to eradicate smallpox, working in the field in Africa during the 1970s. Between 1977 and 1983 he served as director of the U.S. Centers for Disease Control (CDC) under President Jimmy Carter, but he left government service when the Reagan administration began cutting the CDC's budget at the dawn of the AIDS epidemic. His interest in the efficacy of vaccination campaigns led him to the Task Force for Child Survival.

Foege suggested that researchers should focus on a vaccine that would contain all the necessary antigens in a single injection, provide lifelong immunity with a single dose, have no short-term or long-term adverse reactions, and be inexpensive, easily administered, stable at tropical temperatures for months—or even years, and efficacious if administered any time after birth. Foege and others attending the conference agreed that program managers would sacrifice some amount of vaccine delivery in exchange for an increased emphasis on basic research that might one day result in this Holy Grail of vaccines. Most of the Bellagio II attendees understood the urgency. Given the millions of children who were dying from vaccine-preventable deaths—40,000 per week from measles alone—something had to be done.

The Rockefeller Foundation agreed to provide funding to support the initiatives that emerged from the Bellagio conferences. Through the Task Force for Child Survival, for example, the Foundation made grants to strengthen the management structure within the Ministry of Health in Uganda in its fight against measles, whooping cough, polio, tetanus, diphtheria, and tuberculosis.

By the time the task force was disbanded in 1990, basic childhood vaccination rates for six communicable diseases—tuberculosis, measles, diphtheria, pertussis, tetanus, and polio—had been increased from roughly 5 percent in the early 1970s to nearly 80 percent. Universal Childhood Immunization would be recognized as one of the most important global immunization initiatives in decades.

Children's Vaccine Initiative

At the World Summit for Children, mobilized by UNICEF in New York in September 1990, the Children's Vaccine Initiative came together as a partnership between divisions of the Rockefeller Foundation, the U.N., the WHO, and the World Bank. Inspired by the chairman of the Task Force for Child Survival, William Foege, and his 1985 clarion call for a single-dose, multi-antigen vaccine, the initiative resulted from close coordination between the Foundation's Scott Halstead and UNICEF's James Grant and his staff, with strong impetus provided by the Commission on Health Research for Development, chaired by Rockefeller Foundation trustee John Evans. The idea was to create a "Manhattan-type project" for vaccines. Scott Halstead helped spread the idea of a single-dose vaccine among the WHO staff, and was one of the Children's Vaccine Initiative's founding members. These agencies hoped, by working together, to do what none of them could do working alone—advance a single-dose vaccine, from research to production to delivery, for all the world's children.

For the Rockefeller Foundation, this project built on decades of experience with yellow fever, malaria, and other arboviruses, during which the Foundation had learned to work across scientific communities in different countries. Like no other private nonprofit organization, the Foundation had formed close working relationships with the WHO and UNICEF. Because of its role as a major supporter of the Task Force for Child Survival and vaccine research and development in general, the Foundation had also come to be seen by the international community as a leader in the campaign to immunize the world's children.

The Children's Vaccine Initiative was intended to be a "long-term worldwide program to mobilize resources and develop an 'ideal' vaccine for children" that would build on the success of earlier initiatives. Since 1980, for example, the WHO's Expanded Program on Immunization had saved the lives of an estimated two to three million children per year. The Children's Vaccine Initiative sought to save an additional two to three million children per year, and protect an additional five to eight million more from disabilities, through new and improved vaccines. As it turned out, these goals were overambitious.

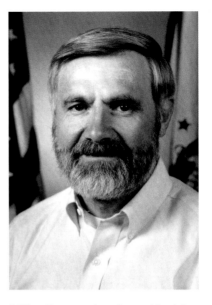

William Foege, an American epidemiologist, served as the director of the U.S. Centers for Disease Control from 1977 to 1983. With several colleagues, in 1984 he formed the Task Force for Child Survival, which helped accelerate childhood immunizations in developing countries. He served as a trustee of the Rockefeller Foundation from 1997 to 2008. (Centers for Disease Control and Prevention.)

The Children's Vaccine Initiative achieved major successes, but for scientists and policymakers there were also disappointments. The scientists involved underestimated the amount of time required to translate their new research into a vaccine. Donor fatigue set in as a result, even as scientists grew frustrated because they felt the program did not receive the research budget it needed to be successful. Meanwhile, according to historian William Muraskin, rivalries between international agencies undermined the political consensus needed to sustain the program. In the end, researchers were not able to develop a single "magic bullet" vaccine.

Despite these disappointments, the Children's Vaccine Initiative consultative group (composed of public, private, governmental, and NGO representatives) made several major contributions to improving the health of children around the world. New vaccines were produced and added to the development pipeline, while the process created by the project for analyzing vaccine quality and supply provided a model for others. The project also highlighted key issues in vaccine development in the age of biotechnology. And it provided valuable political lessons for future vaccine initiatives and funders, including the Bill and Melinda Gates Children's Vaccine Program. Most important, by the time the initiative ended in 1999, vaccines against measles, diphtheria, pertussis, rubella, polio, and tetanus had been delivered to more than 75 percent of the children in the world.

HEALTH SCIENCES FOR THE TROPICS

While the Children's Vaccine Initiative worked to promote the development of new vaccines and the vaccination of children in the developing world, parallel efforts sought to increase the capacity of developing nations to create new vaccines closer to home. In the 1960s and 1970s, the Foundation's University Development Program had invested in facilities and people to train a new generation of medical and scientific professionals. The program—later named Education for Development—ended in the 1970s, but in the mid-1980s, the Foundation created its International Program to Support Science-Based Development, which continued the interdisciplinary effort to transfer technology and expertise from the developed to the developing world.

The Great Neglected Diseases program (see Chapter IX) had further demonstrated that scientists from developing nations could be trained to work in their local environment, rather than move to research centers in the developed world. It also suggested that attacking diseases in the developing world could be more effectively achieved by building research institutions in the developing world. However, the program had fallen short of meeting the Foundation's goal of creating research capacity in tropical countries, and a new strategy was needed. In 1987 the Foundation ended its Great Neglected Diseases program in order to focus more closely on building vaccine capacity in less developed nations.

This new strategy focused on matching institutions in developing nations with those in developed countries so that scientific knowledge and information on infrastructure and support systems for research and development could be transferred at the same time. Thus, in September 1987 the Health Sciences Division launched the program Health Sciences for the Tropics, planned and funded jointly with the WHO, to build partnerships between laboratories in developed and developing nations around the world to better target diseases afflicting the poor. More than 200

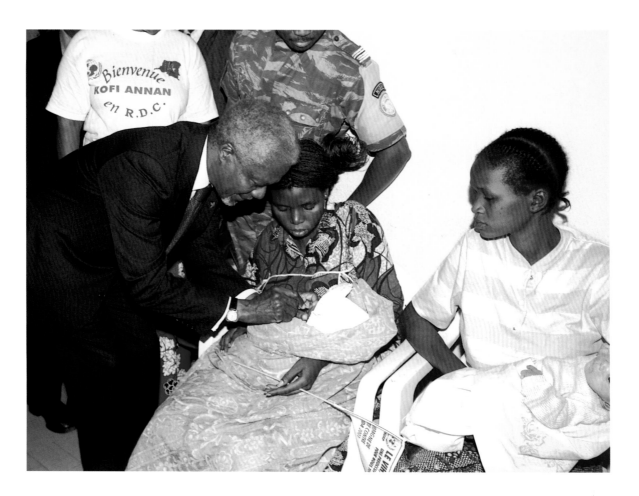

would-be partners applied, hoping to be one of the ten partnerships the Foundation had said it would fund. The applications were so impressive, however, that the Foundation expanded the funding and awarded grants to 40 laboratories, or 20 percent of all applicants. Appropriations in 1987 totaled $1.3 million ($2.7 million in 2013 dollars), awarded to those research facilities judged by an advisory council to have the greatest potential to train or receive training in the prevention and control of amebiasis, Chagas disease, childhood diarrheas, malaria, and schistosomiasis—major diseases of the developing world.

Efforts to vaccinate children against polio and other diseases continued after the end of the Children's Vaccine Initiative in 1999. United Nations Secretary-General Kofi Annan administered a polio vaccine to a baby at a hospital in Kinshasa in the Democratic Republic of the Congo in 2001. (Evan Schneider. United Nations.)

Following its historical pattern, the Foundation worked to build networks of professionals by facilitating the exchange of personnel between institutions, creating an advisory panel, and organizing annual meetings.

During this program the Foundation allocated a total of $7.7 million. In contrast to previous Foundation programs that had allocated finances only to the lead institution in the developed country, Health Sciences for the Tropics provided grants to both of the paired institutions, thus establishing a true partnership. Additional aspects of the program that led to its success included collaborative research projects addressing the developing nation's health issues, along with an exchange of personnel between the developed and developing nations' labs. Finally, as with previous Rockefeller development programs, a hallmark of Health Sciences for the Tropics was a series of scientific meetings and site visits conducted by WHO officers.

These grants helped build capacity in the developing world and strengthened scientific networks. The Foundation supported these networks by helping to cultivate an interest in science within the general population. In Africa, for example, Foundation staff developed a program to popularize science and technology in the schools and cultures. The Foundation also partnered with the Carnegie Corporation and the MacArthur Foundation to support the establishment of the African Academy of Sciences in 1985.

These efforts supported a broader goal to help developing countries become self-sufficient in vaccine research and development. But the Rockefeller Foundation was also increasingly aware that developing countries faced challenges related to the production of vaccines as well.

Technology Transfer Program for Vaccine Production

The Foundation viewed technology transfer for vaccine production as a critical facet of the Children's Vaccine Initiative. In the mid-1980s, many pharmaceutical companies in the developed world were reluctant to teach developing countries how to produce affordable vaccines. By promoting the construction of production facilities in the developing world, the Foundation and its partners hoped to break this pattern of dependency and assure more affordable prices.

Once again, the Foundation's long history provided precedent for a new initiative. During World War Two, the Foundation had helped to establish yellow fever vaccine manufacturing operations around the world. Local manufacturing helped to increase the supply, improve access, and, in some cases, lower prices for immunization. In the mid-1980s, however, without the exigencies of war, this initiative looked daunting.

Successful technology transfer depends on the capacity of recipient countries to absorb, translate, and transmit knowledge within the academic, philanthropic, private-sector, and public-sector institutions that comprise their national research and innovation systems. Vaccine manufacture, in particular, posed substantial risks to investors. A successful vaccine production and distribution campaign, for example, can eradicate a disease, drying up demand and leaving investors with manufacturing plants that might no longer be useful or profitable. Moreover, vaccine production requires a skilled workforce with experience in a broad range of specialty areas, each of which may be specific to the vaccine in question.

The Foundation began its vaccine production technology transfer project by hosting a series of meetings in 1985. These conversations led the Foundation's board to allocate $6.6 million between 1985 and 1993 to this new initiative. With these funds, in Colombia, Japan, and Thailand, the Foundation helped to develop tissue-culture techniques that are useful in the manufacture of vaccines against dengue, Japanese encephalitis, and both human and veterinary rabies. Once these vaccines were created, the Foundation helped developing nations acquire the training methods and facilities needed to test the safety and efficacy of these vaccines with their own populations—a critical first step before local production can begin.

The Foundation also provided grants to make viral vaccine production a generic and technically accessible process available at moderate cost to developing countries. Grants to the Veterinary Products Company of Colombia, for example, helped enable the construction of a new plant to produce a rabies vaccine, the cost of which was reduced by the facility's large-scale manufacturing systems. In some instances, the Foundation also placed staff in recipient countries to assist with the transfer of technology.

Meanwhile the Foundation supported other organizations working in the same arena. Grants to the WHO's regional arm in Latin America—the Pan American Health Organization—helped create vaccine research and development centers in Brazil and Mexico. Epidemiological studies showed that these locations would be ideal for cost-effective manufacturing and distribution. Both countries had strong scientific communities, and the Foundation was already supporting active research on tropical diseases, such as malaria, in these regions.

All of this work to enable vaccine research, development, and production in the developing world complemented the Foundation's ongoing efforts to help strengthen health care delivery. Given the expertise of the Health Sciences staff in population-based, community health, the Foundation's focus increasingly shifted to the strategy and structure of health systems.

Beginning in 1969, for financial and programmatic reasons, the Foundation had started to reduce its field staff operating in foreign countries. Pressure on the Foundation's endowment—combined with a growing realization that many countries were ambivalent, if not opposed, to development initiatives that were not homegrown or locally managed—led to a fundamentally new approach. In 1968 the Foundation had 136 field staff outside the United States. By 1981 this number was down to 34. Without "boots on the ground," the Foundation would focus increasingly on collaborative approaches that would leverage philanthropic dollars and institutional resources.

In the short run, however, the Rockefeller Foundation's reductions in force and overall grantmaking were disconcerting, especially within the context of broader trends in philanthropy. U.S.-based foundations, still the primary donors to global charitable projects, were on the decline. By 1980 less than five cents of every dollar granted by U.S. private foundations went to projects in foreign nations.

Rockefeller Foundation President Richard Lyman predicted that the governments of developed nations would be unlikely to step in and take up the slack in fostering international development. "Governments are notoriously weak at thinking through a problem and its proposed solution before undertaking to act. And they generally have difficulty evaluating the effects of an attempted solution once these become detectable." For these and other reasons, in health care especially, he looked to collaborate with universities and community organizations in less developed countries.

With efforts already underway to strengthen vaccine research and epidemiological networks in the developing world in 1987, the Foundation sought to foster the creation of nonprofit health-management organizations through the formation of a training program for public health managers, who would advise developing nations' governments. A collaborative network was established among Boston-based Management Sciences for Health in the U.S., Jakarta's Yayasan Indonesia Sejahtera, and, in India, New Delhi's Centre for Health Research and Development. This consortium was expected to examine staff-training issues, insurance policies, drug management and delivery methods, and medical information sharing. Unfortunately, in the short run, these nonprofit health-management organizations did not take off, and by 1987 this research capacity model was absorbed by INCLEN.

The nonprofit health-management organizations, and later INCLEN, sought to address the use and abuse of antibiotics; contraception; the quality of family planning programs; and the equitable distribution of medications in developing nations. On the subject of antibiotics, for example, the organizations obtained estimates of use and problems with resistance in various developing countries. The collaborative network then found that much of the information was anecdotal or biased toward one group, and thus was not representative of the nation as a whole. To improve the data, the network recommended a set of empirical guidelines for the diagnosis and management of common conditions requiring antibiotics, which would take into account social, financial, and manpower constraints as well as local findings about the presence of resistant bacteria.

Overall, by the late 1980s, the Foundation had expanded its focus on population-based health care in a number of directions. The work of the Great Neglected Diseases program had been redirected into several vaccine initiatives, including the Task Force for Child Survival and the Children's Vaccine Initiative; the vaccine production technology transfer program for increasing the application of biotechnology in the developing world; and Health Sciences for the Tropics. These efforts delivered not only vaccines that protected millions of people against measles, diphtheria, pertussis, rubella, polio, and tetanus, but also vaccine-production training and technology that would make vaccines more widely available, often at reduced costs. Along the way, the Foundation built and maintained, through conferences and exchanges, a strong network of experts in global health who were cooperating with the WHO, UNICEF, and other multilateral agencies. In the process, the Foundation had asserted its role as a serious and reliable partner in the development of vaccines. The lessons learned in both the research and the development of multilateral partnerships in these vaccine initiatives would prove invaluable at the end of the twentieth century as the world encountered an apparently new and mysterious disease.

"These efforts delivered not only vaccines that protected millions of people against measles, diphtheria, pertussis, rubella, polio, and tetanus, but also vaccine-production training and technology that would make vaccines more widely available, often at reduced costs."

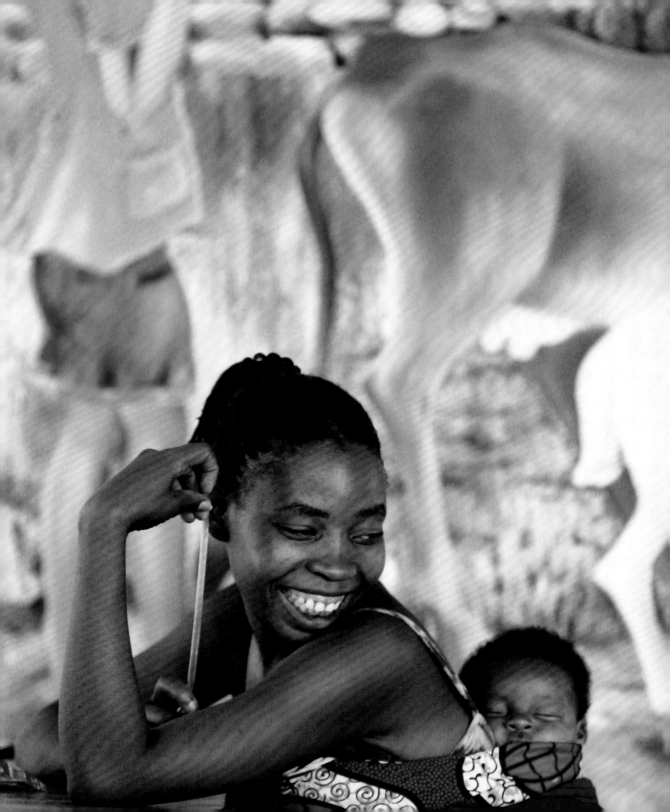

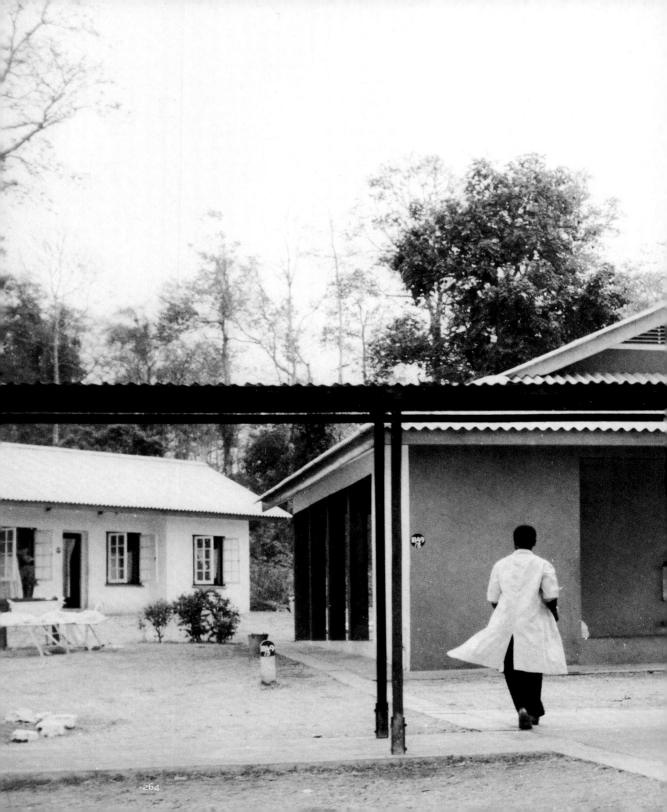

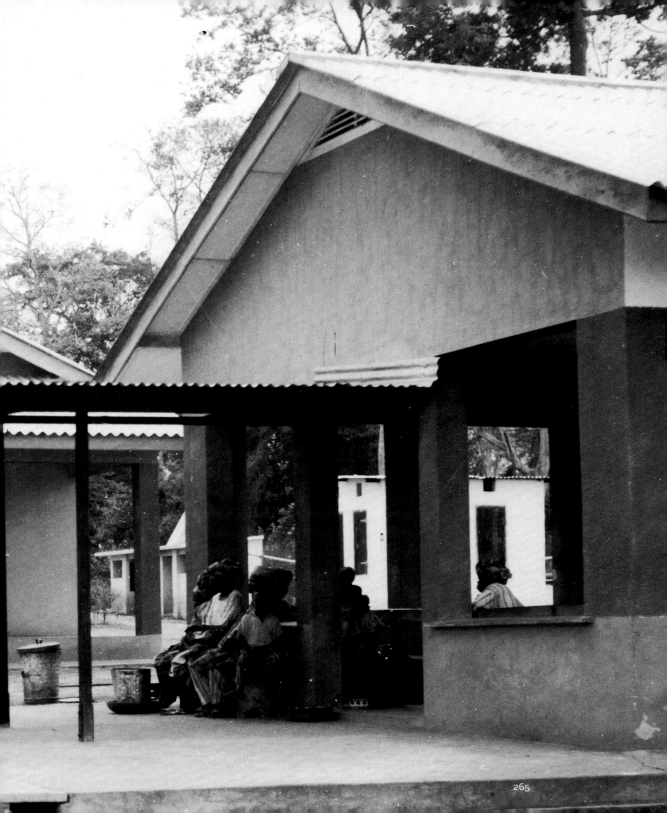

FIGHTING A GLOBAL SCOURGE

In the fall of 1980, Michael Gottlieb, a young immunologist at the University of California, Los Angeles (UCLA) Medical Center, was asked to consult on a strange case of *Pneumocystis carinii* pneumonia complicated by opportunistic infections. The case made no sense. In a young, otherwise healthy patient, the immune system should have been able to fight back. But lab tests revealed that the patient's immune system had collapsed. Nothing Gottlieb and his staff prescribed seemed to stop the spread of infections or restore the immune system. By February 1981, Gottlieb had three other patients under observation. Nothing he did worked. By March the first patient had been hospitalized. He died in May.

Gottlieb reported his observations in the *Morbidity and Mortality Weekly Report* of the U.S. Centers for Disease Control (CDC). Over the next few months other doctors in the United States and Europe reported similar incidents—strange cases of *Pneumocystis carinii* and a rare form of Kaposi sarcoma cancer. The cases were clustered among homosexual men, intravenous drug users, young children who needed blood transfusions, and prostitutes, but one common thread connected all the cases: the patients had devastated immune systems. Epidemiologists were stumped. Were they looking at an environmental cause? A complex of bacterial causes? A virus? How was the mystery agent spread from person to person? By blood? By sexual contact? If it could be

HIV, a retrovirus that inserts a copy of its DNA into the host cell, was first identified in 1983 as the cause of AIDS. Researchers used transmission electron microscopy to record this image of the virus in a tissue sample. (Centers for Disease Control and Prevention.)

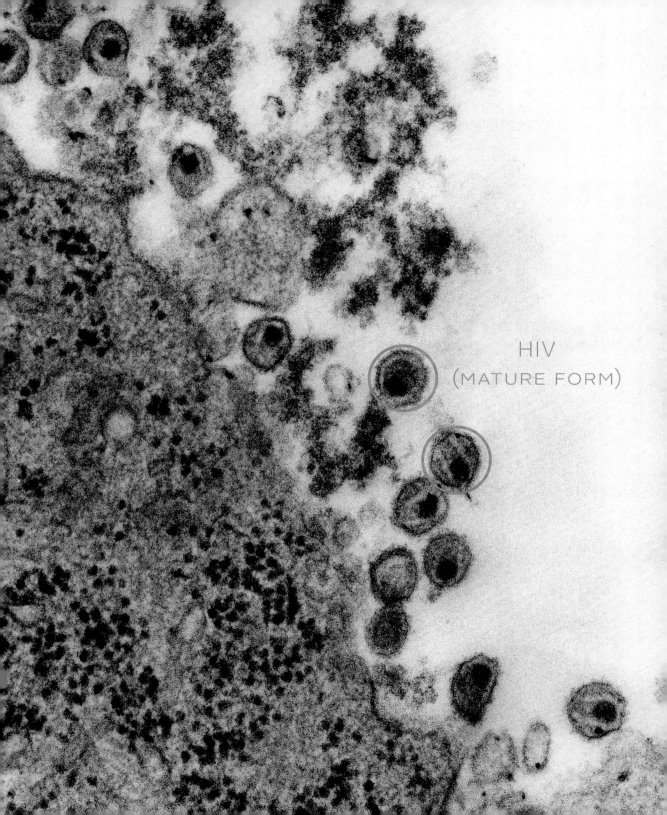

HIV
(MATURE FORM)

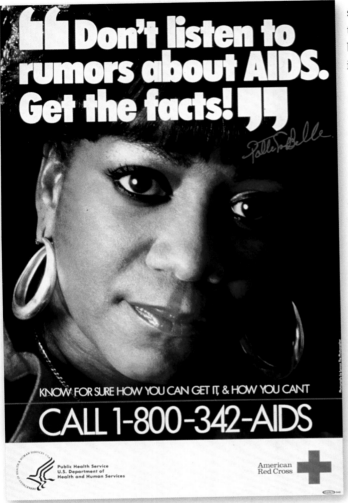

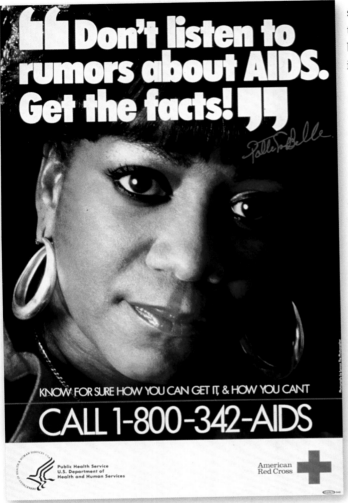
spread by a needle during a blood transfusion, could it be spread by a mosquito? Was it connected in some way to gay lifestyles? Could a husband infect his wife? Could a pregnant woman pass it to her unborn baby? These were unanswered questions in 1981, but the grim reality was that the infection appeared to be 100 percent fatal. No one understood what was happening at the time, but the world was on the precipice of the most devastating epidemic since the "black death" of the fourteenth century.

As it became apparent in the late 1980s that AIDS was a global pandemic, leaders at the Rockefeller Foundation debated its potential role in addressing the crisis. People on every continent were infected, and the epidemic was no longer limited to small clusters of homosexuals or drug addicts or hemophiliacs. In Africa AIDS was rampant. It was killing young mothers and creating thousands of orphans. It also

Pop singer Patti LaBelle helped dispel fears about AIDS in the mid-1980s by working with the American Red Cross and the U.S. Public Health Service to encourage people to "get the facts." (American Red Cross. National Library Medicine.)

cut down people in the prime of their professional careers. Officially, the number of AIDS cases had risen to 60,000 by 1988. Ten thousand cases had been identified in the developing world. But officials at the World Health Organization worried that they were seeing only the tip of the iceberg. They estimated that as many as two million Africans might be infected. In some African countries, life expectancy, after rising for nearly 30 years, was already beginning to drop. With no vaccine and no drug treatment protocol, governments promoted prevention through education campaigns, local diagnostic capabilities, blood bank screening, counseling services, and condom distribution.

Chapter Eleven: Fighting a Global Scourge

Looking for ways to contribute to the fight against AIDS, the Foundation sought to address critical gaps in the research on HIV, the virus that causes AIDS, especially with regard to its relationship to reproductive health. With the Ford and MacArthur Foundations, the Rockefeller Foundation funded the creation of the AIDS and Reproductive Health Network at Harvard. Other AIDS grants supported non-research initiatives like the International HIV/AIDS Alliance, which raised and channeled donor funds to national consortia in developing countries. These national consortia, or "linking organizations," provided small grants and technical support to grassroots NGOs working on AIDS prevention and care. In 1989 the Foundation gave $750,000 ($1.4 million in 2013 dollars) for three two-year grants: a collaborative study with Makerere University in Kampala, Uganda, on heterosexual transmission of AIDS; a collaborative study with the Ugandan Government AIDS Control Program on the effect of health education on transmission of HIV; and a study with the Health Department of Pikine, Senegal, of integrated STD/AIDS prevention and family planning services. Over a 12-year period between 1989 and 2001, the Foundation invested over $20 million in 102 different AIDS grants. But the biggest investment—$9 million—would be in a major effort to develop an AIDS vaccine.

Seth Berkley

A tall, curly-haired, long-distance runner, Seth Berkley reflected the tradition of the progressive, intellectual physician-scientists who staffed the Rockefeller Institute and the Foundation's International Health Division in the early years. He had grown up in a lower-middle-class neighborhood in New York City, studied medicine at Harvard, and in 1984 went to work as a medical epidemiologist at the National Center for Infectious Diseases at the CDC. During his time at the CDC, he spent time in Sudan investigating famine. When he left the CDC in 1986, he joined William Foege's team at the Carter Center in Atlanta.

The AIDS epidemic was raging in Africa, and Berkley was sent to Uganda, where he was instrumental in helping the Ministry of Health establish Uganda's AIDS surveillance system and AIDS Control Program. He became an attending physician at Mulago Hospital in Kampala. From the frontlines of the AIDS epidemic, Berkley became a champion for vaccine research.

In the United States and Europe, a highly organized AIDS activist movement was focused on developing treatments for those already infected. But Berkley's experience in Africa showed that the epidemic was out of control there, becoming a permanent part of the epidemiological landscape. Even if scientists could develop drugs to keep AIDS patients alive, these drugs would be expensive and hard to administer in developing countries, and they did nothing to prevent initial infection. Drugs might help to manage a growing epidemic over time, but they could not stop it. Berkley believed that only a vaccine could beat AIDS.

In 1988 Berkley moved back to the United States to become associate director of Health Sciences at the Rockefeller Foundation and to help lead the Foundation's response to the growing AIDS epidemic. He suggested the idea of an AIDS vaccine initiative, but for the Foundation the prospect of such a massive effort seemed almost overwhelming. The Foundation's resources paled in comparison to those of private sector pharmaceutical companies and publicly funded agencies like the World Health Organization, the Centers for Disease Control, the National Institutes of Health, and the National Science Foundation, as well as dozens of smaller government programs and research universities. Moreover, frustrations at the U.S. National Institutes of Health underscored the challenges. In 1984 U.S. Secretary of Health and Human Services Margaret Heckler had announced that with the support of the federal government a vaccine for AIDS would be ready for testing in two years.

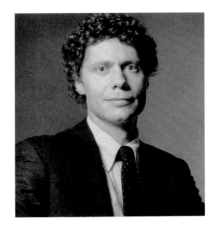

Seth Berkley became associate director for Health Sciences at the Rockefeller Foundation in 1988. He led the effort to launch the International AIDS Vaccine Initiative in 1996, then became CEO of this innovative product-development partnership. (Rockefeller Archive Center.)

Heckler's deadline came and passed. Although the U.S. National Institute of Allergy and Infectious Diseases and its collaborators at the biotechnology company MicroGeneSys launched the first AIDS vaccine trial, it was not successful and many AIDS researchers believed that support for the search for a vaccine was waning within the federal government. Meanwhile other private sector efforts were underway. In 1986, for example, Merck & Co. began work on an AIDS vaccine. And scientists at various biotechnology companies including Genentech were exploring possible routes for the development of a vaccine. But by the mid-1990s, these efforts had not produced fundamental breakthroughs. Critics charged that government and private industry were not doing enough.

At the Rockefeller Foundation, President Peter Goldmark supported the idea of investing in vaccine research. Reflecting on the world's experiences with smallpox, yellow fever, polio, and measles, he wrote: "Never in history has a serious viral public health threat been eliminated without the use of a vaccine." But Goldmark was concerned about the expense, the long time frame for research, and how a vaccine initiative would be organized. It had

Chapter Eleven: Fighting a Global Scourge

taken 47 years to create a vaccine for polio. Berkley and others hoped that with HIV it might take only two decades, but the costs would be enormous and well beyond the means of a single nonprofit foundation.

Berkley and Goldmark believed that somewhere in the intersection of governments, international agencies, the pharmaceutical industry, and non-profit philanthropy, an economic model for vaccine development could be constructed. They became convinced that the Rockefeller Foundation could play a pivotal role, but they needed the board's support.

Berkley took his vaccine development proposal to the Rockefeller trustees and found a powerful ally in Peggy Dulany, the great-granddaughter of John D. Rockefeller. "She talked about why it was important for foundations to get involved in big problems like this," Berkley remembered years later. And as they pushed their ideas forward, these champions within the Foundation formulated a concept that would catalyze a global effort aimed at developing a safe, effective, and inexpensive vaccine that could be made available in the developing world—where the vast majority of new cases were occurring. Along the way, they would also develop an institutional prototype that was able to respond in instances of market failure that would pave the way for new initiatives focused on other diseases that overwhelmingly attacked the poor and vulnerable around the world.

Forging an Alliance

With the trustees' support, the Foundation began to convene meetings of experts and representatives of political entities and international agencies to talk about a vaccine for AIDS. At Bellagio in 1994, the Foundation hosted what *Science* magazine described as the most important and diverse group of experts that had ever been gathered on the subject of AIDS vaccines. It included research scientists and institutional leaders. As Berkley explained, "We brought in U.N. agencies and the World Bank. We also brought some biotech companies and government officials. We tried to bring in a broad cross-section of stakeholders and ask whether a vaccine was possible. The answer was yes, but the scientists believed a new approach was needed. Later, there were meetings on structure and financing, intellectual property, and, most interestingly, meetings of the AIDS community."

Soon after the Bellagio conference, the Rockefeller Foundation organized the Ad Hoc Scientific Committee on "Accelerating the Development of Preventive HIV Vaccines for the World." Meeting at the Val-de-Grâce Hospital in Paris in late October 1994, the committee members recognized that they would

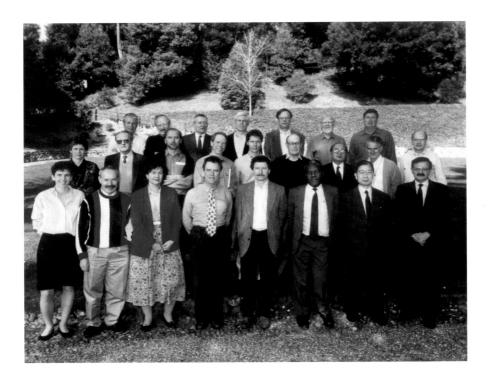

have to mobilize the entire world community, including governments, private companies, NGOs, and international agencies. The effort would need to take calculated scientific and financial risks, with the understanding that failure would often be the result. Berkley asked the participants, for the moment, to forget the current programs in place; to ignore national boundaries, resource constraints, and politics; and to focus instead on the need for a strategic scientific plan.

Experts from around the world gathered at the Rockefeller Foundation's Bellagio Center in 1994 to discuss efforts to develop a vaccine for HIV. Seeds planted during the meeting led to the creation of the International AIDS Vaccine Initiative in 1996. (International AIDS Vaccine Initiative.)

Berkley also brought together leaders from developing countries, some of whom were uneasy with the idea of a new initiative. They wanted to make sure this effort was not going to take away resources needed for treatment. Berkley tried to reassure them.

Despite all of these concerns, the meetings convinced Berkley and others at the Rockefeller Foundation that "without a substantial scientific breakthrough or other large change in the incentive structure it is unlikely that there will be a major effort by the large pharmaceutical industry on its own." To address this situation, the Rockefeller Foundation began to work on developing an innovative public-private partnership to support vaccine research and clinical trials in the developing world.

In September 1995, when AIDS researchers from around the world gathered in Chiang Mai in northern Thailand, the Rockefeller Foundation was the largest U.S. foundation engaged in funding international efforts to fight HIV/AIDS. To oversee this grantmaking, the Foundation had created a program called "HIV in the Developing World." But on the eve of this conference, the Foundation and its partners were preparing to announce a bold new initiative.

At the time, the epidemic in Thailand was ferocious. A million of the nation's 60 million residents had already been infected. The government was aggressively seeking a way to block the spread of the disease, and was preparing to start efficacy trials on a potential new vaccine. But no one was wildly optimistic. In the United States, the Food and Drug Administration had decided that the vaccine the Thais were testing offered too little hope to warrant authorizing a trial. Among the meeting participants, there was a widely shared belief that something more had to be tried.

On the final morning of the conference, Seth Berkley told the assembled group: "The AIDS vaccine effort is foundering. We can't let the effort die." To reinvigorate the search, Berkley said, the Rockefeller Foundation would help launch the International AIDS Vaccine Initiative (IAVI). Berkley suggested that IAVI would follow the "social venture capital" model in which the Rockefeller and other foundations would fund scientific research in collaboration with pharmaceutical companies, as long as the drug companies pledged to distribute vaccines widely to poor nations at a reasonable cost. This approach built on lessons learned in the Great Neglected Diseases program and Children's Vaccine Initiative, but it also reflected the Foundation's long and rich history in global health and other arenas.

On one hand, IAVI continued the tradition of vaccine work begun in the 1910s and carried through in different contexts for nearly eight decades. But it also incorporated lessons learned in completely different arenas. In agriculture, for example, during the Green Revolution of the 1960s, the Foundation had sparked the development of research institutions focused on particular crops and created a worldwide network to share research in agricultural science. These unique international agricultural institutions involved governments, private enterprise, and university scientists. The success of these institutions, many of which thrived long after the Foundation ended its initial support, created a belief within the culture of the Foundation that, with its reputational capital, it could play a key role in bringing others together to launch new institutions targeting emerging problems around the world.

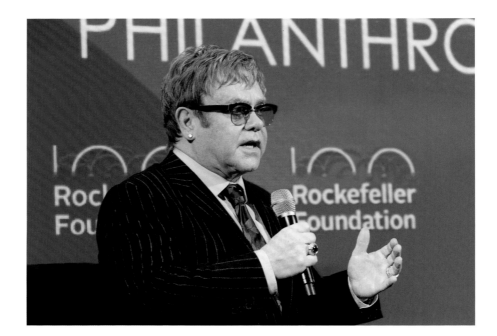

With Berkley named as CEO of IAVI, the Foundation invested $2.5 million in the start-up in 1996. "We started with $100,000 and one employee," he said later, "and were going to influence the world on a topic that was so expensive and so big. This was, to most people, patently ridiculous. Had we just started as an outside organization, we would have had zero chance of doing this." But, as Berkley pointed out, "there was a level of credibility that came from being part of the Rockefeller Foundation." The Foundation's early grants to IAVI, which totaled $8 million in the first decade, provided critical initial capital.

Berkley and the IAVI staff sought partners and donors for the vaccine program, but were careful to avoid undercutting or taking resources away from proven treatment protocols. With the fears of treatment advocates in mind, Berkley cautiously encouraged other organizations to support IAVI's work, but he focused particularly on donors who were not already involved with AIDS.

Invited to a dinner at the home of Bill and Melinda Gates in 1998, Berkley was asked by Bill Gates how charitable dollars could help stop AIDS. Berkley described the IAVI approach to vaccine development. Gates read more about the issue and realized that there was no market incentive to create a vaccine for developing countries because they could not afford to pay the cost of research and development. The Bill & Melinda Gates Foundation agreed to

Elton John received the Rockefeller Foundation's Lifetime Achievement Award at the Foundation's centennial celebration in Washington, D.C., on October 30, 2013. The award recognized the entertainer's efforts to support AIDS care and vaccine development. (Ralph Alswang. Rockefeller Foundation.)

Chapter Eleven: Fighting a Global Scourge

join the Rockefeller Foundation in funding the initiative, providing $1.5 million in 1998 and $25 million in 1999, followed by a five-year commitment of $100 million in 2001.

With Rockefeller and Gates backing for IAVI, other foundations, nonprofits, and agencies joined the initiative, including the Starr and Alfred P. Sloan foundations, Fondation Marcel Mérieux, Until There's a Cure Foundation, the Elton John AIDS Foundation, the U.K.'s National AIDS Trust, and the World Bank. Berkley also galvanized support from the Joint United Nations Program on HIV/AIDS, European governments, and the National AIDS Trust. By February 2001, IAVI had a war chest of $239 million, with a goal of raising $550 million to support research and clinical trials.

The Challenge of HIV

Moving innovative ideas through the scientific process necessary to develop a vaccine for HIV was no easy task. The two traditional approaches to vaccine development sought to engage the immune system in blocking infection and to train the body to recognize and destroy cells infected with a virus. But HIV proved to be elusive. HIV weaves itself into the DNA of target cells, creating a lasting reservoir of infection, and it attacks the very cells that coordinate the immune response to viral infections. The most difficult problem for vaccine researchers, however, was HIV's ability to mutate and outmaneuver the body's immunological response. A highly effective vaccine would need to be able to block or kill hundreds of different versions of HIV.

The first challenge was to isolate and analyze antibodies that might neutralize a broad spectrum of HIV variants around the world. This would require a coordinated international effort, and IAVI organized a network of academic and independent laboratories to conduct the science. In 1998, with Rockefeller Foundation help, this effort expanded to Kenya and South Africa, locating AIDS research, for the first time, in two countries that had been dramatically affected by the epidemic. By 2002 the development of IAVI's international network led to the creation of the Neutralizing Antibody Consortium, an association of individual researchers and their laboratory staffs. When the consortium became sufficiently organized to benefit from regular communication, IAVI established the Neutralizing Antibody Center at Scripps Research Institute in La Jolla, California, to centralize the sharing of information. This new facility worked closely with the Duke Center for HIV/AIDS Vaccine Immunology and Immunogen Discovery created by the U.S. National Institute of Allergy and Infectious Diseases.

In the late 1990s and early 2000s, the search for antibodies proved frustrating and disappointing. Early optimism faded when researchers were unable to find a sufficiently powerful antibody or even trigger further production of less effective antibodies in animals or humans.

In parallel with efforts to identify antibodies, IAVI-funded researchers looked for ways to develop so-called killer T-cells that would attack the virus either alone or in combination with an antibody vaccine. Researchers had high hopes that clinical trials for a vaccine developed by Merck known as HVTN 502 or STEP would induce an immune response, but a series of trials organized by the South African AIDS Vaccine Initiative in 2007 proved the vaccine was ineffective. Meanwhile another group of researchers was pursuing a more traditional path of testing various formulations in animals and people in the hope that one might work, but these efforts also came to naught.

Nevertheless, IAVI-funded researchers continued the search. In 2006 IAVI began a massive effort to sift through an enormous number of specimens from people infected with HIV to find what *Science* writer Jon Cohen called "the rarest of immune system warriors against HIV—antibodies that could thwart almost every known strain of the virus." Scientists had discovered some of these so-called "broadly neutralizing antibodies," but most were able to combat only a few dozen of the hundreds of strains of HIV that had been catalogued.

The IAVI effort began to pay off in 2009. Nearly 28 years after the first HIV/AIDS patients were identified, and more than a decade after IAVI spun itself off from the Rockefeller Foundation, researchers at the Vaccine Research Center of the National Institutes of Health reported two broadly neutralizing antibodies, and quickly discovered many others. Promising research slowly crystallized into candidate vaccines, ready for clinical trials in the field. The Human Immunology Laboratory at Imperial College of Science, Technology and Medicine in London became a central repository for samples collected during clinical trials.

Also in 2009, researchers in Thailand demonstrated for the first time that a vaccine could actually prevent HIV infection. The protection was too weak to be worth licensing, but the scientific threshold had been crossed. With support from the Rockefeller Foundation, IAVI built a network of clinical research centers in central and southern Africa where vaccine candidates could be tested in the local environments in which patients lived, and where epidemiological studies could be conducted. The network required investments in laboratory capacity and the training of researchers.

Over the following four years, IAVI developed 13 HIV vaccine candidates into the early stages of human trials, and conducted 15 observational epidemiological studies in Africa. Although new vaccines continued to be developed, success continued to be elusive. In 2013 Anthony Fauci, the director of the

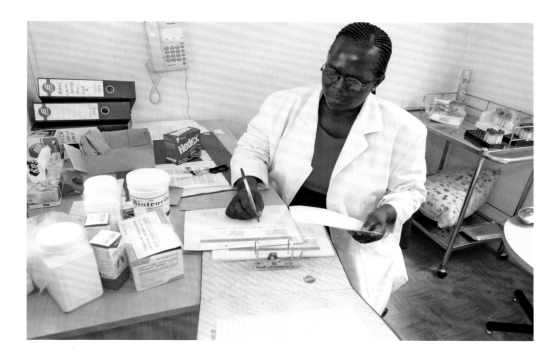

U.S. National Institute of Allergy and Infectious Diseases, reminded those attending the AIDS Vaccine Conference in Barcelona that the quest for an AIDS vaccine was a marathon, and not a sprint. In this race, IAVI had played an important part in setting the early pace.

The Kenya AIDS Vaccine Initiative was created in 1998 with support from the International AIDS Vaccine Initiative (IAVI). It was one of two research facilities established in Africa by IAVI to test promising new vaccines. (Vanessa Vick. International AIDS Vaccine Initiative.)

In the meantime, IAVI's early institutional success had already prompted a revolution in one segment of the business of drug development. IAVI had proved that public-private partnerships could help to fund and promote research and development of vaccines and treatments for the great neglected diseases that affected poor and vulnerable populations around the world. Acting on this proof of concept, the Rockefeller Foundation had launched a whirlwind of new initiatives.

A New Model for Collaborative Innovation

Sharing resources, leveraging credibility, supporting collaboration, and building partnerships typified the Rockefeller Foundation's approach to promoting the well-being of humanity at the end of the twentieth century, especially in arenas that demanded enormous long-term investments to promote fundamental innovations in medical science. In 2000 President Peter Goldmark summarized this approach when he reported that, "Today we

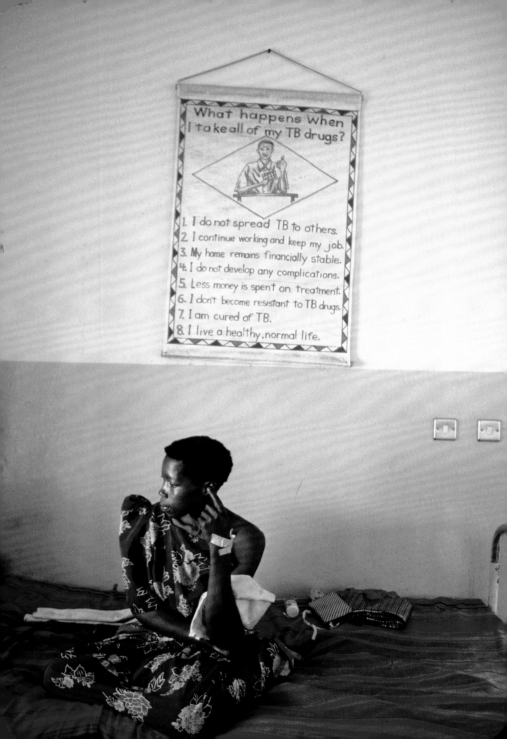

As HIV claimed more and more lives in the developing world, it was linked to a rise in deaths from tuberculosis, particularly in sub-Saharan Africa. Researchers discovered that people infected with HIV were 30 percent more likely to contract TB. In 2000 the Rockefeller Foundation helped create the Global Alliance for Tuberculosis Drug Development. (Jonas Bendiksen. Rockefeller Foundation.)

operate as a catalyst and partner among the myriad public, private and non-governmental organizations engaged in health-equity work."

The first replication of the IAVI model came in 1999 when the Medicines for Malaria Venture (MMV) was established with initial seed money of $4 million from the Rockefeller Foundation; the governments of Switzerland, the Netherlands, and the United Kingdom; and the World Bank, and launched under the umbrella of the WHO Special Program for Research and Training in Tropical Diseases. The venture aimed to discover and develop new effective and affordable antimalarials. The following year, the organization partnered with Glaxo Wellcome, the University of Bristol, and the London School of Hygiene and Tropical Medicine, bringing together a powerful combination of resources and expertise from the public and private sectors. Also in 2000, the Gates Foundation made a five-year commitment to provide $25 million, a commitment that was increased in 2003 to a total of $65 million over ten years. By 2005, well ahead of projections, MMV drugs were moving to clinical trials.

With the successful launch of IAVI and MMV, the Rockefeller Foundation sought to use this new institutional model to accelerate the development of vaccines and treatments for other neglected diseases. A year after helping to launch MMV, the Foundation participated in the creation of the Global Alliance for Tuberculosis Drug Development. Like IAVI and MMV, the alliance operated independently as a small virtual R&D company. Using Foundation money for initial research costs, pharmaceutical companies agreed to make the new drugs, once developed, available at cost to poor people in developing nations in return for guarantees from the ministries of health in those countries that they would purchase a certain number of doses. The Rockefeller Foundation made a long-term commitment of $15 million to help launch the program, and once again it partnered with the Gates Foundation, which added another $25 million. This seed money gave other funders confidence, leveraging another $150 million from foundations and international agencies. "We were able to do that because, when a foundation comes into the game, we kindle interest, add credibility, eliminate initial risk and stick with it for the long haul," Peter Goldmark explained in the Foundation's annual report in 2000.

In 2002 the Foundation provided funding to help launch another unique product development partnership. Pledging $15 million, the Foundation established the International Partnership for Microbicides to fight the spread of HIV with microbicidal foams and gels that could be inexpensively mass produced and used by women to protect themselves from sexually transmitted diseases. Following the pattern of previous initiatives, the Foundation organized a conference in 2000 of major stakeholders from the research community, the pharmaceutical industry, international organizations, advocacy groups, and potential donors. Scientific reports convinced major stakeholders that microbicides might help stem the spread of HIV and empower women whose husbands or partners refused to use a condom. The conversation continued, along with additional research. Finally, after the Foundation's financial commitment, other funders joined the partnership, including the Gates Foundation and the governments of the Netherlands, Ireland, the United Kingdom, Norway, and Denmark, along with the World Bank and the United Nations Population Fund.

As with the development of an AIDS vaccine, early optimism that a microbicide could be developed using basic over-the-counter ingredients was disappointed in the laboratory and in clinical trials. Researchers then shifted to strategies using anti-retroviral drugs, like those used to treat AIDS patients. By 2013 a number of microbicides were either ready for or actually in Phase III clinical trials. Zeda Rosenberg, the founding director of the International Partnership for Microbicides, and her co-investigator Robin Shattock were cautiously optimistic, expressing a "fervent hope that in the near future microbicides [would be] introduced as part of a comprehensive, multicomponent prevention strategy" for HIV.

All of these initiatives brought together the people and organizations in the public and private sectors that were needed to launch a major new initiative to attack a major disease. In 2008 a study by Julian Reiss and Philip Kitcher published by the London School of Economics (LSE) showed that these public-private partnerships were becoming essential to the development of new drugs and treatments for neglected diseases. The LSE report identified 47 similar collaborations covering 75 percent of all drug development for neglected diseases. Eighteen new drugs for neglected diseases were in clinical trials as a result of work performed by these partnerships, and two drugs were undergoing registration.

Many of these projects soon realized, however, that, as with AIDS, the development of vaccines or fundamentally new approaches to the treatment of great neglected diseases demanded patience and enormous amounts of capital. The LSE report noted that between 2000 and 2008, more than $100 billion annually had been spent on research and development in biomedicine, but the total expenditures by public-private partnerships focused on neglected diseases in the four years between 2000 and 2004 totaled only $76 million. Even when these partnerships were able to successfully develop new drugs, more money was needed for Phase III clinical trials—sometimes hundreds of millions of dollars. Nevertheless, these public-private partnerships had fundamentally changed the innovation system for the development of treatments to benefit the poorest communities in the world. By venturing in at the point where the risk of failure was the highest and sustaining new research and development to the point where new drugs had a much higher potential for success, the Rockefeller Foundation and its partners had planted and germinated the seeds of innovation for larger multinational and governmental organizations to sustain and grow.

The Role of Medical Research

Thus, in the first decade of the twenty-first century, the Rockefeller Foundation returned to its roots: working with governments and universities to blend cutting-edge scientific research on vaccines with community-based medicine in order to effectively deliver vaccines and treatment therapies to large segments of the vulnerable population. These initiatives reflected both the hookworm campaign's emphasis on community medicine in the Southern United States and the Rockefeller Institute's emphasis on scientific research. In many ways, these initiatives aligned with the highest aspirations of Johns Hopkins' William Welch and Frederick Gates, who hoped that new scientific discoveries would ultimately lead to improvements in the well-being of mankind.

"This is like building a cathedral," Ariel Pablos-Méndez said in describing the Foundation's role in the early days of the Global Alliance for Tuberculosis Drug Development. "It will take more than a group of people. It will take several generations to see it through. But this is the foundation. This is the blueprint." Pablos-Méndez carried primary responsibility for launching these partnerships after he joined the Rockefeller Foundation in 1998. And like Wickliffe Rose before him, he understood that while scientific research represented a critical aspect of the effort to promote public health, investments in research had to be matched with improvements in health systems. The victims of AIDS could not wait for a vaccine; they needed immediate treatment. Building health systems to meet their needs demanded ingenuity and innovation as well. Most of all, it demanded a basic recognition that public resources deployed for health care should provide the maximum benefit to the largest number of people. This was the idea of "equity" that increasingly infused the Rockefeller Foundation's efforts in health in the twenty-first century.

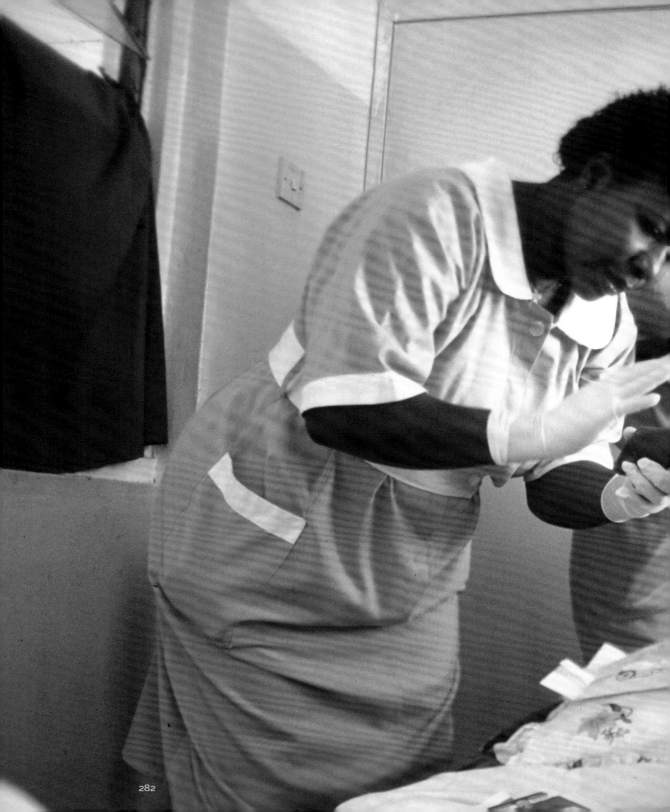

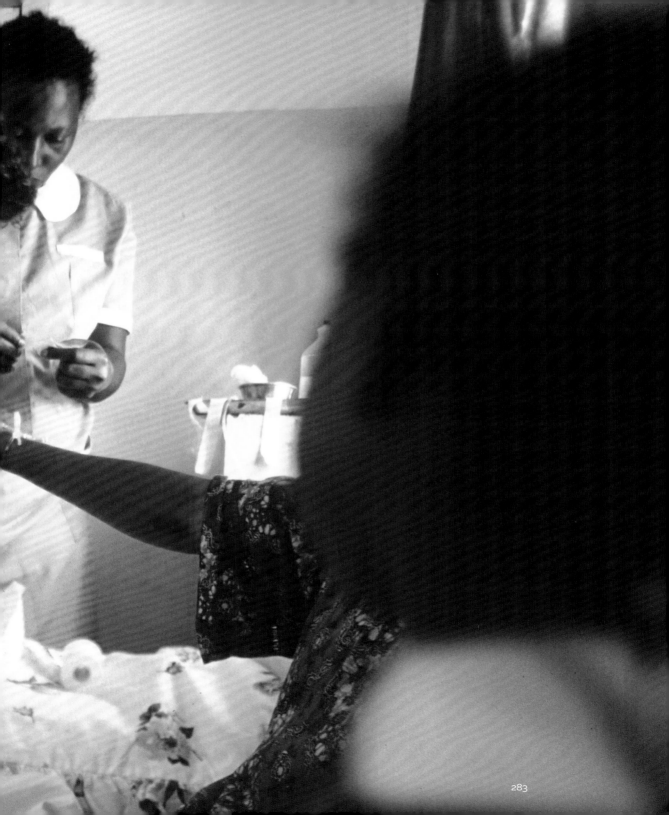

HEALTH SYSTEMS
THAT WORK FOR ALL

O n February 10, 2003, the WHO office in Beijing received a mysterious email describing a "strange contagious disease" in Guangdong Province, China. One hundred people had died in just one week. The next day the Chinese Ministry of Health reported an outbreak of acute respiratory syndrome. Laboratory tests had confirmed that the victims were not infected with influenza. They had succumbed, rapidly, to an atypical form of pneumonia. Three days later Chinese authorities reassured the WHO that no new cases had been diagnosed and the outbreak was under control. Unfortunately, it was not.

On February 21, a physician at Zhongshan University, who had been treating patients with the unknown respiratory infection in Guangdong, flew to Hong Kong for a wedding. He had been feeling under the weather for almost a week, but he did some shopping with his brother and checked into a room on the ninth floor of the Metropole Hotel. The next day he collapsed from respiratory failure and was admitted to a local hospital. The mystery disease had escaped China to Hong Kong. Two days later, an elderly female tourist checked out of her room in the Metropole Hotel and flew home to Toronto, Canada. She was feeling fine.

Canadian officials were already on the alert. In the wake of AIDS, officials at the World Health Organization, the Centers for Disease Control, the Rockefeller Foundation, and national health agencies throughout Europe and Asia had scrambled to cobble together an international early-warning

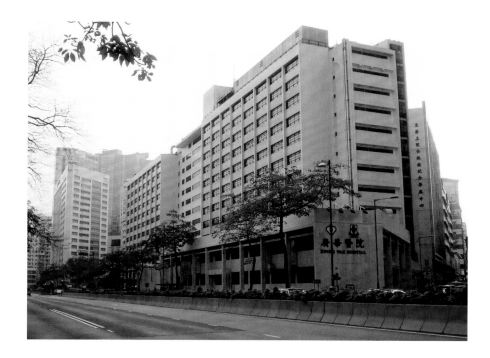

system—the Global Outbreak and Alert Response Network. The system included constant Internet monitoring of disease outbreaks throughout the world. Epidemiologists working with the Canadian Global Public Health Intelligence Network had received an Internet report through ProMED-mail, a project founded in 1994 with

Two of the earliest SARS patients in Hong Kong were admitted to Kwong Wah Hospital, where doctors struggled to identify this new and virulent disease. (Chong Fat.)

support from the Rockefeller Foundation, that hospital staff were infected with a mysterious pneumonia in Guangzhou, China. The report triggered heightened concern within the WHO and in Canada. But nothing in the report said anything about the Chinese doctor in the hospital in Hong Kong, or the elderly Canadian tourist who had just arrived home.

On February 26, a 48-year-old Chinese-American businessman was admitted to a French hospital in Hanoi, Vietnam, with an acute respiratory infection. He had recently spent a few days in Hong Kong—in a room on the ninth floor of the Metropole Hotel. Now he was in intensive care, tended by a Vietnamese hospital staff and Dr. Carlo Urbani, an Italian physician who worked for the WHO. Unaware of the reports coming out of China, Urbani suspected that his patient had avian flu.

Events escalated over the next few days, and the WHO realized that the Guangdong mystery disease had not been contained. On March 4, the Chinese doctor in Hong Kong died. On March 5, the woman in Toronto died, and five members of her family were admitted to the hospital with symptoms of infection. Seven health care workers in the Hanoi hospital where Dr. Urbani was tending to the Chinese-American businessman became sick. Urbani himself fell ill on a flight to Bangkok, where he was scheduled to give a presentation at a medical conference. He was immediately hospitalized.

By March 12, events began to cascade. The number of Hanoi hospital staff who were sick soared to 26. Five were in critical condition. The WHO issued a global alert. The next day the businessman died in Hanoi. The Ministry of Health in Singapore reported "atypical pneumonia" in three young, previously healthy women just returning from Hong Kong. They had all stayed on the ninth floor of the Metropole Hotel. Singapore was the fifth nation to report cases of "atypical pneumonia." Back in Canada, the 44-year-old son of the Toronto tourist died in the hospital.

On March 15, a young Singapore physician, who had treated patients with the mystery disease and subsequently attended a medical conference in New York, became sick on his flight home to Singapore. His plane was diverted to Frankfurt, Germany, where he was hospitalized. The United States and Germany became countries six and seven. On March 29, Dr. Carlo Urbani died in a hospital in Thailand—country eight.

The WHO mobilized an international response. One month after receiving the first notification from the Chinese, it established a network of eleven laboratories in nine countries to try to determine the cause of the illness and to develop a diagnostic test. In historical terms, the decision was very quick. It was even more remarkable that, just one month later, the WHO labs were able to announce that they had isolated the causative agent, a coronavirus "unlike any other human or animal member of the coronavirus family."

Around the world, governments were also taking action. First Singapore, then Hong Kong and China, announced school closures and quarantines. The WHO established guidelines for controlling the epidemic: early identification and isolation of patients; vigorous contact tracing; management of close contacts between patients and friends, relatives, and co-workers; and public education and information that would encourage early reporting of suspect cases. By the mid-summer of 2003, the WHO was reporting 8,000 cases in 37 countries. The epidemic had hit health care workers the hardest. It had spread worldwide in the early days of the outbreak, before epidemiologists understood what they were up against, and the accompanying fear had had a major impact on the global economy. But by early July the epidemic had been contained.

In many ways the campaign against what came to be known as SARS—Severe Acute Respiratory Syndrome—was a triumph of modern epidemiology and international cooperation. Although 775 people died from SARS, the death toll was far lower than what it might have been. International surveillance had worked. Inspired by the results, leaders in the international health community and at the Rockefeller Foundation, having invested in disease-spotting networks for years, looked for ways to make the system even more responsive.

For the Rockefeller Foundation, this effort reflected a further return to the values articulated by Wickliffe Rose—the creation of a public health system that emphasized the efficient allocation of resources to maximize benefits for the broadest number of people. In other words, a system committed to the idea of health equity.

HEALTH EQUITY

I n the earliest days of the Rockefeller Foundation, men like Frederick Gates and Wickliffe Rose had imagined a future where access to health care would not depend on a patient's ability to pay. The Foundation's efforts to eradicate hookworm or disease-bearing mosquitoes; develop vaccines for yellow fever, influenza, or AIDS; or enlist support in the fight against great neglected diseases or for childhood immunization had all been undertaken primarily to benefit poor and marginalized communities around the world. In the later years of the twentieth century, however, the Foundation made health equity more explicit in its communications and its programming.

The new emphasis on health equity began in the early 1990s, after a report issued by the Commission on Health Research for Development drew renewed attention to disparities in health care. Entitled *Health Research, Essential Link to Equity in Development*, the 1990 report estimated that illnesses affecting a small minority of the world population—around 10 percent— were receiving nearly 90 percent of the resources in health care.

The Rockefeller Foundation's efforts to promote selective primary health care in the 1980s (see Chapter VIII) had sought to address this imbalance. In 1993, however, the Foundation furthered this work by creating its Population-Based Health Care program within the Health Sciences Division. The goal of the program was to increase the quality and equity of health outcomes with preventative and accessible care by 2005 in developing countries. The Foundation allocated 17 percent of its budget to the challenge.

Foundation President Peter Goldmark drew further attention to the problem of inequity in the 1994 annual report when he noted that global consumption patterns of Western-style industrialized nations and those of developing countries were inclined toward what he termed "unsustainable" levels. "The consequences of failing frameworks and systems," for Goldmark, "become more painful, and the need for purposeful adaptation on a global scale more urgent."

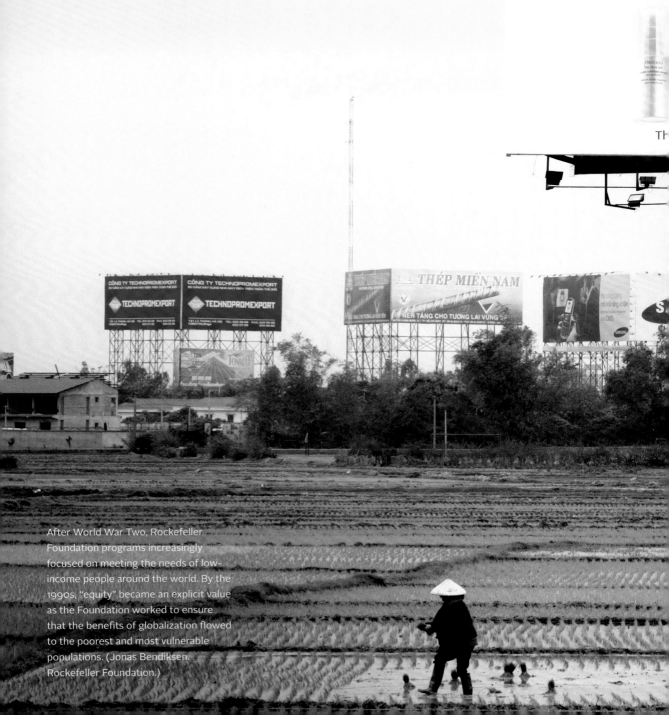

After World War Two, Rockefeller Foundation programs increasingly focused on meeting the needs of low-income people around the world. By the 1990s, "equity" became an explicit value as the Foundation worked to ensure that the benefits of globalization flowed to the poorest and most vulnerable populations. (Jonas Bendiksen. Rockefeller Foundation.)

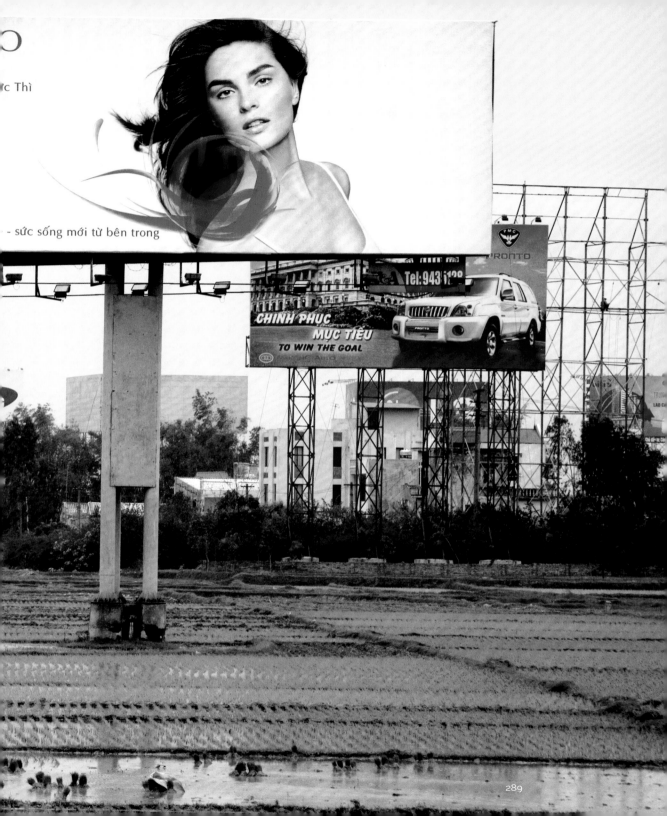

The Foundation envisioned a balanced sharing of world resources to include health, food, and human rights, and advised various agencies and governments on the development of equitable policies to achieve this end.

In 1997 the Rockefeller Foundation began a major review of its Health Sciences programs with an eye to advancing understanding of health equity, promoting equity-oriented health research and development, and strengthening the capacity of health systems to reduce inequities in health. This effort was led by Tim Evans, the director of Health Sciences, and the Foundation's new Vice President for International Programs, Lincoln Chen. Chen was a Harvard-trained physician who had earned his M.P.H. at the Johns Hopkins School of Public Health and worked with the Ford Foundation in India and Bangladesh for 14 years. He then taught at the Harvard School of Public Health and served as the director of the Harvard Center for Population and Development Studies.

As they worked to reframe the Health Sciences Division, Evans, Chen, and others at the Foundation were heavily influenced by lessons learned in the Great Neglected Diseases program and the Children's Vaccine Initiative. They also recognized the potential for a new wave of health risks linked to global climate change, violent behaviors, and drug-resistant infectious diseases. Early grants to the Global Health Equity Initiative (GHEI), a multi-faceted project that incorporated more than 100 researchers in 15 countries around the world, also provided important insights. By comparing health systems and outcomes in non-industrialized nations, GHEI's researchers hoped to highlight best practices and create an incentive for health care reform.

These conversations and initiatives were underway in 1998 when Gordon Conway, an ecologist and well-known expert in agricultural development, succeeded Peter Goldmark as president of the Rockefeller Foundation. As in the past, the change of leadership led to a thorough evaluation of the Foundation's programs. This review affirmed the increasing emphasis on equity as a major theme for the Foundation's work. Conway dramatically highlighted the issue in the millennial annual report, which was titled "Toward a More Equitable World." Life expectancy in Japan exceeded 75 years, while in Sierra Leone it was about 25 years. Treatments for HIV/AIDS available in developed countries meant that infected individuals could expect to live for 20 years with the disease, while in Southern Africa HIV/AIDS was contributing to a dramatic drop in life expectancy for the entire population. As Conway pointed out, poverty and ill health went hand in hand.

The review of the Foundation's programs led by Conway, the trustees, and senior staff made increasing health equity the primary goal of the Foundation's health program. To achieve this goal, the Foundation devoted new resources to improving the delivery of health services to the poor by strengthening the capacity of the health systems that served them. A new grant program called Resourcing Public Health paid particular attention to issues related to AIDS care in the developing world, disease surveillance, training frontline public health workers, and addressing issues related to reproductive health. Another program focused on Strengthening Global Leadership in health care to promote systemic reform. All of these initiatives were based on the idea that well-led, well-organized systems would manage information to foster timely insights into emerging health care crises. These insights and discoveries would then accelerate the process of innovation and improve the care and treatment of patients and communities in developing countries.

Disease Surveillance

Disease surveillance networks emerged as a critical tool in this effort to strengthen and transform health systems. Since the early days of the hookworm campaigns at the beginning of the twentieth century, the Rockefeller Foundation had considered data and information systems to be essential in the fight against disease and the campaign for public health. Persis Putnam, the Foundation's indomitable statistician in the early days, had worked to make reliable data a key component of the Foundation's public health initiatives. In 1976 the Foundation had established the Health Information Systems grant program. The goal of this venture had been to make it easier for researchers and clinicians to locate relevant information within the entire corpus in a rational, systematic manner.

As the science of epidemiology advanced, Foundation staff realized that available biomedical information was growing at an exponential rate, making it harder for general health care providers to remain current in their medical training. While scientific literature had doubled approximately every 15 years during the first half of the twentieth century, for example, the Foundation feared that as Russian and Chinese scientists advanced—along with those from developing nations—the doubling might occur as quickly as every three years. Under the Health Sciences Division, beginning in 1978, the Great Neglected Diseases program created a biomedical research network that focused on the major diseases of the tropical world, with the goal of developing better tools for prevention and treatment.

In the ensuing years the Foundation supported library programs to set up electronic information databases as well as provide free access to information to researchers and clinicians. Other projects included an international classification system for primary care health problems

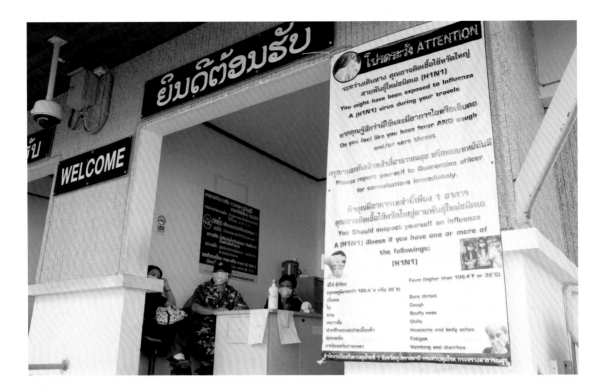

and a qualitative literature evaluation system. The Foundation also funded several meetings and conferences at Bellagio and the New York Public Library focused on such matters as data falsification and information overload in medical education, among other topics. Aware of the growing number of scientists in less-developed nations, the Foundation sponsored a conference in 1984 and published a report dealing with how best to incorporate the scientists' research into existing databases.

The Mekong Basin Disease Surveillance Network, established in 1999, supported collaborative efforts by national ministries of health to share information about changing patterns of infectious disease. At the Mukdahan crossing between Thailand and Laos, officials screened for diseases like "swine flu," caused by the H1N1 virus. (Patrick de Noirmont. Rockefeller Foundation.)

All of these initiatives supported the idea that decreasing the cycle time of information would lead to greater innovation, improvements in practice, and saved lives. But in 1985, after studying the utilization patterns of various scientific journals by researchers and clinicians, the Foundation recognized that information gaps in developing nations handicapped health workers. The Foundation sponsored an experimental program to provide a majority of the relevant medical publications (about 80 percent) to four major universities in Colombia, Egypt, Indonesia, and Mexico. The success of this program led to a new effort extending the dissemination strategy to ministries of health in other developing nations over the next several years. An increasing focus on the importance of timely and relevant data and information also fueled the Foundation's interest in epidemiology and the development of the International Clinical Epidemiology Network (INCLEN) (see Chapter IX).

CREATING INDEPTH

In early 1990, Steve Sinding came to the Rockefeller Foundation from the U.S. Agency for International Development (USAID) to serve as director of the Population Sciences program. Sinding hired demographer Cheikh Mbacké as an associate director, and asked him to visit sub-Saharan Africa as part of an overview of the Foundation's population work with demographic surveillance systems.

The systems had been created to address a basic weakness in the epidemiological approach. To understand the patterns of disease in poor communities and the extent to which health services were reaching them, researchers needed good data on population. But for the nearly one billion people living in the world's poorest countries in the 1990s, this data was either inadequate or nonexistent.

With support from the Rockefeller Foundation as well as other philanthropies and multilateral agencies, advanced laboratories for research on diseases like avian influenza were increasingly located in developing nations around the world, closer to the populations they served. (World Bank.)

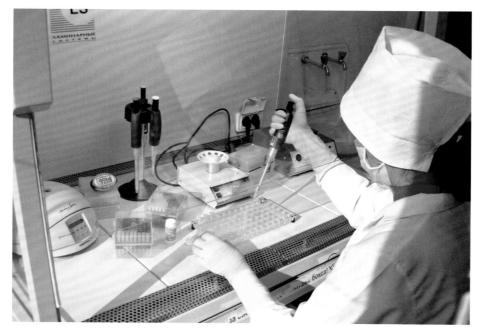

With Rockefeller Foundation support, a number of local initiatives had been launched to create demographic surveillance systems to provide better information on populations in developing countries. But Sinding, Mbacké, and others at the Foundation recognized a need to begin linking these efforts, and helped organize a number of informal and formal meetings that eventually led to the establishment of the INDEPTH Network in 1998.

The INDEPTH Network initially incorporated 17 field sites (each based on a geographically defined population), drawn from 13 countries, primarily in Africa. The network sought to provide a platform for a wide range of health system innovations as well as research studies and social, economic, behavioral, and health interventions. It hoped to provide evidence-based information for decision making at the policy level, foster evidence-based planning and the reassessment of priorities, strengthen the sites themselves, and encourage collaboration.

The Foundation believed that the longitudinal design of INDEPTH research and the data collected by its member sites would lead to a greater understanding of the root causes of poverty in more than two-dozen communities in Africa and Asia. The overarching goal of the Population Sciences program was to harness resources for population and reproductive health, and officers anticipated that the new network would spur funding in those fields.

The Foundation's support for INDEPTH over the years mirrored internal programmatic changes. As grantmaking in Population Sciences gradually wound down, INDEPTH grants under Health Equity focused less on reproductive health and more on other health issues. With the passing of time, Foundation officers identified other programmatic intersections. The Africa Regional Office, for example, supported work related to intervention research, AIDS, and resource development as part of its Information for Development portfolio. In all, 13 grants and more than $4.7 million were awarded for INDEPTH activities.

INDEPTH working groups focused on the relationship between individual- and household-level socioeconomic factors and the inequality of health outcomes. They looked at cause-specific mortality in developing countries, along with fertility, reproductive health, malaria infections and deaths, and the prevalence and prevention of HIV/AIDS. Statisticians associated with the project also tracked migration and urbanization.

The success of the INDEPTH Network attracted other funders, including the Wellcome Trust, whose evaluators believed that INDEPTH provided a unique model for health care-related demography in the developing world.

The Rockefeller Foundation hoped that demographic and disease surveillance projects could play an essential role in empowering frontline health care workers, especially those in developing countries who were working to provide care to people affected by HIV/AIDS. In the 1990s, as part of its continuing effort to train and support these workers, the Foundation launched a new initiative in Africa that would bring health care training opportunities to the communities that needed them most.

Disease Surveillance Networks

INCLEN's success led to the creation of disease surveillance networks in many parts of the developing world. One of the first, the Mekong Basin Disease Surveillance (MBDS) Network, was established at a meeting in Bangkok in 1999 and funded by the Foundation in partnership with the WHO, both of which were concerned by an increase in the number of new varieties of infectious disease in the region. The MBDS Network, in turn, provided funding for a collaborative program among ministries of health in the Greater Mekong Subregion, and would eventually serve as a model for a much larger and more ambitious program designed to have a global impact. The MBDS Network also provided the member countries assistance in acquiring

In the Rufiji demographic surveillance district in Tanzania, part of the INDEPTH Network, a health care worker at a district dispensary collected data on the prevalence of certain diseases. (Jonas Bendiksen. Rockefeller Foundation.)

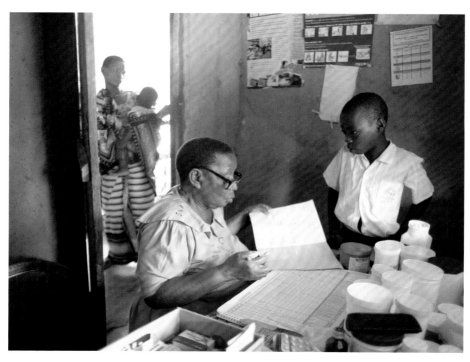

technology, creating a network of medical professionals, and developing the human resources to achieve the goals of the project—to collect, analyze, and disseminate information about changing patterns of infectious diseases in the area. (See *Innovative Partners: The Rockefeller Foundation and Thailand*.)

In the wake of the SARS outbreak in 2003, the MBDS Network provided the model for a new initiative called Disease Surveillance Networks, launched by the Rockefeller Foundation in 2007 as part of a broader effort under the leadership of the Foundation's new President Judith Rodin, to be described later. The new initiative encouraged the development of sub-regional networks of countries and disease specialists to enhance surveillance of and response to national, regional, and global outbreaks of disease that have particularly dire consequences for the world's poorest populations. The effort was prompted by the appearance of a host of new infectious diseases in addition to SARS—HIV/AIDS, Ebola, avian influenza, and H1N1 influenza (Swine Flu)—that could cause pandemics.

The Disease Surveillance Networks (DSN) Initiative employed a multi-pronged approach to its mission. It sought to increase individual and institutional capacity for detecting outbreaks of new diseases and to enhance the ability to respond to them. It also worked to improve connections among disease surveillance networks around the world. As part of this effort, the Rockefeller Foundation again worked to develop a new field of zoonotic disease health researchers and clinicians by funding collaboration among specialists in animal health, human health, and environmental health in the One Health initiative.

To cope with pandemic diseases, it is essential that they be identified quickly and confined to a particular locality in the best way possible. Establishing surveillance networks has proved difficult because of the fragility of health systems, the poor mechanisms for responding to outbreaks, and unreliable coordination. Still, there are local initiatives that contribute to the larger objectives of the DSN. For Thailand and the Lao People's Democratic Republic, for example, officials have established a cross-border site between Mukdahan, Thailand, and Savannakhet, Laos. Representatives of district and public health offices regularly share information through e-mails, websites, conferences, and personal communication (especially during outbreaks) about 18 diseases of concern to the region. This effort has involved the cooperation of doctors, public health officials, and animal specialists, and has greatly reduced the spread of disease.

The Rockefeller Foundation also provided support for the global network Connecting Organizations for Regional Disease Surveillance (CORDS), which began in 2012. The objective is to encourage closer collaboration, knowledge transfer, and sharing of best practices among surveillance networks across the world—the Mekong region, Eastern and Southern Africa, South Asia, the Middle East, and Eastern Europe.

The DSN Initiative represented one part of a multi-faceted approach to transforming health systems around the globe and increasing collaboration and trust among policymakers and health care professionals. Meanwhile treating the people affected by great neglected diseases and emerging viruses like HIV had prompted the Foundation and others to look for new ways to train and serve affected populations.

PUBLIC HEALTH SCHOOLS WITHOUT WALLS (PHSWOW)

I n 1991 Seth Berkley had established a pilot program in Zimbabwe conceived as a "two-year, degree-granting curriculum that stressed the competencies required for solving on-site problems." Known as "Public Health Schools Without Walls," the program was accomplished through apprenticeships with the Ministry of Health, the University of Zimbabwe Department of Community Medicine, and the International Clinical Epidemiology Network Unit, with assistance from visiting public health faculty. At the time, there was not a single graduate-level public-health training program available in Southern Africa.

PHSWOW's curriculum focused on the technical, managerial, and leadership skills needed to operate largely decentralized health systems, like those in Africa. It concentrated on practical problem-solving skills, and emphasized a process of lifelong learning. Students spent 25 percent of their time in classroom instruction. The rest of their work was in the field and emphasized maternal as well as child health, including family planning, nutrition, and immunization along with diarrheal and respiratory diseases. The trainees would also respond to the growing AIDS crisis and help children cope with the loss of parents and particularly mothers.

In many ways, the PHSWOW program represented an extension of INCLEN, but without the need to send trainees abroad. Rather, they could be trained in the area where they would work upon graduation. But the network and partnership aspect of INCLEN continued within PHSWOW as a means of development. This strategy echoed a major theme in the Rockefeller Foundation's initiatives in the late twentieth century: increase the capacity of developing nations to respond to health and development issues by locating research facilities and investing in human capital close to the communities that needed help.

Based on its success, PHSWOW was later extended to Uganda, Ghana, and Vietnam. Two cohorts of students had graduated from the Zimbabwe program by 1997. In Uganda a large percentage of the graduates remained in

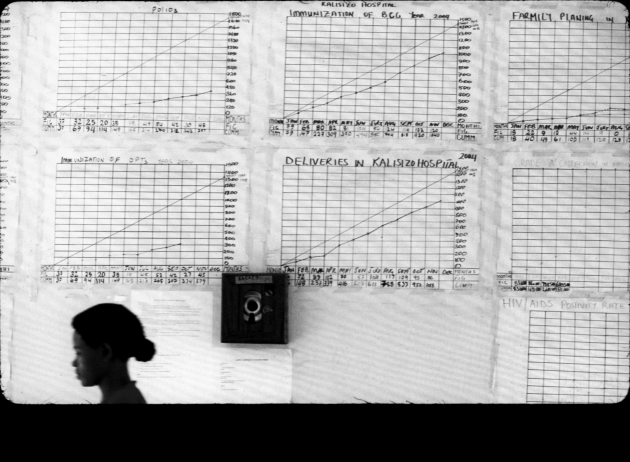

Health care workers trained through the Public Health Schools Without Walls program provided services to rural clinics and hospitals in Zimbabwe, Ghana, Vietnam, and Uganda. (Jonas Bendiksen. Rockefeller Foundation.)

their home areas, and over 85 percent of the nation's 120 districts had graduates working within them. The Foundation also extended the program into a network of affiliations throughout Africa—known as the Network of African Public Health Institutions—to more widely disseminate related knowledge and materials.

A 2001 reevaluation of the PHSWOW programs in Africa tied outcomes directly to the growing HIV/AIDS epidemic, suggesting that the crisis might help transform the management of public health. The evaluators also reported that the PHSWOW program had had a substantial impact on health systems, especially at the district level, by lowering the barriers between the academic programs and the ministries of health. The authors noted that PHSWOW graduates were at the forefront in responding to major public health crises such as the Ebola outbreak in Uganda and plague outbreaks in the Matabele region of Zimbabwe. Leadership provided by PHSWOW graduates in the Zimbabwe Ministry of Health's disease surveillance program had an impact on disease control in the country, and helped to provide health care to the poorer communities, especially for women who were at the heart of many challenges facing developing nations and who were increasingly seen as pivotal to efforts to stem the spread of HIV.

Empowering Women

The Foundation's driving philosophy of reforming health systems to provide a more equitable allocation of resources served no group better than women of the developing world. The Foundation's approach toward addressing the unmet needs of these women included three foci in which the Foundation works effectively: underwriting research initiatives, advocating at various decision-making levels for pro-women policy changes, and forming public-private partnerships.

In 1990 sub-Saharan Africa lost twice as many women while they were pregnant, or during delivery, as did the global population. The Foundation soon spearheaded the "Mobilization for Unmet Demand," including as one of its nine central goals the "availability of high-quality reproductive health and family-planning services to all women in the developing world."

In 1994 the Foundation awarded a grant to support the International Conference on Population and Development in Cairo, which "succeeded in reaching a broad global consensus on the direction that should be taken in developing policies and programs in the field of family planning and women's reproductive health." The Program of Action that emerged from the conference included a "call for a dramatic increase in high-quality reproductive health care and family planning services" that would put women's rights and their health needs at the center of development programming.

That same year, the Foundation convened another Bellagio conference under the aegis of its Population Sciences program to "discuss how private/ public sector cooperation can advance the woman-centered agendas." The conference led to a new collaboration with the Mellon Foundation and USAID to "create a consortium for collaboration in contraceptive research," which the Foundation supported with a $1.3 million grant. Armed with studies that showed that by eliminating all unwanted pregnancies, population growth could be reduced by nearly 20 percent, this new public-private consortium—known as the Contraceptive Research and Development Program—provided a way for private industry to contribute toward public agencies working on contraceptives research. It became one of several precursors to the public-private model that would be developed for AIDS, malaria, tuberculosis, and microbicides. In 1995 the Foundation's Population Sciences program also laid out a ten-year plan and appropriated $14.7 million toward mobilizing available resources for voluntary family planning and reproductive health services.

Caring for People Infected with HIV

I n the 1990s, the AIDS crisis brought into sharp relief all of the Foundation's efforts to promote health equity through demographic and disease surveillance systems as well as improved training for health care workers in the developing world. They also helped promote fundamental innovations in patient care that reflected the Foundation's long-term commitment to community and population-based medicine.

The Foundation's work on HIV/AIDS patient care had begun in August 1987, when its AIDS Task Force met to study the reasons for the relatively equal distribution of HIV infection between the sexes in Africa. In those early days, much of the Foundation's funding was channeled to organizations seeking to understand and prevent the spread of the disease. As the epidemic grew, however, some staff looked for ways the Rockefeller Foundation could do more. In April 1989 Jane Hughes, an expert on adolescent health, wrote to President Peter Goldmark and Vice President Kenneth Prewitt with a detailed analysis of the challenges of HIV/AIDS in developing countries, as well as the possible solutions on which the Foundation might work. Hughes's recommendations led the Foundation to incubate and launch an international effort to raise and channel donor funds to developing countries for HIV/AIDS initiatives.

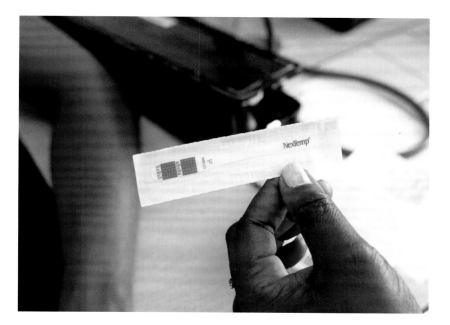

These efforts came to fruition in December 1993 when the Foundation brought together nine major donor agencies in Paris to form the International HIV/AIDS Alliance, with the goal of providing money and technical assistance to developing-country NGOs engaged in HIV/AIDS prevention and care. The donor groups—which included the European Union, the Organisation for Economic Cooperation and Development (OECD), and the WHO—pledged more than $5 million for the project's first three years. These funds helped national coalitions in developing countries act as linking organizations, channeling small grants and technical assistance to grassroots NGOs working on AIDS prevention and care.

In Kenya researchers associated with the International AIDS Vaccine Initiative conducted vaccine trials and related epidemiological research in partnership with researchers around the globe. (Sokomoto Photography. International AIDS Vaccine Initiative.)

At the end of the 1990s, after more than a decade of involvement with HIV/AIDS in Africa, the Rockefeller Foundation had established a Working Group for AIDS Exploration to determine whether the Foundation was appropriately addressing the still-mounting crisis, especially in Africa. This self-reflection stemmed partly from the realization that the impact of AIDS went far beyond health, that it was a multidimensional problem for economic and social development.

This review had led to a pivotal international meeting in Kampala in 2001, which emphasized AIDS care in the fight against the epidemic in Africa. Organized by the Foundation in cooperation with the Joint Clinical Research Centre in Kampala, Uganda, the conference on "AIDS Care in

Africa: The Way Forward" was attended by nearly 200 African as well as international scientists and citizens from academia, multinational agencies, and governmental research councils and institutes, including bilateral donors, private foundations, and NGOs. Some of the world's leading AIDS scientists also attended, including two of the most distinguished—Anthony Fauci and Luc Montagnier.

Attendees came because the fight against the AIDS epidemic in Africa had reached a crucial moment. The revolution in antiretroviral drug treatment for HIV/AIDS, launched in 1995, had previously bypassed the more than 25 million Africans infected with the virus, but falling drug prices meant that many Africans would now have access to effective treatment for the first time.

A convening of key players at a critical moment once again helped foster coalition building and an innovative strategy. At the Rockefeller Foundation, the conference led to a new focus on AIDS work in Africa under the rubric of a program called Nenda Mbele (Go Forward with Care). Distinguished from "treatment," which emphasized medical approaches to disease, the concept of "care" included not only medical therapy but also the core dimension of humanistic relationships. The conference helped to establish the African Dialogue on AIDS Care (ADAC) with the goal of enhancing clinical research capacity and ensuring coordination, standard setting, ethical review, resource mobilization, and the policy relevance of research. ADAC hoped to become a broker for the continent's interests related to AIDS care.

The conference also led the Rockefeller Foundation to play a catalytic role in the Development of AntiRetroviral Therapy in Africa (DART) trial, which was sponsored and funded by the U.K. Medical Research Council with additional funding from the U.K. Department for International Development and the Rockefeller Foundation. The Foundation granted more than $1.6 million in 2005 and 2006 to the University of Zimbabwe in Harare and the Joint Clinical Research Centre in Kampala, Uganda, for participation in a multi-center clinical trial to assess the safety and effectiveness of two strategies for the use of antiretroviral drugs against HIV/AIDS in sub-Saharan Africa.

Like IAVI, DART included a key role for pharmaceutical companies and the private sector. Antiretroviral drugs given to trial participants were donated by GlaxoSmithKline, Gilead Sciences, Abbott Laboratories, and Boehringer Ingelheim. These companies also provided funding for some of the studies that were part of the DART trial. The results presented at the International AIDS Society Conference 2009 in Cape Town showed that, irrespective of group, the survival rate in the DART trial was among the highest reported from any trial, study, or antiretroviral therapy program in Africa. In fact, the success of antiretroviral therapy played a key role in the larger campaign, funded by the Rockefeller Foundation, to revolutionize primary care and HIV/AIDS treatment in Africa's poorest communities.

Women, Children, and HIV

For a number of years in the mid-1990s, the Foundation had supported efforts to address mother-to-child transmission of HIV. The Foundation had sponsored a workshop on the topic in November 1994, hosted by the Network of AIDS Researchers of Eastern and Southern Africa. Twenty-four researchers and program implementers attended, addressing questions about vertical transmission as well as counseling and community- and home-based care. The workshop helped to develop collaborative linkages among researchers in the region and to trigger new research, training, and intervention-related activities. Insights gained from this conference, from other HIV/AIDS initiatives, and from the Foundation's efforts to empower women in Africa fed a growing interest in mother-to-child transmission.

In the United States, Wafaa El-Sadr, a Columbia University physician and medical researcher focused on AIDS in Harlem, was developing an approach that combined treatment and prevention by working with whole families, not just infected individuals. Her goal was to lower mother-to-child transmission, and this meant ensuring the continued health of the mother as well as of her partner(s). Tim Evans and Ariel Pablos-Méndez of the Foundation's Health Equity program were interested in El-Sadr's work. They believed that the Foundation needed to do more to address the terrible impact of HIV/AIDS on poor communities around the world.

Conversations and meetings with El-Sadr and her team at Columbia University led to new insights. Based on her experience and research, El-Sadr believed strongly that treatment and prevention had to go hand in hand, which meant that HIV/AIDS programs needed to address the whole family and not just the individuals known to be infected. Her approach fit well with the Foundation's long-term work on family planning, women's education, and public health, especially in Africa. As a result of this dialogue, the Foundation committed to exploring the possibilities of a treatment and prevention program that could be applied throughout the developing world.

New grantmaking guidelines established at the beginning of the new millennium pushed the Foundation to deepen its commitment to fighting AIDS. It also recognized, echoing insights that reached all the way back to Wickliffe Rose, that AIDS interventions could lead to efforts to address broader shortfalls in health and social systems.

With Foundation funding for Columbia University's Mailman School of Public Health, El-Sadr's team developed the framework for the Mother-to-Child Transmission project (MTCT-Plus) and sent out requests for proposals for implementing the concept at the community level. Obtaining and distributing drugs was a key part of the program and it presented major challenges, requiring complex negotiations with pharmaceutical companies and state health services as well as local pharmacists and physicians. Along with the life-saving drugs, women and especially pregnant women were provided with general and maternal health care. They were also offered education on prevention and staying healthy. Most important, they were encouraged to bring in their partners and families, however those were defined, in order to learn about maintaining health and reducing the chances of infecting anybody else. Despite early skepticism, clinics, hospitals, and NGOs around the world sent in applications. These institutions understood the value of addressing HIV/AIDS on a community level.

MTCT-Plus was a new kind of medical program and thus a hard sell, but it offered a model for HIV care in resource-limited settings that could be replicated and scaled up.

Wafaa El-Sadr, a Columbia University physician who led the Division of Infectious Diseases at Harlem Hospital Center, pioneered new approaches to AIDS care. With Allan Rosenfield, the former dean of the Columbia University Mailman School of Public Health, she established the Mother-To-Child-Transmission Plus (MTCT-Plus) Initiative. (John D. and Catherine T. MacArthur Foundation.)

Effective implementation of MTCT-Plus required current, integrated, and accurate information on participants that could be easily accessible to caregivers. In order to facilitate this access, the Rockefeller Foundation funded the Electronic Medical Records program at Moi University and the Mosoriot MTCT-Plus Health Centre, both in Kenya. The Medical Records System was aimed at developing a simple stand-alone information system that could be used on individual computers as part of an integrated, paperless, web-based network that would enable more effective monitoring and management of larger numbers of patients through a centralized data repository. These technological innovations provided real-time capture of data critical to the care of HIV/AIDS patients and the management of HIV/AIDS care programs.

By 2006 MTCT-Plus had established care and treatment programs at 14 sites in sub-Saharan Africa. It had enrolled approximately 12,560 individuals, including 4,985 children receiving HIV/AIDS care along with 3,045 adults and 423 infants or children. The project's work was groundbreaking on a number of levels. It made a strong case for early diagnosis, demonstrating why virologic tests of HIV-exposed infants were important during the first months of life. The project also initiated peer-based programs for supporting adherence in antiretroviral treatment clinics, and it illustrated the essential role that a team approach could play in HIV/AIDS prevention and treatment by emphasizing the importance of an entire care team—from the receptionist to the lab technician.

The success of MTCT-Plus changed the mindset of many funders and other organizations working on HIV/AIDS by demonstrating that it is possible to provide treatment and prevention together in poor communities. In fact, the visible effects of treatment, evident to families and community members, provided hope and reinforced the message of prevention. As El-Sadr posits, no prevention campaign could make a dent if people felt that they were already doomed.

TRANSFORMING HEALTH SYSTEMS

The MTCT-Plus Initiative, in combination with the Foundation's other work on health issues in Africa and the developing world, underscored the critical importance of building and maintaining effective health systems. In 2005 Judith Rodin, the president of the University of Pennsylvania and the first woman to lead an Ivy League university, succeeded Gordon Conway as president of the Rockefeller Foundation. Rodin's research career at Yale had focused on behavioral medicine and health psychology and she had joint appointments in the departments of Medicine, Psychiatry, and Psychology at Yale. Through her training and research, she understood that even significant treatment breakthroughs in drugs and vaccines could not be successful without functioning health systems. Rodin built on the Foundation's pattern of success in establishing public-private collaborations to tackle the toughest issues in health care.

In 2008 the Foundation launched a new initiative called Transforming Health Systems, which aimed "to catalyze system strengthening activities that create broader access to affordable health services in developing countries." Transforming Health Systems recognized that past efforts in

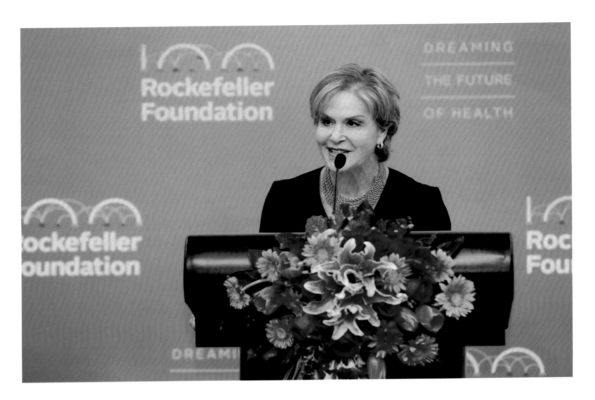

When Judith Rodin became president of the Rockefeller Foundation in 2005, she accelerated the Foundation's efforts to transform health systems and ensure that new technologies would benefit the poor in developing nations. At the Foundation's Global Health Summit in Beijing in January 2013, she urged world leaders to "dream the future of health for the next 100 years." (Rockefeller Foundation.)

public health had tended to combat specific diseases or to launch population-specific initiatives, but had paid relatively little attention to health systems. The new initiative targeted leverage points in the health systems of developing countries, including financing models, the training of health policymakers, potential contributions of knowledge and resources from the private sector, and building interoperable health information systems that contributed to health delivery.

A primary goal of the Transforming Health Systems initiative was the promotion of universal health coverage as a way to ensure that sudden or chronic illness did not impose catastrophic costs on low-income families and people had access to care when they needed it. By advocating for universal health coverage globally and building capacity in developing countries, the Foundation demonstrated to policymakers that universal health coverage was financially and operationally feasible and desirable. Consistent with its past, the Foundation hoped to promote fundamental innovation and collaboration to improve the quality, access, and affordability of health services.

Transforming Health Systems contributed to a number of innovative projects and sparked important political commitments. The Joint Learning Network, for example, was formed in 2009 by a group of developing countries eager to learn techniques from one another that would help improve the effectiveness and efficiency of their health systems. The network facilitated knowledge exchange and joint problem solving among practitioners and policymakers in ten low- and middle-income countries in Africa and Southeast Asia. The Rockefeller Foundation provided resources to strengthen the network's ability to share information, monitor quality, and work toward universal health coverage.

The Foundation's leadership and advocacy gained traction, and by December 2012, the United Nations General Assembly passed a resolution on universal coverage and WHO Director-General Margaret Chan called universal health coverage "the single most powerful concept that public health has to offer." Through the Transforming Health Systems initiative, the Foundation partnered with the WHO, the World Bank, UNICEF, civil society organizations, and governments to support implementation of health reforms leading toward universal health coverage in individual countries and regions and around the world.

In 2008 the Foundation convened "Making the eHealth Connection," a global summit to look for ways to deploy information technology to reduce the cost of health care in the developing world and continue to improve patient care with good epidemiological, demographic, and other information systems. A month-long series of conferences at the Foundation's Bellagio Center brought together more than 200 leaders from the health, financial, and technology sectors. Out of the Bellagio series, the Foundation forged new alliances and launched a partnership with the United Nations Foundation and the Vodafone Foundation to create the mHealth Alliance to champion the use of mobile technologies to improve health throughout the world.

Indeed, at the dawn of the Rockefeller Foundation's second century, new technology seemed to President Rodin to promise a revolution in health care delivery and the hope of greater access for the poor. In many ways, this new emphasis on systems echoed the aspirations of Frederick Gates and Wickliffe Rose more than a hundred years earlier. They had imagined that science and organization would combine to prevent disease before it emerged, and cure it when necessary. As the Rockefeller Foundation celebrated its centennial in 2013, finding the balance between these two goals remained a driving force.

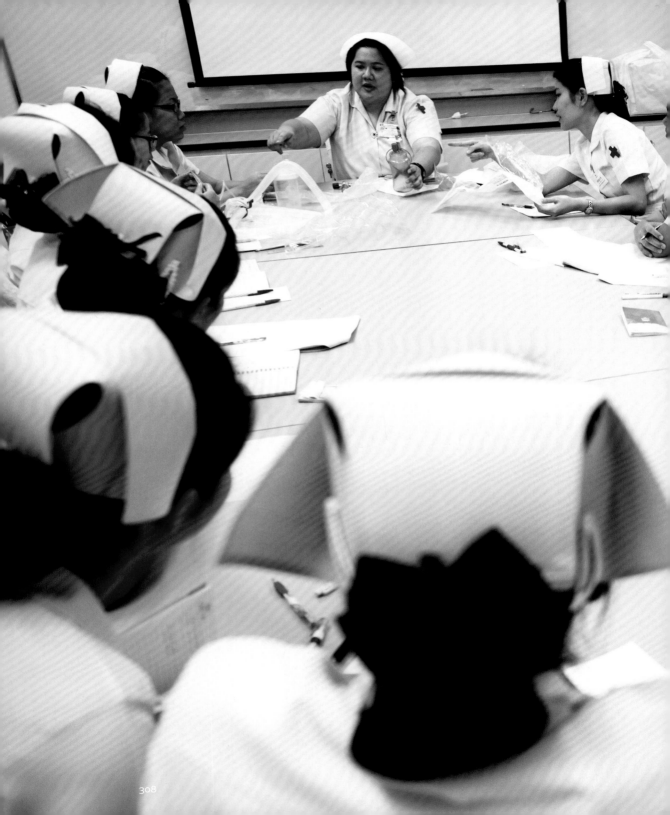

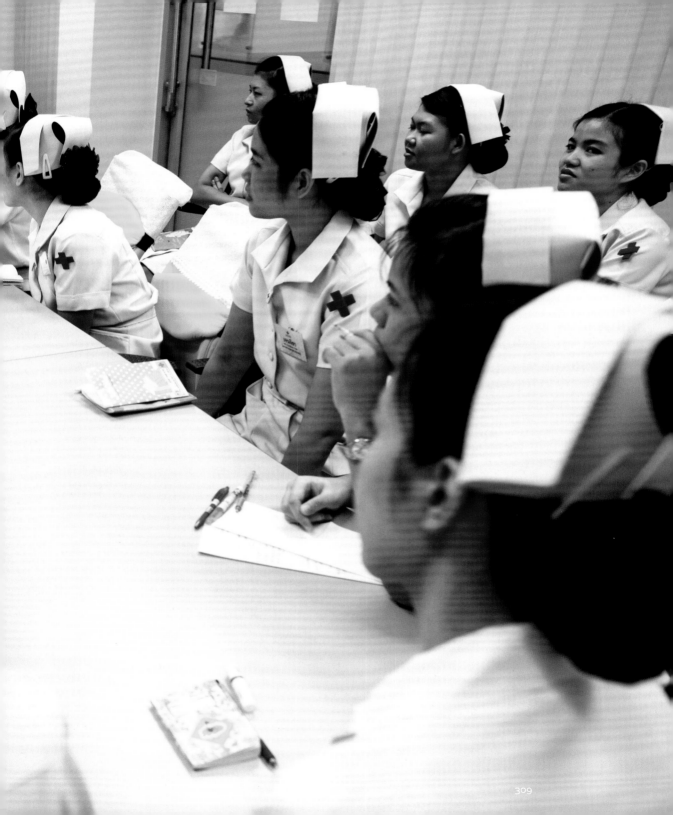

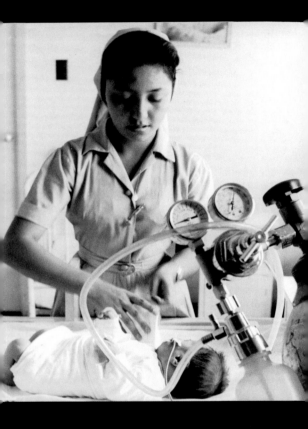

killed and caring professionals were at the heart
f the system of public health that Wickliffe Rose
nd others at the Rockefeller Foundation envisioned
n the early twentieth century. Breakthroughs
n therapy, driven by scientists and engineers in
esearch laboratories, have empowered these
rofessionals just as William Welch envisioned.
Rockefeller Archive Center.)

CONCLUSION

Over the course of a century, Rockefeller philanthropies have initiated and supported numerous programs in basic science, medical education, and public health in the United States and around the globe in order to do the most good with its available resources. Each new initiative was, in part, the outgrowth of an ongoing debate among Foundation trustees and division directors over the proper balance between backing specific cures for disease and promoting broader issues such as community health, agriculture, and care of the environment.

John D. Rockefeller Sr. set the tone for the Foundation's overarching mission with his 1913 mandate to promote the well-being of humanity throughout the world. The leaders who followed him achieved his vision through a variety of programs, the nature and scope of which were shaped by personal experiences and predilections and the eras in which they lived. But certain themes in the Foundation's work have abided over the decades. First and foremost, its leaders have been pioneers and field builders.

In the arena of public health, they almost single-handedly envisioned, designed, and built the field. They saw that the development of medical science alone could not address the health needs of vast numbers of the planet's citizens without an understanding of the way people and societies work. Thus the Foundation has long focused on capacity building as well, whether that meant empowering county health workers in the American South in the twentieth century or trainees in the Public Health Schools Without Walls in Africa in the twenty-first.

Trustees and staff have often been divided over how much emphasis to place on research versus the application of knowledge in the field; this was the essential tension that confronted William Welch and Wickliffe Rose in 1915.

Nevertheless, the Foundation has remained committed to the importance of the scientific discovery of new knowledge, as championed by Welch and others, even as it has understood, with Rose, that villages, towns, and cities must be able to obtain and deliver new drugs, as well as crucial information about effective treatment and prevention to those who need them if the payoff from research is to be realized in improvements to human health. Working in the rural communities of China in the 1920s or the growing cities of Latin America and Africa in the 2000s, the Foundation has recognized throughout its history that successful philanthropy in health, as in agriculture and education, depends on engaging and empowering local citizens.

Successful philanthropy in health also depends on the ability to establish partnerships and collaborations. The Rockefeller Foundation has collaborated with local, regional, state, and national agencies and organizations as well as governmental, non-governmental, and quasi-governmental bodies. More recently it has worked with for-profit entities such as biotechnology firms and multinational pharmaceutical corporations. Every relationship was formed in the Foundation's pursuit of improvements in both specific and broad areas of health—from recommending educational campaigns in the Southern United States that would dispel myths about hookworm in the 1910s and 1920s to setting up limited partnerships with pharmaceutical companies to bypass vaccine bottlenecks in the 1990s. Such endeavors sought to create an "entering wedge," as Rose would say, to leverage Rockefeller assets to better serve the health of affected populations.

Before World War Two, when the International Health Division maintained extensive field operations in countries around the world, and when few other philanthropic organizations were engaged in international work, the Foundation's partnerships were often with government.

After World War Two, with the rise of international agencies like the U.N. and the WHO, these partnerships reflected broad-based coalitions among different interests. In recent decades, engaging the private sector through projects like the International AIDS Vaccine Initiative has increased the complexity as well as the potential impact of these initiatives.

When Wallace Buttrick chose Wickliffe Rose to lead the Rockefeller Sanitary Commission in 1910, he recognized that a background in education was as important to public health as a knowledge of science. Throughout the Rockefeller Foundation's history, education has played a critical role in increasing the capacity of local health care systems to meet local needs and in empowering people to take care of themselves. Indeed, education has been a mainstay of the Foundation's approach, either in part or in whole, to many world problems.

Fundamentally, however, the Foundation's philanthropy has always sought to drive innovation, which, as John D. Rockefeller knew, addresses the root causes of problems. It leads to new treatments, new systems, and new approaches to organizing and deploying resources in ways that are scalable and can address the needs of many people.

Today, as developed and developing nations seek to provide effective, efficient, and equitable health services—and to transform the systems that provide them—questions of how best to achieve these goals remain an urgent part of the public and political debate. In the history of the Rockefeller Foundation there are lessons to be learned about the issues that drive this debate. There are also models to be adapted and deployed for a new era. Most important, the Foundation's history shows that in the creative tension between preventing disease and seeking cures, fundamental innovation moves forward, driven by humanity's longing for the security of health and well-being.

Health and Well-Being has been an inherently collective project that would have been impossible without the contributions of many people.

The book is part of the Rockefeller Foundation's Centennial initiative. At the Rockefeller Foundation, President Judith Rodin inspired the project concept. The Foundation's Centennial team, including Michael Myers, Carolyn Bancroft, and Charlanne Burke, helped envision and shape the entire work, providing support and input, including reviewing drafts and giving essential feedback. Bob Bykofsky and Elizabeth Pena in Records Management facilitated research of recent materials. Kathy Gomez collected photographs highlighting the Foundation's recent work. In the General Counsel's office, Shari Patrick and Erica Guyer provided legal guidance. Many other people at the Foundation read manuscript drafts, including Neill Coleman, Heather Grady, Robert Marten, Carey Meyers, Natalie Phaholyothin, Hilary Tabish, and Jeanette Vega. Their work is greatly appreciated. Teneo Strategy kept us on track for the duration of the project. Many thanks to Michael Coakley, Andy Maas, and Max Dworin for their tireless work.

None of this would have been possible without the staff at the Rockefeller Archive Center. Jack Meyers, RAC's president, and James Allen Smith, its vice president, welcomed our team and provided continuous institutional support. Barb Shubinski and Teresa Iacobelli, the RAC's Rockefeller Foundation Centennial Research Fellows, generously coordinated with us, sharing ideas and research. The reference team applied their considerable skill to our efforts. Thanks to Michele Hiltzik, assistant director and head of reference, for her heroic efforts to help us find images, and to James Washington for scanning so many of these illustrations. Archivists Nancy Adgent, Bethany Antos, and Tom Rosenbaum were especially helpful with this book.

Many people contributed to the creation of this book, offering both inspiration and assistance. Professor Louis Galambos shared his insights from his work on the history of research on AIDS vaccines. Special thanks to Professor Leo Ribuffo, Department of History, Columbian College of Arts and Sciences, George Washington University, Washington, D.C., for his continued support throughout my professional career. The Pentagram team, including Michael Gericke and Matt McInerney, skillfully crafted the series, according each member book its own identity.

The Vantage Point team contributed immeasurably. Lois Facer managed photographs, helped with research, and provided administrative support. Claire Wilkens and Amanda Waterhouse helped select photographs. Madeleine Adams suggested changes to structure and helped with the overall flow of the text. Sam Hurst facilitated writing and content development, helping to add color to key sections. Susan Abrahamson provided invaluable assistance with some of the more scientific passages. Ernie Grafe's diligent and thoughtful fact-checking and copyediting helped strengthen the book immeasurably. Amanda Waterhouse proofread the entire set of galleys. Mindy Johnston and Leigh Armstrong handled photo rights management. Craig Chapman and Vivian Jenkins compiled the index. Eric Abrahamson offered invaluable editorial and intellectual feedback throughout the writing-process, helping to give this book focus, direction, and depth. He also provided patient guidance and tireless motivation, and established a shared vision that helped us complete this book.

Any errors or omissions are entirely my own.

Angela Matysiak, Ph.D., M.P.H.

	Description	Creator. Source.
52	Sanitary Privies are Cheaper than Coffins (ca. 1920).	Source: National Library of Medicine.
54	Schoolchildren, Knotts Island, North Carolina (1913).	Source: Rockefeller Archive Center.
56-57	Yellow Fever Commission, São Luis, Brazil (1925).	Source: Rockefeller Archive Center.
59	Moving Picture Unit, South Carolina (1920).	Source: Rockefeller Archive Center.
60	World map showing scope of RF activities in Public Health, Medical Education and War Work, 1917 Annual Report (1917).	Source: Rockefeller Archive Center.
61	The first dose of Thymol ever given on foreign soil by the International Health Commission, British Guiana (1913).	Source: Rockefeller Archive Center.
63	Office of the International Health Commission at Bagotville, British Guiana.	Source: Rockefeller Archive Center.
64	Laboratorio Antianemico. Departamento de Uncinariasis, Cali, Colombia (ca. 1926).	Source: Rockefeller Archive Center.
67	Soutenez-la! Poster for anti-tuberculosis campaign, Paris, France.	Source: Rockefeller Archive Center.
68	Poster for the Grande Conférence sur la Tuberculose, Rouen, France (1919).	Source: Rockefeller Archive Center.
70	Mosquitoes, sample no. 2, Yazoo City, Mississippi (1923).	Created by Yazoo County Health Department. Source: Rockefeller Archive Center.
71	Searching for *Anopheles* larvae, ditch R-11 cane fields, Puerto Rico (1920).	Source: Rockefeller Archive Center.
72	A general view of the exhibit of the International Health Board, Rio de Janeiro, Brazil (1922).	Source: Rockefeller Archive Center.
75	American and Brazilian Directors in Brazil (1921).	Source: Rockefeller Archive Center.
76-77	Baby girl waits (ca. 2005).	Photo by Jonas Bendiksen. Source: The Rockefeller Foundation.

	Description	Creator. Source.
109	William Osler at work on *The Principles and Practice of Medicine* at Johns Hopkins Hospital, Maryland (ca. 1891).	Source: National Library of Medicine.
110	U.S. Marine Hospital No. 21, Stapleton, New York.	Source: National Library of Medicine.
112	First Board of Directors of The Rockefeller Institute for Medical Research, Founders Hall, New York (1909).	Source: Rockefeller University, Rockefeller Archive Center.
114-115	"Vivisection. The critics and the criticized" (1914).	Illustration by Udo J. Keppler. Source: Library of Congress.
117	Oswald T. Avery (ca. 1920).	Courtesy Tennessee State Library and Archives. Source: National Library of Medicine.
118	A. Maurice Wakeman at work in the lab, Accra, Ghana (1928).	Source: Rockefeller Archive Center.
120	Hideyo Noguchi with Johannes Bauer, Accra, Ghana (1928).	Source: Rockefeller Archive Center.
122	Telegram from Noguchi to Russell (1928).	Source: Rockefeller Archive Center.
123	Max Theiler (1951).	Photo by Pach Brothers. Source: Rockefeller Archive Center.
124	Station Hospital, Ft. Jay, Governors Island, New York (1942).	Photo by U.S. Army Signal Corps. Source: Rockefeller Archive Center.
126	Wilbur A. Sawyer, Yellow Fever Laboratory, Rockefeller Institute, New York (1935).	Photo by Thomas P. Hughes. Source: National Library of Medicine.
128	Exterminator using hand flint-gun to treat *labranchiae* breeding place near Iglesias, Sardinia, Italy (1947).	Source: Rockefeller Archive Center.
130	Preparing a liquid suspension of spores of *Penicillium notatum* for use as inoculum (1944).	Photo by Merck & Co., Inc. Source: Rockefeller Archive Center.
132-133	Polio vaccination campaign, Darfur, Sudan (2011).	Photo by Olivier Chassot. Source: United Nations photo #465120.
135	Raymond Fosdick.	Photo by Kaiden Keystone Photos. Source: Rockefeller Archive Center.

	Description	Creator. Source.
159	Health education class, Woodrow Wilson High School, Washington, D.C. (1943).	Photo by Esther Bubley. Source: Library of Congress.
160-161	Infant surrounded by protective malaria bed net, Ghana (2006).	Photo by Arne Hoel. Source: World Bank.
163	UN 16th plenary session, San Francisco (1945).	Photo by McCreary. Source: United Nations photo #159673.
164	A group of students at the University of Toronto School of Nursing from Brazil, China, Philippine Islands, and the U.S., Canada.	Source: Rockefeller Archive Center.
166	Segnalatori searching for larvae in a shallow well, Sardinia, Italy (1947).	Source: Rockefeller Archive Center.
167	Letter from John Kerr to Fred Soper (1946).	Source: Rockefeller Archive Center.
169	U.S. army decontamination sprayer converted for DDT, Taiwan (1949).	Source: Rockefeller Archive Center.
172	Mexico malaria field report (ca. 1950).	Source: Rockefeller Archive Center.
174-175	A nurse at the Jorge Lingan health clinic weighs baby boy as father looks on, Lima, Peru (2013).	Source: World Bank.
177	Street scene, Hong Kong (ca. 1950).	Source: Rockefeller Archive Center.
179	Clinic in Ipoh, Malaysia (1968).	Source: Ford Foundation Archives, Rockefeller Archive Center.
182	Indian farmers sift wheat to remove any traces of soil, Karnal, India.	Photo by Raghubir Singh. Source: Ford Foundation Archives, Rockefeller Archive Center. Copyright 2014 Succession Raghubir Singh.
184	Universidad del Valle Escuela de Enfermeria - Estado Actual de la Construccion, Colombia (1963).	Source: Rockefeller Archive Center.
185	Carnet de Salud, Candelaria, Colombia (ca. 1966).	Photo by Joe D. Wray. Source: Rockefeller Archive Center.
186	Medical students taking rural health surveys, Thailand (ca. 1968).	Photo by Joe D. Wray. Source: Rockefeller Archive Center.

	Description	Creator. Source.
216-217	A Hmong woman and her baby in the village of Sin Chai, Vietnam (2011).	Photo by Kibae Park. Source: United Nations photo #491903.
219	Sterling Wortman.	Source: Rockefeller Archive Center.
220	Kenneth Warren (ca. 1989).	Source: Rockefeller Archive Center.
221	Residents and refugees receive vaccinations against smallpox and typhus, Koje Island, Korea (1951).	Photo by Gordenker. Source: United Nations photo #188010.
223	Graph from "A Study of Pulmonary Tuberculosis Sex and Death Ratios for Tennessee" (ca. 1927).	Graph by Persis Putnam. Source: Rockefeller Archive Center.
224	Village Health Survey, Ibadan, Nigeria (1959).	Source: Rockefeller Archive Center.
225	Snail culture room, National Institute of Health, Maryland.	Source: National Library of Medicine.
227	Studying the parasite, Institute for Schistosomiasis Research, Cairo University, Egypt.	Photo by D. Henrioud/WHO. Source: National Library of Medicine.
228	NTD Control Program Office, Freetown, Sierra Leone (2013).	Photo by Romina Rodríguez Pose. Source: Overseas Development Institute.
231	Staff and students of Asian and Pacific Centre for Clinical Epidemiology, the University of Newcastle, Australia (1986).	Source: University of Newcastle.
232	Dr. John Evans and long-time colleague and friend Dr. David Sackett, internationally acclaimed epidemiologist, share a special moment at the Reception following Dr. Evan's lecture and discussion to celebrate his Henry G. Friesen International Prize in Health Research. Drs. Evans and Sackett were two of the pioneers of problem-based learning at McMaster.	Photo by Mike Lalich. Source: McMaster University http://www.fcihr.ca/prize/friesen-prize-institutional-visits/friesen-prize-institutional-visit-john-evans-mcmaster-university.
235	Scott Halstead.	Source: Rockefeller Archive Center.

	Description	Creator. Source.
272	Bellagio conference on HIV/AIDS vaccine initiative, Italy (1994).	Source: International AIDS Vaccine Initiative
274	Elton John, Washington, DC (2013).	Photo by Ralph Alswang. Source: The Rockefeller Foundation.
277	Worker at a Kenya AIDS Vaccine Initiative (KAVI) clinic, Kenya (2005).	Photo by Vanessa Vick. Source: International AIDS Vaccine Initiative.
278	"What happens when I take all of my TB drugs?" (ca. 2005).	Photo by Jonas Bendiksen. Source: The Rockefeller Foundation.
282-283	Patient care (ca. 2005).	Photo by Jonas Bendiksen. Source: The Rockefeller Foundation.
285	Kwong Wah Hospital, Hong Kong (2008).	Photo by Chong Fat. Source: Wikimedia Commons.
288-289	Rice fields and billboards, Vietnam (ca. 2006).	Photo by Jonas Bendiksen. Source: The Rockefeller Foundation.
292	Mukdahan Port entry, Thailand (2009).	Photo by Patrick de Noirmont. Source: The Rockefeller Foundation.
293	Laboratory specialist working on avian influenza (2008).	Source: World Bank.
295	District dispensary, Rufiji, Tanzania (2006).	Photo by Jonas Bendiksen. Source: The Rockefeller Foundation.
298	Wall charts, Kalisizo, Uganda (2005).	Photo by Jonas Bendiksen. Source: The Rockefeller Foundation.
301	Disposable thermometer, Kenya (2011).	Photo by Sokomoto Photography. Source: International AIDS Vaccine Initiative.
304	Wafaa El-Sadr (ca. 2008).	Source: Courtesy of the John D. and Catherine T. MacArthur Foundation.
306	Judith Rodin.	Source: The Rockefeller Foundation.
308-309	Team of nurses, Thailand (2012).	Photo by Athit Perawongmetha. Source: World Bank.
310	Nurse and baby, Candelaria, Colombia (1961).	Source: Rockefeller Archive Center.

OTHER BOOKS IN
THE ROCKEFELLER FOUNDATION CENTENNIAL SERIES

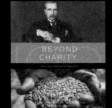

BEYOND CHARITY: A CENTURY OF PHILANTHROPIC INNOVATION

The creation of the Rockefeller Foundation in 1913 was in itself a marked innovation in the development of modern philanthropy. Foundation staff, trustees, and grantees had to learn by doing. The topical chapters in *Beyond Charity* explore the evolution of the Foundation's practice from the board room to the field office. For professionals or volunteers entering the field of philanthropy, each chapter offers an opening essay that highlights abiding issues in the field. The vivid stories and fascinating characters that illuminate these themes make the history come to life.

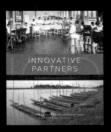

INNOVATIVE PARTNERS: THE ROCKEFELLER FOUNDATION AND THAILAND

For nearly a century, the Rockefeller Foundation and its Thai partners have been engaged in an innovative partnership to promote the well-being of the people of Thailand. From the battle against hookworm and other diseases to the development of rice biotechnology and agriculture, the lessons learned from this work offer powerful insights into the process of development. On the occasion of its centennial in 2013, the Rockefeller Foundation has commissioned a history of this innovative partnership.

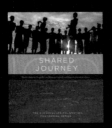

SHARED JOURNEY: THE ROCKEFELLER FOUNDATION, HUMAN CAPITAL, AND DEVELOPMENT IN AFRICA

In every society, development depends on investment in institutions and individuals. Wickliffe Rose, an early leader in the Rockefeller Foundation, called this "backing brains." But developing human capital is a risky proposition. This intriguing history explores the challenges and triumphs in the Rockefeller Foundation's efforts to invest in the people of Africa over the course of a century.

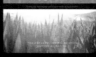

FOOD & PROSPERITY: BALANCING TECHNOLOGY AND COMMUNITY IN AGRICULTURE

John D. Rockefeller recognized in his early philanthropy, even before the creation of the Foundation, that agricultural productivity is key to increasing overall wealth and health in the poorest of rural communities. Embracing the promise of science, the Rockefeller Foundation focused on the discovery of new technologies to enhance food production. But technology was never enough. New techniques and tools had to be adapted to local cultures and communities. This engaging book explores lessons learned from the Foundation's efforts to improve this most basic, but still so complicated, arena of human endeavor.

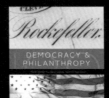

DEMOCRACY & PHILANTHROPY: THE ROCKEFELLER FOUNDATION AND THE AMERICAN EXPERIMENT

Many argued in 1913 that Rockefeller wealth seemed poised to undermine the democratic character of American institutions. Under the shadow of public concern, the trustees of the Rockefeller Foundation launched programs to strengthen American political institutions, promote equal opportunity in a plural society, and reinforce a shared sense of national identity. The relationship between democracy and philanthropy has been constantly tested over the last century. *Democracy & Philanthropy* offers insights and anecdotes to guide the next generation of American philanthropists.

To find out more about how to receive a copy of any of these Centennial books, please visit www.centennial.rockefellerfoundation.org.